A Practical Guide to
Joint & Soft Tissue Injections

Fourth Edition

James W. McNabb, MD

Private Practice—Family Medicine
Full Circle Family Medicine of Piedmont HealthCare
Mooresville, North Carolina

Francis G. O'Connor,
MD, MPH, FACSM, FAMSSM

Professor
Department of Military and Emergency Medicine
Uniformed Services University of the Health Sciences
Bethesda, Maryland

. Wolters Kluwer

Philadelphia • Baltimore • New York • London
Buenos Aires • Hong Kong • Sydney • Tokyo

Acquisitions Editor: Colleen Dietzler
Development Editor: Thomas Celona
Editorial Coordinator: Christopher George Rodgers
Editorial Assistant: Victoria Giansante
Marketing Manager: Kirsten Watrud
Production Project Manager: Justin Wright
Design Coordinator: Stephen Druding
Art Director, Illustration: Jennifer Clements
Illustrator: Body Scientific
Manufacturing Coordinator: Beth Welsh
Prepress Vendor: SPi Global

Cataloging-in-Publication Data available on request from the Publisher

ISBN: 978-1-9751-5328-1

DEDICATION

This book is dedicated to those who make our work possible. We especially want to thank and recognize the understanding and support given by our wives, families, colleagues, staff, and patients.

Foreword

There are few opportunities in the typical day of a busy clinician's practice where we can offer immediate improvements in pain or discomfort to patients. Providing a joint or soft tissue injection is one of those. While a therapeutic injection may not alleviate the discomfort completely, it usually offers some relief. With improvement in symptoms often comes hope … and a reinforcement of the doctor–patient relationship. And, is not that what practicing the art of medicine is all about?

Since corticosteroids may take a while to work, they may not offer immediate relief, but perhaps there will be resolution in the future? However, after performing intra-articular steroid injections for many years, often without mixing with lidocaine, I'm convinced that even steroids alone can offer immediate improvement. Is this the power of using a needle (needling) or the power of suggestion on my part when giving the injection? Does it really matter? That is part of the art of medicine—another topic and another discussion for another day among clinicians fortunate enough to offer and perform joint and soft tissue injections in their practice.

Such immediate relief for a patient is often immediately gratifying to a busy clinician, often adding a spark to the day. That is part of the reason why so many clinicians enjoy performing such injections. At the same time, teaching other clinicians to perform joint and soft tissue injections is also immediately gratifying. Watching a colleague learn how to properly perform an injection procedure is what it is all about for busy clinician educators. And that is what the authors of this fourth edition have been doing for at least a collective 50 years (it may be more years than that, but that's all that they are willing to admit). In addition, joint and soft tissue injections do not take much time to perform for clinician educators worried about the total numbers of patients seen/encounters per half day.

A Practical Guide to Joint & Soft Tissue Injections, an award-winning text now in its fourth edition, has become the standard for those performing joint or soft tissue injections. It is the Bible, Torah, Koran, etc., for joint and soft tissue injections. Whether the clinician is new to a procedure or technique, perhaps has not performed one in a while, or perhaps wants to brush up on the latest evidence regarding a particular procedure or technique, this work is a valuable resource. What should probably be called McNabb's Joint and Soft Tissue Injections is the go-to reference.

For this edition, James McNabb is joined by Fran O'Connor, a legend in the field of Primary Care Sports Medicine and Musculoskeletal Ultrasound. Significant additions include several facial/head nerve blocks to provide anesthesia and treat headache disorders, treatment of intersection syndrome, hamstring tendon/ischial bursa, gluteal pain syndrome, Baker's cyst and midfoot joint injections. In addition, auricular battlefield acupuncture, barbotage, tendon brisement, fenestration, nerve hydrodissection, capsular hydrodilatation/hydroplasty, dry needling, and percutaneous tenotomy with debridement have been added. This edition has been exhaustively researched and is also the most evidence-based of all editions. But such evidence must be tempered by experience, knowledge, and common sense. This writing team brings at least 50 years of experience, knowledge, and common sense to performing and teaching these procedures.

Some of the most significant recent technological advances in joint and soft tissue injections have been in the areas of musculoskeletal ultrasound, viscosupplements, and orthobiologics. Relatively inexpensive handheld ultrasound units are now becoming widely available. These interface with smart phones and other small devices to offer portability and ease of access at the bedside whether that is in the outpatient office, hospital ward, emergency room, urgent care, long-term care facility, sports sideline, or other setting. This book thoroughly demonstrates the use of ultrasound to assist with joint and soft tissue injections. It also covers the latest medical evidence related to viscosupplements and orthobiologics. Having taught and written extensively about procedures myself, this book also offers a dream I have not yet fulfilled: videos of each procedure being performed. These are all original videos and all of the photos are of real patients.

Musculoskeletal conditions are one of the most common reasons for going to clinicians' offices. With a global pandemic exploding around us, spending time in gratitude is a survival skill. There is evidence that such time will contribute to our well-being. We should all reflect on our privilege to benefit the lives of our patients. Using McNabb and O'Connor's *A Practical Guide to Joint & Soft Tissue Injections* provides a tangible opportunity for us to improve the quality and comprehensiveness of our care.

Grant C. Fowler, MD
Professor and Chair
Department of Family and Community Medicine
TCU/UNT Medical School and John Peter Smith Hospital
Senior Physician Executive
Primary Care and Geriatrics Service Line
John Peter Smith Healthcare System
Fort Worth, Texas

Preface

I write this at a moment in time that is truly unique. It is now about 6 months after the COVID-19 coronavirus pandemic impacted the United States and completely disrupted not only medical care but also our society. On the medical front, we are much more concerned about the remaining stock of personal protective equipment, conducting parking lot car visits on ill patients, and embracing telemedicine. However, our patient's need for competent care with their other medical concerns including musculoskeletal, dermatologic, and others remains unchanged. For insight into my practice at this time, my son Bryce created the short film—Plague on the Practice (https://www.youtube.com/watch?v=vavhuJ2teLE&t=3s). You are invited to view it. I am indeed fortunate to enjoy a professional career with a full-time practice of direct patient care at Full Circle Family Medicine of Piedmont HealthCare in North Carolina. I truly regard myself as a simple country doctor but also teach and write when I have time.

When planning this fourth edition, it became evident that there is an increasing need to address the common gap in education regarding musculoskeletal issues, MSK ultrasound, the use of orthobiologics, and other advanced and adjunctive injection techniques. It is my pleasure and great privilege to know COL(Ret) Francis G. O'Connor, MD, MPH, FACSM, FAMSSM. Trained as a family physician, he is widely recognized as a leader in sports medicine education and research. Dr. O'Connor is professor and past chair of military and emergency medicine at the Uniformed Services University of the Health Sciences. We have worked together for many years as a result of our mutual faculty appointments with the American Academy of Family Physicians and the National Procedures Institute. Dr. O'Connor brings unique knowledge, a set of procedural skills, and teaching mastery regarding these issues. It was only natural that we combine resources, and I am very proud to introduce him as coauthor of this updated and greatly expanded text.

While teaching musculoskeletal and dermatology courses, we have both found that primary care providers' learning needs include procedures that extend beyond traditional musculoskeletal injections. For this reason, we continue to take this project in a different direction from traditional injection textbooks. The result of this collaboration represents the spectrum of useful, straightforward, effective, medical procedures that can be performed with simple, inexpensive equipment in a variety of medical settings. Although written from the perspective of practicing family physicians in busy offices, these procedures cross specialty lines. They may be employed in settings as diverse as outpatient offices, urgent care centers, nursing homes, emergency rooms, and inpatient facilities. This text is also used for teaching purposes in medical schools and residency training programs.

With this fourth edition, Dr. O'Connor and I have expanded the focus of this project to include practically every needle-based procedure that can be performed in the primary care setting, with the exceptions of spinal injections and aesthetic procedures. This text is meant to serve as an extensively researched, evidence-based, yet, practical guide for those clinicians who wish to learn and apply the techniques and finer details of these useful procedures.

The last 10 years have seen a significant expansion of basic science knowledge, discovery of important medication toxicities, introduction of orthobiologics, increasing adoption of musculoskeletal ultrasound, and documentation of different techniques to improve patient care. We strongly advise that every provider using this text please read, study, and understand all of the information contained in the initial sections of this text BEFORE attempting to perform ANY of the procedures documented in the individual injection technique chapters.

The challenge of writing this new work is to build on the success of the previous editions by expanding content and stimulating thought, while keeping the text truly relevant and accessible to practicing clinicians. The entire edition has been reorganized and rewritten to incorporate recent information, expand injection procedures, and add even more value. New sections added by Dr. O'Connor include Orthobiologics, Musculoskeletal Ultrasound, and Advanced and Adjunctive Techniques. These new sections are critical to the success of this edition. The section on Skin Anesthesia has been expanded to include a new technique to perform digital blocks and add more nerve blocks so that various headache conditions may be effectively treated. The remaining sections have been reorganized, completely updated, and expanded. This fourth edition now includes a total of 68 individual injection topics.

Other features that add value include updated CPT and ICD-10 codes. Examples of informed consent, aftercare instructions, and procedure documentation are found in the appendices. We are grateful to Wolters Kluwer Health for their continued commitment to improving the quality of this work by creating beautiful anatomic drawings that are consistent across all chapters.

High-definition videos that demonstrate the performance of each procedure by both landmark-guided and ultrasound-guided techniques (where available) are included as part of this text. These are all case-based films that have been recorded in real-time in our offices on actual patients, not models. Each gave their permission to use the images to advance medical education. A unique feature is that all of the videos are taken from the operator's viewpoint. The videos solidify learning after the user reviews the background information, local anatomy, landmarks, and techniques for each procedure.

I would like to acknowledge the following people and organizations who taught, encouraged, and helped me write this text. This project is a culmination of 35 years of private practice and teaching. First, I must again thank my wife, Liz, for her support during my medical education, training, years of practice, teaching, and finally during the research and writing of this text. Without you I could never have done this. The leadership and faculty of family medicine residency training programs at the University of Wyoming–Casper, Scottsdale HealthCare in Arizona, and Cabarrus Family Medicine in North Carolina were instrumental in allowing me to expand my knowledge base, develop sports medicine and procedural curricula, and build expertise in evidence-based medicine. My office staff has been great—putting up with my demands and politely getting out of my way when I rush down the hall with "another great idea" or carrying video camera equipment. Without the confidence of my patients, I would not have been able to achieve mastery of these techniques—for that I remain privileged to serve as your family physician. I must acknowledge the opportunity to teach the Joint Injections workshops for the American Academy and North Carolina Academy of Family Physicians and the Dermatologic Procedures workshops for National Procedures Institute over the last 20 years. Many thanks are directed to workshop participants for their involvement and honest feedback. Deserved recognition is extended to teaching faculty who have provided encouragement, support, and stimulated my thinking. These physicians include Drs. Grant Fowler, Roy "Chip" Watkins, Kevin Burroughs, Gerald Admussen, Stuart

Forman, and, of course, Francis O'Connor. Finally, a big thank you to those at Wolters Kluwer Health, in particular, Thomas Celona—Development Editor, and Colleen Dietzler—Acquisitions Editor. They have treated us with the utmost professionalism, support, and patience during the extremely long process of writing this fourth edition. To all involved, and so many more unintentionally left unnamed—thank you, be healthy, and stay safe!

James W. McNabb

Contents

Videos

 Videos of the following procedures can be found in the companion eBook edition.

ADVANCED AND ADJUNCTIVE TECHNIQUES
Auricular Battlefield Acupuncture
Barbotage
Tendon Brisement/High-Volume Injection
Fenestration (Percutaneous Tenotomy)
Nerve Hydrodissection
Capsular Hydrodilatation/Hydroplasty
Myofascial Trigger Point Dry Needling
Tenotomy With Debridement

SKIN ANESTHESIA
Direct Local Injection
Field Block Injection
Digital Nerve Block
Facial Nerve Blocks
Supraorbital and Supratrochlear Nerve Blocks
Infraorbital Nerve Block
External Nasal Nerve Block
Mental Nerve Block
External Ear Field Block
Greater Occipital Nerve Block
Headache Nerve Blocks

SKIN AND SKIN STRUCTURES
Chalazion
Keloid Scar
Common Warts
Granuloma Annulare and Other Thin, Benign, Inflammatory Dermatoses
Prurigo Nodularis and Other Thick, Benign, Inflammatory Dermatoses

HEAD AND TRUNK
Temporomandibular Joint
Suprascapular Nerve
Scapulothoracic Syndrome
Sacroiliac Joint

UPPER EXTREMITIES

LOWER EXTREMITIES

Introduction

James W. McNabb

The performance of joint and soft tissue injections and aspirations is a valuable skill that can be mastered by primary care physicians and qualified medical providers. These procedures can help relieve pain and improve function for the patient, while at the same time empowering the clinician, improving continuity of care, and decreasing health care costs. It is essential that these techniques be used thoughtfully and precisely—only after making the correct dermatologic or musculoskeletal diagnosis. This can be quite challenging at times but is no more difficult than diagnosing and treating any of the other many medical conditions that the primary care physician encounters on a daily basis. Learning how to confidently make an accurate diagnosis of these conditions is beyond the scope of this text.

Our primary consideration is the welfare of the patient. We must always endeavor to provide the best medical care at the least risk of harm. This can be achieved by developing a cognitive knowledge base along with an accompanying set of complementary procedural skills. In addition, our focus must remain on providing a positive patient experience. This starts with active patient engagement and shared decision-making. It then is incumbent on us as providers to provide a safe and supportive environment while ensuring a pain-free procedural experience. Patient satisfaction from a positive experience along with an excellent clinical outcome is our primary goal.

An important concept is that aspiration and injection therapy is not an end in itself. It is only one treatment option. The withdrawal of fluid or the precise deposition of a therapeutic agent is a temporary measure that generally should be used as adjunctive therapy to other modalities. In many conditions, corticosteroid injection therapy used alone has been demonstrated to give only short- to intermediate-term pain/functional relief, with no difference in long-term results. In these cases, initial injection treatment in combination with other treatment modalities and activity modification gives patients optimal long-lasting results. Additional therapeutic options may include relative rest, compression, splinting/casting, ice, heat, ultrasound, stretching, physical therapy, acupressure, administration of other medications, or even surgery. The performance of aspirations or injections alone, without correcting the underlying factors, is likely to result in recurrence if used without complementary treatments.

In this text, the following primary learning objectives are identified:

- Describe the indications and contraindications for each procedure.
- Review the current evidence-based medical literature.
- Select appropriate equipment/products for each procedure.
- Illustrate pertinent anatomic landmarks for each procedure.
- Perform injections and/or aspirations safely and effectively.
- Properly code the procedures.

Foundation Concepts

James W. McNabb

"The good physician treats the disease; the great physician treats the patient who has the disease."

—William Osler

THOUGHTFUL CONSIDERATION

The evaluation and treatment of musculoskeletal conditions is an integral aspect of primary medical care. With improved understanding of anatomy, biomechanics, pathophysiology and modern treatment options, the primary care provider can be empowered to make positive contributions to musculoskeletal patient care. Long gone should be the days when patients were treated with an oral nonsteroidal anti-inflammatory medication (NSAID) and benign neglect with the hope that the condition would heal itself. This text may be used to further understanding of techniques useful in the treatment of the most common musculoskeletal disorders as well as select skin conditions and anesthetic nerve blocks. As with any medical procedure, performing injections and aspirations places a great responsibility on the clinician. All invasive procedures should be done with a clear differential diagnosis and treatment plan in mind. They should never be performed indiscriminately.

Primum non nocere or "first, do no harm" is one of the fundamental principles of medical care. Therefore, the physician is obligated to consider the indications, contraindications, weight of evidence in the medical literature, expected benefits, possible side effects, anticipated outcomes, diagnostic certainty, his or her personal experience with the procedure, clinical experience, biases, the patient's response to previous interventions, and respect for the patient's values before making a decision on whether or not to perform any injection. This shared decision-making is a very complex process that requires thoughtful contemplation and a conversation with each patient. Furthermore, it is imperative that the clinician use common sense and know his or her limits before performing any medical procedure. In some cases, following a discussion with the patient, it may be preferable to use an alternative approach or request specialty consultation, rather than performing any invasive procedure. Put another way, just because one can do a procedure doesn't mean that one should do the procedure.

WHEN TO REFER TO A SUBSPECIALIST

Although the majority of patients with musculoskeletal disorders can be competently managed by primary care providers, there will be situations where referral to subspecialist colleagues is desirable and necessary. Standard indications include instances when there is uncertainty regarding the correct diagnosis, the provider feels uncomfortable performing a procedure, the expected response to treatment has not occurred, there are structures involved that are not easily accessible (especially spine, hip or sacroiliac joints), procedure attempts have been unsuccessful, possible septic arthritis, suspected inflammatory polyarthritis, recurrent monoarthritis unresponsive to treatment, or undiagnosed chronic monoarthritis. In these instances, the patient may be referred to a sports medicine specialist, rheumatologist, orthopedic surgeon, interventional radiologist, or pain specialist. If an acute septic joint is suspected, the patient requires emergent inpatient hospitalization for joint drainage, debridement, irrigation, intravenous antibiotics, and possibly an infectious disease consultation in the case of an atypical infection.

STANDARD MEDICATION MANAGEMENT

Musculoskeletal disorders are commonly encountered in practice by primary care providers. Traditionally, many of these have been treated using oral medications. However, the prescriber must be aware of their adverse reactions and potential toxicities. The most effective pain management strategies are often multimodal. In addition to drug treatment, psychosocial interventions to reduce anxiety, as well as physical strategies such as physical therapy, acupressure, and TENS, can reduce pain, improve pain coping skills, and restore function.

Recent clinical guidelines regarding the management of acute pain from non-low back, musculoskeletal injuries in adults were published by the American College of Physicians (ACP) and American Academy of Family Physicians (AAFP) in 2020.[1] The recommendations in the guidelines are based on a systematic review of the comparative safety and efficacy of drug and nondrug management of acute pain lasting less than 4 weeks. The review included 207 trials that enrolled 32,959 participants and evaluated 45 treatments. Their strongest recommendation with overall moderate-certainty evidence supports the first-line use of topical NSAIDs with or without menthol gel. This was the only intervention that documented positive effects in all three areas of pain relief, improvement in physical function, and patient satisfaction with treatment. No serious gastrointestinal or renal adverse events have been observed in trials. However, confirmation of the cardiovascular safety of topical NSAIDs still warrants further observational study.[2]

Oral nonselective NSAIDs and selective cyclooxygenase-2 (COX-2) inhibitors are a very commonly employed class of medication for use in the treatment of inflammatory conditions. However, many of the musculoskeletal conditions treated by primary care clinicians do not actually involve active inflammation in their pathogenesis. Nevertheless, these medications are commonly employed. The ACP/AAFP guidelines noted above give a conditional recommendation with moderate-certainty evidence to oral NSAIDs to reduce or relieve symptoms, including pain, and to improve physical function, or with oral acetaminophen to reduce pain.[1]

Unfortunately, NSAIDs and COX-2 inhibitors have side effects that extend beyond their well-recognized gastrointestinal side effects, hepatotoxicity, nephrotoxicity, edema, increase in blood pressure, and exacerbation of congestive heart failure. A meta-analysis of 754 trials in 353,809 patients with greater than 233,798 pt years of follow-up was reported in 2013. COX-2 inhibitors and diclofenac were found to increase major vascular events by a third—primarily due to an increase in coronary events. Ibuprofen significantly increased major coronary events. Naproxen, however, was not found to increase the incidence of major vascular events. A high-quality meta-analysis of 4 studies including 61,460 cases was published in 2017 in the BMJ. This showed that all NSAIDs, including naproxen, were found to be associated with an increased risk of acute myocardial infarction. Risk of myocardial infarction with celecoxib was comparable to that of traditional NSAIDs. Risk was greatest during the first month of NSAID use and with higher doses.[3] All NSAIDs double the risk of heart failure and increase the risk of upper GI complications.[4] A nationwide cohort study determined that even short-term treatment with most NSAIDs is associated with an increase in the risk of death and recurrent myocardial infarction in patients with prior MI. Therefore, neither short- nor long-term treatment with NSAIDs is advised in this population. Any NSAID use should be limited from a cardiovascular safety point of view.[5]

Two large European population-based studies show that traditional NSAIDs and COX-2 inhibitors increase the incidence of atrial fibrillation.[6,7] This is especially noted with recent use within 30 days of onset of atrial fibrillation. Since NSAIDs inhibit cyclooxygenase enzymes expressed in the kidneys, it is thought that this mechanism causes fluid retention, increases blood pressure, and leads to enlargement in both end-diastolic and end-systolic dimensions of the heart. Alternatively, because NSAIDs are used as anti-inflammatory drugs, the underlying inflammatory conditions and pain they treat may be associated with their cardiac effects.

A large systematic review and meta-analysis published in 2015 showed that NSAIDs and COX-2 inhibitors also nearly double the risk of venous thromboembolism.[8] It is postulated that inhibition of the COX-2 enzyme inhibits synthesis of prostacyclin leading to platelet activation and also stimulates the release of thromboxane causing platelet aggregation.

Although mild to moderately effective for pain relief, acetaminophen toxicity occurs on a frequent basis. From 1990 to 1998, there were 56,000 emergency room visits, 26,000 hospitalizations, and 458 deaths on average per year related to acetaminophen-associated overdoses.[9] In 2007, the Centers for Disease Control estimated 1,600 cases of acute liver failure each year of which acetaminophen-related was the most common.[10] In 2014, 50,396 single exposures to acetaminophen alone and 22,951 single exposures to acetaminophen combinations were reported to the National Poison Data System.[11] In 2014, the U.S. FDA withdrew approval of all combination drug products containing more than 325 mg acetaminophen per tablet, capsule, or other dosage unit. A boxed warning emphasizing the potential for severe liver injury and a warning highlighting the potential for allergic reactions (e.g., swelling of the face, mouth, and throat, difficulty breathing, itching, or rash) were added to the label of all acetaminophen prescription drug products. Other reported side effects include anaphylaxis, acute renal tubular necrosis, anemia, thrombocytopenia, nausea, rash, and headache. A systematic literature review of eight studies by Roberts and colleagues, 4 showed an increase in cardiovascular adverse events (AE), 1 documented gastrointestinal AEs or bleeds, 3 showed renal AEs, and 2 reported increases in all-cause mortality.[12] In 2013, the FDA published a news release informing the public of the potential of rare, but severe skin reactions reported in individuals following acetaminophen ingestion. These reactions include Stevens-Johnson syndrome, toxic epidermal necrolysis, and acute generalized exanthematous pustulosis. All of these skin conditions are potentially fatal and can occur with even first exposure.[13]

Oral corticosteroid bursts are frequently prescribed. However, they may pose significant risks that are unrecognized by many practitioners. In a 2020 population-based study from Taiwan, over 15 million patients received oral steroids for a median duration of 3 days. The incidence of GI bleeding increased by a factor of 1.8, sepsis doubled, and heart failure increased by 2.4 times the controls. These adverse events were noted within 5 to 30 days after steroid initiation.

A Cochrane Database systematic review in 2019 downgraded the benefit of tramadol. Compared to placebo, tramadol alone or in combination with acetaminophen probably has no important benefit on pain or function in people with osteoarthritis. Moderate quality evidence shows that adverse events probably cause substantially more participants to stop taking this medication.[14]

According to the 2020 ACP/AAFP guidelines,[1] opioids including tramadol should not be prescribed for managing acute pain from non–low back musculoskeletal causes, except in cases of severe injury or when first-line therapies are not effective. This class of medication is associated with little to no benefit in patients with acute non–low back pain. There are substantial harms, such as the potential for longer-term addiction and overdose. Avoiding prescribing opioids for acute musculoskeletal injuries to patients with past or current substance use disorder, and restricting duration to 7 days or less and using lower doses when they are prescribed, are potentially important targets to reduce rates of persistent opioid use.[15] A number of adverse events, including serious events, are associated with the medium- and long-term use of opioids for chronic noncancer pain. A Cochrane review published in 2017 showed that the absolute event rate for any adverse event with opioids in trials using a placebo as comparison was 78%, with an absolute event rate of 7.5% for any serious adverse event.[16] Based on the adverse events identified, clinically relevant benefit would need to be clearly demonstrated before long-term use could be considered in people with chronic noncancer pain in clinical practice.

Duloxetine, a serotonin and norepinephrine reuptake inhibitor, is often used for adjunctive treatment of chronic musculoskeletal pain. It has been shown to produce modest to moderate relief of pain, functional improvement, better mood regulation, and improvement in quality of life. This medication is usually well tolerated with mild adverse events in the treatment of osteoarthritis and chronic low back pain. Side effects include nausea, fatigue, dizziness, and dry mouth. A recent review confirmed low cardiovascular risk.[17]

Glucosamine and chondroitin sulfate are over the counter dietary supplements that are commonly taken by patients in an effort to reduce pain from osteoarthritis. Unfortunately, despite their popularity, the data showing any benefit are weak, and the data showing efficacy are conflicting. A meta-analysis of 18 articles published in 2018 by Orgata found a marginally favorable effect of glucosamine on pain and a small, nonsignificant effect on knee joint function.[18]

Given the relatively low efficacy and considerable toxicity of standard pharmacologic oral medications to control pain and progression of common musculoskeletal disorders, it is incumbent on medical practitioners to consider the use of other treatment options that may be more effective and pose less toxicity. There is often a good response to conservative measures of weight loss, relative rest, acupressure,[1] and utilization of devices such as casts, splints, orthotics, TENS units, extracorporeal shock wave therapy, and others. Formal physical therapy is also quite helpful in those patients who are able to fully participate but is commonly underutilized.[19] Other treatment options include many of the needle-based injection and aspiration procedures in this text.

INDICATIONS FOR INJECTIONS AND ASPIRATIONS

There are many indications for performing injections and aspirations. From a diagnostic standpoint, the introduction of local anesthetic solution into a joint or soft tissue structure to temporarily decrease pain may allow the clinician to perform a more comprehensive examination. Pain limits the musculoskeletal examination through voluntary or involuntary guarding of the affected area. Muscle spasm commonly develops in response, further limiting the range of motion of the area examined. Providing effective pain relief allows the clinician to adequately examine the area of interest. This is essential in order to determine the integrity of underlying structures including muscles, tendons, ligaments, and cartilage.

Important clinical management decisions may be made based on the results of a diagnostic injection. For example, a patient may present with acute shoulder pain. Upon examination, she complains of moderately severe pain, holds the shoulder at her side, and is unable to demonstrate shoulder abduction. The clinical question may be whether she has a complete tear of the shoulder rotator cuff complex or if impingement of the rotator cuff under the acromion is the cause of her pain. The clinician may elect to perform a subacromial space injection of 1 to 2 mL of 1% mepivacaine. If after 1 min, the patient is able to demonstrate full range of motion including unrestricted abduction, then this "impingement test" indicates that pain was the limiting factor in her inability to abduct the shoulder. Consequently, there is not a complete tear of the rotator cuff structures. She may be able to continue to receive conservative care directed by the primary medical provider without specialty referral at that particular time.

Fluid may also be obtained upon aspiration of a joint or soft tissue space. If so, then it should be grossly examined for color, clarity, and the presence of blood. Normal synovial fluid is clear and transparent. The fluid may contain blood that indicates a hemorrhagic cause—most commonly acute trauma. It may also be yellow due to xanthochromia from the breakdown of hemoglobin leaking from inflamed synovium. The clarity of the fluid may be altered by the presence of white blood cells. Crystals and cellular debris can also decrease clarity. The information obtained from the microscopic examination of the fluid in order to assess it for cells, crystals, bacteria, and blood is critically important and is discussed in a following section.

Therapeutically, there are many reasons to perform injections and aspirations. Removal of fluid itself from a joint can result in significant pain relief and restore joint range of motion. With relatively small joints such as the elbow, this can occur with the removal of as little as 3 to 5 mL of fluid. In a large knee joint, the clinician may remove as much as 100 to 150 mL of fluid in chronic conditions!

Indications for therapeutic injections include crystal arthropathies, synovitis, rheumatoid arthritis, other nonseptic inflammatory arthritides, osteoarthritis, and osteoarthrosis. Soft tissue indications include bursitis, tendonitis, tendinosis, epicondylitis, trigger points, ganglion cysts, neuromas, nerve entrapment syndromes, and fasciitis. With inflammatory joint and soft tissue conditions, therapeutic effect is often achieved by the precise placement of a corticosteroid/local anesthetic mixture.

Injections of corticosteroids may also be given directly into lesions in patients with skin diseases as diverse as hypertrophic scars, keloids, lichen planus, lichen simplex chronicus, psoriasis, prurigo nodularis, alopecia areata, and discoid lupus.

Injection of local anesthetics into skin structures and around nerves temporarily eliminates pain. This is clinically important in order to allow the performance of otherwise painful surgical procedures.

CONTRAINDICATIONS TO INJECTIONS AND ASPIRATIONS

While understanding the indications of aspirations and injections is important, it is perhaps even more valuable to recognize the situations in which these procedures should not be performed. Absolute contraindications include performance of a procedure on an uncooperative patient, history of true allergy to the proposed injected medication, injection through infected tissues, and injection of corticosteroid into critical weight-bearing tendons. In particular, the injection of steroid into and around the Achilles, patellar, and quadriceps tendons may result in catastrophic rupture of these vital structures. Recovery from such rupture is often difficult, prolonged, and incomplete.

Many relative contraindications exist. These are variable and may apply only to certain patients or situations. Some of these include procedures near critical structures such as arteries, veins, nerves, or pleural surfaces. Also, caution must be exercised in patients with coagulation disorders, allergy to the preservative in the injected solution, immuno-compromised states, brittle diabetes, history of avascular necrosis, previous joint replacement at the injection site, excessive anxiety concerning the procedure, and in patients who may not follow postprocedure instructions.

Patients receiving corticosteroids may experience activation of latent disease or an exacerbation of infections caused by amoeba, *Borrelia burgdorferi* (Lyme disease), *Candida, Cryptococcus, Mycobacterium, Nocardia, Pneumocystis, Strongyloides* (threadworm), *Toxoplasma, or others.*

The Society of Interventional Radiology consensus guidelines stratify musculoskeletal percutaneous procedures as having a low risk of bleeding.[20] However, there are many clinical situations where the risk of bleeding may be increased. A review of each patient's comorbidities, medications, and coagulation parameters should be considered prior to proceeding with a procedure. Coagulopathies such as hemophilia and von Willebrand disease predispose patients to bleeding complications including hemarthrosis and compartment syndrome. Certain conditions such as cirrhosis, chronic liver disease, chronic kidney disease, and vitamin K deficiency can increase the possibility of bleeding. In addition, anticoagulant, antiplatelet, and NSAIDs all increase bleeding risk. The patient's coagulation profile including prothrombin time/INR, partial thromboplastin time (PTT), and platelet count may need to be evaluated and any corrections made prior to an invasive procedure.

In patients treated with anticoagulants, the practitioner must weigh the risk of bleeding associated with a needle-based procedure against the possibility of thrombosis occurring if anticoagulation therapy is withheld or reversed. Patients taking the oral anticoagulant medication, warfarin, do not represent an absolute contraindication to injection or aspiration. In the journal *Arthritis and Rheumatism* in 1998, Thumboo reported the results of a prospective cohort study of 32 joint and soft tissue injections and aspirations involving patients attending a rheumatology clinic taking warfarin with an INR less than 4.5. Patients followed up for 4 weeks after the procedure showed no significant hemorrhages.[21] This has also been the author's experience in many more patients (unpublished). In 2015, Foremny and colleagues stratified musculoskeletal procedures into those cases with low and high bleeding risk. When performing procedures with a low risk of bleeding such as joint injections or aspirations, aspiration of fluid collections (hematomas or abscesses), peritendinous injections, and peripheral nerve blocks, anticoagulation does not need to be held (for INR ≤ 3.0). Furthermore, holding clopidogrel is not recommended for these procedures, and platelet count of over 20,000/μL are considered adequate.[22] No clinical trials involving injection procedures have been reported to date on patients receiving antiplatelet drugs, thrombolytics, fibrinolytics, low molecular weight heparin, or the newer oral anticoagulant medications including direct thrombin inhibitors (dabigatran and others) and factor Xa inhibitors (rivaroxaban, apixaban, and others). Data on the safety of the performance of injection procedures in patients taking warfarin should not be extended to these anticoagulation agents.

SPECIAL MEDICAL CONDITIONS

Several medical conditions deserve special consideration. Diabetes is a very common and increasingly prevalent medical condition in the primary care patient population. Because of the frequent association with obesity, these patients place mechanical and metabolic stress on joint and soft tissues that may be amenable to treatment using therapeutic injections. Although there is concern that blood glucose levels may rise significantly, studies show that the transient elevation is usually not clinically significant. A single intraarticular steroid injection into the knee produces acute hyperglycemia for 2 or 3 days in patients with diabetes who otherwise have good glucose control.[23,24] Intra-articular steroid injections into the shoulder may briefly raise postprandial (but not mean) glucose levels with larger and repeated doses.[25] The rise in blood sugars can usually be well controlled with carbohydrate restriction, continuation of the usual diabetes treatment regimen, and close monitoring of blood sugars for a few days following injection. However, the presence of diabetes may make treatment using injected corticosteroids less effective.

Concern has been raised regarding the performance of injections in patients taking oral anticoagulants including aspirin, NSAIDs, antiplatelet agents, warfarin and newer oral anticoagulant medications including direct thrombin inhibitors (dabigatran and others) and factor Xa inhibitors (rivaroxaban, apixaban, and others). This issue was discussed above in the section on Contraindications.

Septic arthritis is a medical emergency. A joint infection is a very serious condition with dire consequences to the integrity of the joint and surrounding structures. All efforts must be made to diagnose septic arthritis as soon as possible and provide emergent hospitalization. The patient requires treatment including surgical drainage with irrigation of the affected joint, administration of intravenous antibiotics, and pain control. This is best done in a coordinated fashion by the primary care physician with an orthopedic surgeon, and possibly an infectious disease subspecialist. Common organisms causing joint infections are *Streptococcus/Staphylococcus* species, *Neisseria gonorrhoeae,* and, increasingly, methicillin-resistant *Staphylococcus aureus.*

Rheumatoid arthritis presents unique challenges to the primary care provider. This is a destructive, rapidly progressive inflammatory arthritis. Lytic enzymes quickly degrade the joint surfaces, synovium, and supporting structures unless the process is interrupted and controlled. Joint and soft tissue injections play an important role in medical care because they can be used to deliver relatively small doses of corticosteroids locally in the affected joint(s) to augment the overall systemic management of this condition.

Management of pain involving joint replacement devices demands special consideration. Pain involving a joint replacement often occurs because the normal biomechanics are altered. Other causes of pain may include excessive postoperative scar tissue, poorly fitting, or loose components of prostheses. Simple injections of corticosteroids or other substances often do not lead to meaningful improvement in the patient's pain and certainly do not correct any underlying biomechanical abnormality. There is also the possibility that an injection may be complicated by an infection of the prosthetic joint with catastrophic outcomes. In these patients, it is usually more prudent to not perform injections and to refer the patients back to their orthopedic surgeon for management of this challenging problem.

COMPLICATIONS

Complications from needle-based procedures used in injections and aspirations fall into two categories—systemic and local. Systemic complications include vasovagal reactions, local anesthetic-related complications, and corticosteroid-related complications. Patients can develop allergic reactions including anaphylaxis. Other serious toxicities of local anesthetics may involve cardiac arrhythmias and seizures—but usually with inadvertent intravascular administration of doses far in excess of the amounts used with soft tissue and joint injections. Systemic complications linked to corticosteroid injections include vascular flushing, elevated blood sugar levels in patients with diabetes, impaired immune response, psychological disturbances, hypothalamic pituitary adrenal axis suppression, irregular menses, abnormal vaginal bleeding, and osteoporosis. Patients receiving corticosteroid therapy are also at increased risk of infections or reactivation of an old infection due to potentially decreased immune resistance with an inability to localize infections. This risk of infection exists with any pathogen (viral, bacterial, fungal, protozoan, or helminthic) at any location of the body. Infections may be mild or severe, and the risk for complications increases with corticosteroid dose. In addition, corticosteroid therapy may mask the signs and symptoms of an active infection.

Local dermal complications of corticosteroids may include subcutaneous fat atrophy, dermal atrophy, and skin depigmentation. These are most noticeable after injection of superficial structures but can also be seen after an intraarticular injection. This is presumably due to inadvertent superficial injection of corticosteroid or reflux of corticosteroid along the needle track back into the subcutaneous fat or dermis. It can take up to 2 months for skin effects to manifest. Skin depigmentation normalizes in most patients over a period of 1 year.[26] Although skin atrophy usually resolves, effects lasting longer than 5 years have been reported.[27] The extent and duration of such skin complications is likely related to the solubility and concentration of the corticosteroid preparation. Interestingly, normal saline infiltration has been shown to rapidly reverse local corticosteroid skin atrophy.[28] Other local complications may involve bleeding, infection, osteonecrosis of juxta-articular bone, ligament rupture, or tendon rupture. Intratendinous corticosteroid injection can lead to tendon rupture.[29–31] This is likely to occur through the inhibition of tenocyte proliferation[32] and the reduction in the strength of isolated collagen fascicles. Pneumothorax has been reported as a complication of trigger point injections of back muscles.[33] Injuries to the radial artery can occur with attempted aspiration of large volar wrist ganglion cysts.[34]

Postinjection flare is a local phenomena commonly believed to be due to a reaction to steroid crystals in the soft tissue and/or synovial space. The reaction occurs 6 to 24 h following corticosteroid injection. Although the flare has been attributed in the past to crystalline corticosteroids, this is controversial and has no support in the medical literature. A clinically identical reaction occurs from chemical synovitis due to preservatives including methylparaben.[35,36] Multidose vials of plain lidocaine, lidocaine with epinephrine, and bupivacaine all contain 1 mg of methylparaben. If a patient has a history of a "steroid flare" or "lidocaine allergy," single use vials of 1% lidocaine that do not contain a preservative might be carefully used instead. In either case, an acute postinjection reaction can be managed by the use of oral NSAIDs and ice application after a repeat aspiration confirms that there is no infection.

There has been increasing concern following recent reports of toxicity of amide local anesthetics on chondrocytes. This effect has been reported with lidocaine, bupivacaine, and ropivacaine in in vitro studies[37,38] and confirmed with in vivo trials.[39,40] Of these, bupivacaine and ropivacaine may be the least toxic agents.[40] The evidence suggests that there is a greater risk for chondrolysis with longer exposure to a high concentration of local anesthetic, such as with the use of a continuous infusion of anesthetic via a pain pump following orthopedic surgery.[41] However, toxic late cellular and metabolic changes are seen even after a single injection of local anesthetic in animal models.[38] Some studies suggest that the preservatives and the pH of the local anesthetic solution may also play a role in chondrotoxicity.[42]

Intra-articular injection of local anesthetics differs from that of continuous intra-articular infusion. Chondrocyte toxicity to the anesthetic directly correlates with the length of exposure to the product. The uptake and clearance of the anesthetic in the joint or soft tissues is dependent on several factors related to the physiochemical properties of the local anesthetic and local blood flow. Uptake tends to be delayed for local anesthetics with high lipophilicity and protein binding.[43] Of the amide local anesthetics, bupivacaine has the greatest values for these properties and probably has the longest residence time in tissues.[44] In a systematic review of the effects of a single dose of local anesthetics on cartilage in 2017, Kreuz and colleagues included 12 studies with 4 different anesthetics. They found a toxic effect on chondrocytes and cartilage that increased in a type-, dose-, and time-dependent fashion, especially on osteoarthritic cartilage. In this review, bupivacaine and lidocaine were more chondrotoxic than mepivacaine and ropivacaine.[45]

There is now early evidence that corticosteroids may also have deleterious effects on cartilage. In 2017, McAlindon and colleagues published the results of a randomized clinical trial in JAMA.[46] They injected the knees of 140 patients with symptomatic knee osteoarthritis with corticosteroids every 3 months and measured the volume of knee cartilage with MRI scans. They showed that at the end of 2 years, there was a loss of 0.29 mm of cartilage thickness in patients injected with triamcinolone versus 0.13 mm in the saline group, with no significant difference on knee pain severity between treatment groups.

SAFETY

In order to ensure patient and operator safety, the following procedures should be followed. First, the local anatomic landmarks must be defined. This assures the provider that the needle is being advanced with knowledge of the underlying structures. Next, always use universal precautions to avoid inadvertent contact with blood and body fluids. Personal protective equipment must be used. For almost all injections and aspirations, the use of nonsterile exam gloves is sufficient. In almost all clinical outpatient situations, it is unnecessary to use sterile gloves or sterile drapes while performing these procedures—as long as medical antiseptic technique is strictly followed.

In order to decrease the chance of needle stick injury, there are a variety of safer sharps needle systems available for use. It is the practitioner's responsibility to utilize one of these safer designs to avoid injury and maintain compliance with OSHA regulations. After use, all sharps must be placed immediately in a puncture-resistant sharps container. Filled sharps containers are then disposed in accordance with state regulated medical waste rules.

Medical antiseptic techniques are always used when performing invasive procedures. Common commercially available antiseptic products include 10% povidone–iodine–aqueous and 2% chlorhexidine–alcohol solutions. Both are broad spectrum antiseptics with activity against Gram-positive bacteria, Gram-negative bacteria, fungi, and enveloped viruses. Chlorhexidine–alcohol has been shown to be significantly more effective than povidone–iodine in preventing postoperative superficial and deep surgical site infections.[47,48] In patients undergoing neuraxial blockade procedures, alcohol-based chlorhexidine–alcohol significantly lowers the incidence of insertion site colonization compared with the use of povidone iodine.[49] These studies are consistent with others demonstrating superior clinical efficacy of chlorhexidine versus povidone–iodine in reducing the bacterial concentration in the operative field in foot-and-ankle surgery.[50,51] Further, chlorhexidine gluconate is not inactivated by blood or serum proteins, whereas this occurs with iodophors.[52,53] Lower postoperative infection rates with chlorhexidine–alcohol is thought to be related to chlorhexidine's more rapid action, persistent activity, and residual antimicrobial effect.[54] Antiseptics should be allowed to dry according to the manufacturer's recommendation.

Using a medical aseptic technique does not imply that the procedure needs to be done in a sterile operating room environment. However, it does require that the provider takes the necessary precautions to ensure a minimal chance that infectious organisms are carried into the tissues by the needle. When performing injections and aspirations, the operator must always follow the antiseptic, "no-touch" technique. This procedure does not allow for any contact of the injection site after sterile preparation of the skin. Following identification of the local landmarks, the injection site is marked with ink. Then, an impression in the skin is made at that site by applying firm pressure with the retracted tip of a ballpoint pen. Next, the injection site is cleansed with alcohol, followed by application of an antiseptic agent. After these steps are completed, there is no further contact or touching of the site with any nonsterile objects. The only object that comes into contact with this site is the tip of the sterile needle.

It is important to use needles and syringes for only a single patient. These must never be used on other patients. If, single dose (single-use) medication vials are used, then they must only be used for only one patient. Because these vials do not contain preservative, they can never be reused, even at a later time with the same patient. The rubber stopper on a medication vial must be cleaned with alcohol prior to piercing. Medication vials are entered with a new needle and a new syringe, even when obtaining additional doses for the same patient.

Always attempt to aspirate before injecting any substance into tissues. This will confirm that the needle tip is not inside a blood vessel. Performing this simple maneuver ensures that inadvertent intravascular injection of the injection solution does not occur.

Place the injection *within* a joint or bursa and *around* a tendon. An injection into the substance of a tendon is likely to weaken that structure. Rupture may follow—especially if it is a weight-bearing tendon such as the Achilles, patellar, or quadriceps tendons. Also, avoid injecting directly into nerves. Such an injection is often evident since the patient usually reports pain, paresthesias, or numbness at the instant of needle contact with a nerve. In this case, simply withdraw the needle slightly and attempt to reposition it before proceeding with the injection.

After the injection has been completed, sterile gauze is used to wipe the site and if necessary, apply direct pressure. Finally, a sterile adhesive dressing is applied. The needles are immediately disposed in a puncture-resistant sharps container. Following the procedure, the patient should remain in the office for a period of time in which the office staff observes the patient for any signs of systemic or local reactions.

ANATOMY

It is critical that the clinician has a complete understanding of the three-dimensional anatomy and the structure's function in each area that is selected for injection and/or aspiration. A thorough knowledge of the target area brings a deeper understanding of the pathologic process causing the patient's symptoms. This makes the physical examination maneuvers meaningful. Finally, it enables the provider to develop a list of alternative diagnostic possibilities. With this knowledge, the physician is able to take the next step. He or she can understand structural relationships beneath the surface of the skin. The physician is then able to think in three dimensions. While advancing the needle, it is important to "visualize" the location of the needle as it passes through the anatomic structures. Performing these thought processes enables the clinician to clinically determine the location of the needle tip in "real time." This results in improved clinical outcomes through the accurate placement of a therapeutic product or the insertion of a large-bore needle for fluid aspiration. Complications from needle trauma are also minimized by avoidance of critical structures.

LANDMARKS

For each injection or aspiration procedure, the physician must identify the pertinent local anatomic landmarks. These are areas that represent underlying bony prominences or easily identifiable soft tissues. The landmarks are specific to each injection site. After identification, the structures should be marked on overlying skin with ink by using either a ballpoint pen or a surgical marker. Next, the entry site for the needle is indicated with ink. Then an indentation in the skin is created by applying firm pressure over the ink mark using the retracted tip of a ballpoint pen. An indentation must be done since aseptic preparation of the area will remove ink marks. This process gives the clinician a visual frame of reference and standardizes the procedure from one patient to the next. No matter how much experience a physician has with a procedure, the process of identifying and marking the landmarks and entry site should not be skipped. After committing the landmarks to a surface drawing, the patient is instructed not to move that area of the body. Repositioning may change the relationships between the skin markings and the underlying anatomy.

TOPICAL ANESTHESIA

Providing the patient a pain-free experience is the responsibility of the primary care provider.[55] In select injections, such as the posterior approach to the subacromial space, techniques such as stretching/pinching the skin and other dermal stimulation may give adequate distraction to the patient so that pain from needle insertion is not experienced.

Painless local anesthesia via percutaneous needle introduction can be achieved by use of either skin cooling or application of a topical local anesthetic agent. A topical vapocoolant spray can be used to give rapid onset of brief, but effective, skin numbness. These skin refrigerants cause a brief period of noncytotoxic cooling of the epidermis. This provides up to 30 s of local anesthetic effect, which blocks the pain associated with needle injections. The mechanism of action for anesthesia is to decrease nerve conduction velocity of the A-delta fibers and C fibers of the peripheral nervous system, thus interrupting nociceptive input to the spinal cord. A meta-analysis by Zhu and colleagues in 2018 documented that vapocoolant spray significantly decreases pain during intravenous cannulation when compared with placebo spray or no treatment in both adults and children.[56]

The classic vapocoolant agent, Gebauer's Ethyl Chloride®, is available in glass bottle and metal can containers. Both vessels are held 3 to 9 in. away from the treatment area in a well-ventilated space. The bottle is held upside down, while the Accu-Stream 360 canister may be held in any position. The stream of Ethyl Chloride is sprayed continuously to the site for 3 to 7 s from the bottle and 4 to 10 s from the can, or until the skin just turns white—

whichever occurs first. The needle is then immediately inserted into the skin. Extra caution must be exercised when using Ethyl Chloride® as this product is flammable. It should never be used in the setting of open flames or sparks—including cautery units, hyfrecators, electrosurgical machines, radiofrequency devices, intense pulsed light generators, or lasers.

Alternatively, Gebauer's Pain Ease® (a proprietary mixture of 1,1,1,3,3-pentafluoro-propane and 1,1,1,2-tetrafluoroethane) is available both as a medium stream spray and as an aerosolized mist spray. These products are distributed in pressurized metal cans and are nonflammable products. Both Pain Ease® products are administered at a distance of 3 to 7 in. from the target site by holding the can in an upright position. They are sprayed for 4 to 10 s until the skin begins to frost. Do not spray for longer than 10 s. The medium stream produces a pinpoint stream in a smaller target site. The fine droplets of mist are dispersed in a 3-cm diameter circular pattern. Adequate local anesthesia for needle injection or minor surgical procedures lasts up to 30 s. Pain Ease® is not carcinogenic or teratogenic and, thus, may be used safely in pregnancy when used as directed. Furthermore, this product offers advantages over Ethyl Chloride®, including a larger field of anesthesia and lack of "running" of liquid down the skin (with use of the mist spray) and no fire hazard. In contrast to Ethyl Chloride® which is only approved for use on intact skin, Pain Ease® may also be used on minor skin wounds, and intact mucous membranes. With prolonged contact, both Ethyl Chloride® and Pain Ease® may damage polyvinylchloride coverings used to upholster examination tables. Barrier pads used during injections effectively keep the vapocoolant fluid from contact with the upholstery.

Ethyl Chloride® and Pain Ease® do not claim to be sterile, but the products have passed the Microbial Limit Test in accordance with the United States Pharmacopeia. These tests are designed to demonstrate that a substance is free from *Staphylococcus aureus*, *Escherichia coli*, *Pseudomonas aeruginosa*, and *Salmonella* species. Those tests also measure total bacteria, mold, and yeast growth.[57] A 2012 study showed that Ethyl Chloride® may be an effective disinfectant alone and may improve skin disinfection when used with povidone–iodine compared to povidone–iodine alone.[58] Thus, there does not appear to be a need to wipe the field with an antiseptic agent again following the application of a topical vapocoolant spray.

EQUIPMENT

It is highly recommended that medical providers organize all of the equipment and supplies needed to perform injections and aspirations. Organizing them presents the materials conveniently to the practitioner. This decreases the amount of time required to gather all of the necessary items. It also reduces the possibility of inadvertent medical errors. Organizing all equipment/supplies should be done well before the procedure is performed. Based on provider or organization preference, four options can be utilized.

1. A dedicated cabinet
2. An injection tray
3. An injection cart
4. Injection packs

A cabinet works well in a setting where the provider consistently works out of the same room. It keeps the supplies centralized and visible but requires collection of the various components at the time a procedure is performed. A large plastic tray or an injection cart provides a portable option for organizing materials. These may work well in a large clinic or teaching setting. Another option is to create "injection packs" that include all of the supplies used universally in these procedures.

After many years of performing these procedures, the author's preferred option in his private medical office is to store materials in a central location. Then, individual injection packs are organized by medical office assistants prior to patient visits. These are placed with associated medications and various syringe and needle options inside a secure cabinet in each examination room. When a patient presents with a condition that requires an injection or aspiration, a pack is simply retrieved from the cabinet and placed on the counter in the examination room. The author uses those materials but is also free to select other syringe sizes and/or needle lengths from the cabinet. At the time of the injection, the author or his staff fills the injection syringe with the appropriate medication(s) and secures the correct needle. This preprocedure organization enhances office efficiency and reduces the possibility of a medical mistake.

Items that should be collected and organized (Fig. 2.1):

- Gloves—nonsterile examination gloves
- Barrier "chucks" pads—nonsterile
- Alcohol pads
- 10% povidone–iodine pads or 2% chlorhexidine–70% alcohol pads
- Gauze pads—nonsterile
- Adhesive bandages
- Hemostat surgical clamp (optional)
- Syringes
  - 3 mL
  - 5 mL
  - 10 mL
  - 20 mL
  - 60 mL
- Needles
  - 20 gauge—1 in. blunt tip fill needles—for drawing medications and aspiration of small joints
  - 18 gauge—1 ½ in.—for aspiration of large joints and bursa
  - 25 gauge—5/8, 1, 1 ½, and 2 in.—for injections
  - 20 gauge—3 ½ in. spinal needles—for deep injections/aspirations
- Pain Ease® mist or medium stream vapocoolant spray
- Lidocaine: 1% plain
- Mepivacaine: 1% plain
- Bupivacaine: 0.5% plain
- Steroid of choice (usually triamcinolone 40 mg/mL)
- Viscosupplementation agent of choice (ordered as needed)

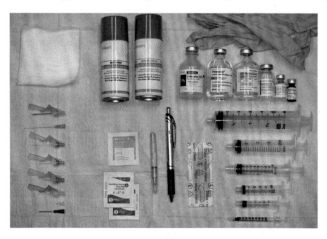

FIGURE 2.1 ● Equipment for injections and aspirations.

LANDMARK-GUIDED INJECTION TECHNIQUE

When performing injections and/or aspirations, it is important that the medical provider follows a standardized routine. This helps organize the clinician, prepares the patient, and reduces the possibility of procedural omissions. The following steps should be done in the order presented:

1. Determine the medical diagnosis and consider relevant differential diagnoses.
2. Consider all contraindications to the procedure.
3. Discuss the proposed procedure and alternatives with the patient and/or responsible party.
4. Obtain written informed consent from the patient and/or responsible party.
5. Collect and prepare the required materials.
6. Correctly position the patient for the procedure.
7. Identify and mark the anatomic landmarks and injection site with ink. (Do not allow the patient to move the affected area from the time that the marks are placed until after the procedure is completed.)
8. Press firmly on the skin with the retracted tip of a ballpoint pen to further identify the injection site.
9. Put on clean examination gloves.
10. Prepare clean skin with an alcohol pad followed by either a 10% povidone–iodine pad or a 2% chlorhexidine–70% alcohol pad. Then allow this to dry according to the manufacturer's recommendations.
11. Provide local anesthesia as indicated through use of tactile distraction, vapocoolant spray (Pain Ease®), and/or injected local anesthesia.
12. Using the no-touch technique, introduce the needle at the insertion site and advance it precisely into the treatment area.
13. If using ultrasound guidance, follow the instructions regarding technique in the ultrasound section (optional).
14. Aspirate synovial or bursa fluid (optional) and send it for laboratory examination if indicated. If injecting corticosteroid solution or viscosupplement immediately following aspiration, do not remove the needle from the joint or bursa. In this case, grasp the needle hub firmly (with a hemostat clamp if necessary), twist off the original syringe, and then immediately attach the second syringe that contains the corticosteroid.
15. Inject the proper corticosteroid solution or viscosupplement into the target site. Always aspirate before injection to avoid intravascular administration. Do not inject the medication against resistance.
16. Withdraw the needle.
17. Apply direct pressure over the injection site with a sterile gauze pad.
18. Apply a sterile adhesive bandage.
19. Provide the patient with specific postinjection instructions.

SYNOVIAL FLUID ANALYSIS

The acquisition of a sample of synovial fluid for microscopic analysis is the primary objective of arthrocentesis. Examination of the fluid can provide information critical to the diagnosis of the condition that has caused the joint effusion.[59,60] This is especially important in the case of acute monoarthritis in which either septic or crystal arthritis may be present. After arthrocentesis has been successfully performed, the appearance of the fluid is observed. Normal synovial fluid is clear and transparent. The gross appearance of the fluid should be noted. This provides a quick clinical estimation of the amount of inflammation present in the joint. Totally transparent fluid originates in normal joints and is observed with noninflammatory conditions such as osteoarthritis. The degree of turbidity generally parallels the amount of inflammation. Most turbid to purulent synovial fluid usually occurs in septic joints, but exceptions are not uncommon. Next, the fluid is either immediately examined under a microscope or transferred as quickly as possible to a laboratory capable of providing diagnostic testing. When the specimen is sent for synovial fluid analysis, it is placed in a glass tube anticoagulated with liquid ethylenediaminetetraacetate (EDTA). Do not use tubes that contain heparin, oxalate, or lithium since these anticoagulants confound crystal analysis. However, for best practices, contact the local laboratory to determine the preferred method for transportation of the fluid. Fluid submitted for culture is transferred from the syringe to appropriate culture media. A general bacterial culture medium is appropriate for most cases of septic arthritis. However, gonorrhea is a common cause of septic monoarthritis. If this is suspected, then transport it in Thayer–Martin medium under carbon dioxide. Cultures from other sites including the pharynx, cervix, urethra, and rectum are necessary if gonococcal disease is suspected. Plate the specimen for growth in Sabouraud dextrose agar if a fungal infection is a consideration.

In the past, a number of tests for glucose, pH, and lactic acid were routinely performed, but evidence-based investigation has disproved their value. Traditionally, joint effusions have been classified as normal, noninflammatory, inflammatory, septic, and hemorrhagic. The absolute cell count is the major discriminating factor between an inflammatory fluid and a noninflammatory fluid. Fluids with cell counts less than 2,000 cells/mm^3 are likely to be noninflammatory, and inflammatory fluids generally have more than 2,000 cells/mm^3. The differential leukocyte count may add further information. Noninflammatory fluid generally contains less than 50% polymorphonuclear cells (PMNs) and an inflammatory fluid considerably more. The only clinically useful synovial tests in the setting of septic arthritis are the WBC count, percentage of PMNs, Gram stain, and culture.

Crystal analysis can be performed in any office equipped with a microscope. A single drop of fluid is placed on a clean slide and examined under a cover slip. Crystals can be observed with plain microscopy and preliminary identification made for crystals, WBCs, and bacteria. A polarizing light microscope provides the gold standard for crystal identification. This is usually present only in a referral laboratory. Monosodium urate crystals found in gout appear needle-shaped and are strongly negatively birefringent when examined under polarization. Calcium pyrophosphate dihydrate crystals are found in pseudogout. These are strongly refractile, short, rhomboid-shaped, and weakly positively birefringent. The presence of intracellular crystals is an even more specific predictor for gout or pseudogout (Table 2.1).

AFTERCARE

Immediately following the aspiration and/or injection procedure, apply pressure to the sterile bandage, covering the site. Once the provider is assured that the patient is stable and is not at risk of falling, the patient should be brought down from the examination/procedure table. Gentle massage and slow range of motion should be encouraged to enable distribution of the corticosteroid throughout the joint space or soft tissues. After discharge from the office, patients should be advised to look for and immediately report any adverse reactions. Of primary importance is recognizing the early signs of infection. Therefore, any swelling, redness, increased warmth, proximal red streaking, or fever greater than 100°F should be reported immediately.

TABLE 2.1

Synovial Fluid Properties

	Appearance	Viscosity	Cells/mm³	% PMNs	Crystals
Normal	Transparent	High	<180	<10%	None
Osteoarthritis	Transparent	High	200–2,000	<10%	None
Rheumatoid arthritis	Translucent	Low	2,000–50,000	Variable	None
Psoriatic arthritis	Translucent	Low	2,000–50,000	Variable	None
Reactive arthritis	Translucent	Low	2,000–50,000	Variable	None
Gout	Translucent to cloudy	Low	2,000–50,000	>90%	Needle-like + birefringence
Pseudogout	Translucent to cloudy	Low	2,000–50,000	>90%	Rhomboid-like + birefringence
Septic arthritis	Cloudy	Variable	2,000–50,000+	>90%	None
Hemarthrosis	Red	Low	2,000–50,000	<10%	None

Patients often experience complete resolution of pain following injection with a local anesthetic. Because of pain relief and absence of negative feedback, there is an increased risk of further injury to the treated area. They should be informed that the initial pain relief is provided by the injected local anesthetic and that its effect will only be temporary. In the case of plain 1% lidocaine, pain relief can be expected to last only about 1 h. The anti-inflammatory effect of the injected corticosteroid product usually has a 24 to 48 h onset of action. Thus, patients should be informed that the pain is expected to return in about an hour and decrease again in 1 to 2 days.

Additional instructions may be given following aspiration and/or injection. The patient might be directed to apply ice to the affected area. However, there is no evidence that this is beneficial. NSAIDs may be prescribed depending on the clinical situation— but with full knowledge and considerations of the side effects and potential toxicities discussed earlier in this chapter. Studies have shown that immobilization of the affected area is not necessary,[61,62] but reduced usage and activity modification are often helpful. A compressive elastic wrap or splint may be desired, but again, there is no literature support for routinely splinting injected areas in the medical literature. An aftercare patient education handout that outlines the most common possible adverse reactions and specific instructions is a useful document (see Appendix 2).

DOCUMENTATION OF THE PROCEDURE

A very important step in the provision of medical services is the full and accurate description of the events that occurred before, during, and after the procedure. This serves not only as the official medical record but also as a billing record and a legal document. The note should affirm that discussion of the proposed procedure and the alternative treatments occurred, possible complications were discussed, and all questions were answered. The note must include the fact that written informed consent was obtained. Then, it should document patient position, anesthesia, supplies used, and the physical steps involved in performing the procedure. The record should also include any pertinent findings, complications encountered, and the patient's postprocedure condition. Finally, a list of patient instructions, treatment plan, and follow-up care should be documented and signed by the medical provider and any supervisors if necessary.

See the example of documentation for a knee joint aspiration and injection in Appendix 3. This may be modified as needed to meet the needs of the specific aspiration/injection procedure, patient, provider, and medical organization. A review of this document by legal counsel prior to implementation is recommended.

BILLING AND CODING

In order to receive appropriate payment, it is essential that the clinician assigns the proper code(s) for the procedure(s) performed. This ensures fair payment for the work done at the visit and reimbursement for any eligible supplies. A complete description of the procedure(s) performed during the patient encounter must be documented in the medical record in order to support the level of coding. At the time of publication, the following Current Procedural Terminology (CPT®) 2021 codes are employed to bill for skin, perineural, and musculoskeletal injections and aspirations:

CPT 2021 defines small joints as those in the fingers and toes. Temporomandibular, acromioclavicular, sternoclavicular, wrist, elbow, ankle, and olecranon bursae are defined as intermediate joints or bursa. Large structures are the glenohumeral joint, sacroiliac joint, hip joint, knee joint, and the subacromial bursa.

According to their definitions, the CPT codes 20550, 20551, 20600, 20605, and 20610 are used once for each tendon, joint, or bursa injected. If more than one tendon, joint, or bursa is injected at a visit, then the codes are listed multiple times for each separate structure that is injected. In addition, the modifiers −51 or −59 should be used to indicate when multiple procedures are performed. Usually −59 is used to code for multiple injections at different sites, but the specific modifier used is determined by the preference of each insurance carrier. Note that trigger point injection CPT codes 20552 and 20553 are used only once each session, regardless of the number of injections performed. CPT 2021 gives specific instructions when reporting multiple ganglion cyst aspirations/injections. In this case, the code 20612 is used and the modifier −59 appended.

CPT 2021 does not specifically define codes to be used for corticosteroid injections of either the ulnar nerve in cubital tunnel syndrome or with the entrapment of the deep branch of the radial nerve (posterior interosseous nerve). The author feels that until CPT descriptors change, the code 64450 (injection, anesthetic agent, other peripheral nerve, or branch) most accurately reflects the procedure performed in these conditions.

Medicare and most commercial insurance companies apply the multiple surgery rule when paying for multiple injections. They generally pay 100% for the first procedure, 50% for the second, and 25% for third and subsequent procedures.

Diagnostic codes must also be submitted in order for an insurance company to justify payment for the injection/aspiration procedure. These codes follow the standard International Classification of Diseases (ICD) system. In each of the injection chapters of this book, the most commonly used ICD-10 (http://www.cdc.gov/nchs/icd/icd10cm.htm) codes are listed.

J codes are utilized to charge for the injected medication/device used during the procedure. Therapeutic injectable products, such as corticosteroids and viscosupplementation agents, are billed in addition to the injection administration codes (Table 2.2). The J codes are not used for local anesthetics since their use is considered a necessary part of the procedure much like the needle and syringe. The charge is reflected as the number of units used during the procedure. For instance, the J code for Kenalog® is expressed in 10 mg units. If

TABLE 2.2

2021 CPT Codes for Injection Procedures

- 11900—Intralesional injections (1–7 lesions)
- 11901—Intralesional injections (>7 lesions)
- 20526—Injection, therapeutic, carpal tunnel
- 20550—Injection(s), single tendon sheath, or ligament, aponeurosis (e.g., plantar "fascia")
- 20551—Injection, single tendon origin/insertion
- 20552—Injection(s), single or multiple trigger point(s), 1 or 2 muscles
- 20553—Injection(s), trigger point(s), 3 or more muscles
- 20600—Arthrocentesis, aspiration and/or injection, *small* joint or bursa; without ultrasound guidance
- 20604—with ultrasound guidance, with permanent recording and reporting
- 20605—Arthrocentesis, aspiration and/or injection, *intermediate* joint or bursa; without ultrasound guidance
- 20606—with ultrasound guidance, with permanent recording and reporting
- 20610—Arthrocentesis, aspiration and/or injection, *major* joint or bursa; without ultrasound guidance
- 20611—with ultrasound guidance, with permanent recording and reporting
- 20612—Aspiration and/or injection of ganglion cyst(s), any location
- 27096—Injection of SI joint using anesthetic agents and/or steroid, with imaging guidance and permanent recording
- 64400—Injection, anesthetic agent; trigeminal nerve, any division or branch
- 64402—Injection, anesthetic agent; facial nerve
- 64405—Injection, anesthetic agent; greater occipital nerve
- 64418—Injection, anesthetic agent (nerve block), diagnostic or therapeutic procedures on the somatic nerves
- 64450—Injection, nerve block, therapeutic, other peripheral nerve or branch
- 64455—Injection(s), anesthetic agent, and/or steroid, plantar common digital nerve(s) (e.g. Morton's neuroma)
- 68200—Subconjunctival injection
- 76942—Ultrasonic guidance for needle placement with imaging supervision and interpretation with permanent recording

the injection is done with 40 mg of Kenalog, then the patient is charged 4 units of J3301. The most common current J codes used for injection are listed in Table 2.3.

An evaluation and management (E&M) code can be billed if the documentation of the visit supports the necessity and completeness of the evaluation. This requires the −25 modifier and may be used only if there is a "significant, separately identifiable evaluation and management service by the same physician or other qualified health care professional on the same day of the procedure or other service".[63] Otherwise, only the CPT code and associated J code can be used if the evaluation is not performed or does not meet those conditions.

INFORMED CONSENT

As with any invasive procedure, informed consent must be obtained from the patient. For the purpose of documentation, this should be done in a written format. The patient must also have an adequate opportunity to ask questions including a discussion of alternative methods of diagnosis and treatment. An example of an informed consent form is included in Appendix 1.

TABLE 2.3

2021 HCPCS J Codes for Injectables

J-Code	Material	Unit (mg)
J3301	Kenalog®	10
J3303	Aristospan®	5
J1020	Depo-Medrol®	20
J1030	Depo-Medrol®	40
J1040	Depo-Medrol®	80
J0704	Celestone Soluspan®	6
J1094	Decadron-LA®	1
J7318	Durolane®	60
J7320	Genvisc-850®	25
J7321	Hyalgan®	20
J7321	Supartz®	25
J7322	Hymovis®	24
J7323	Euflexxa®	20
J7324	Orthovisc®	30
J7325	Synvisc®	16
J7325	Synvisc-One®	48
J7326	Gel-One®	90
J7327	Monovisc®	88
J7328	Gelsyn-3®	34
J0585	Botulinum toxin type A	1
J0587	Botulinum toxin type B	1

EVIDENCE-BASED MEDICINE

Intra-articular and soft tissue corticosteroid injections are common procedures performed by primary care physicians. They are accepted interventions and are frequently used to treat various musculoskeletal conditions. Although significant therapeutic efficacy is claimed from over 50 years of published research, a closer examination of the literature yields less convincing evidence of significant long-term improvement of specific, measured outcomes. The available data support short-term benefit from injected corticosteroids. There is currently insufficient high-quality data to provide a definitive answer on the efficacy of corticosteroid injections. However, lack of discrete medical evidence does not necessarily mean that these procedures are ineffective. Even gold standard, evidence-based, medical resources such as Cochrane Database of Systematic Reviews suffer from performing meta-analysis on studies with data that are themselves flawed. New investigations that are methodologically sound are needed to measure outcomes of corticosteroid injections given for the treatment of specific conditions.

REFERENCES

1. Qaseem A, McLean RM, O'Gurek D, et al. Nonpharmacologic and pharmacologic management of acute pain from non-low back, musculoskeletal injuries in adults: A clinical guideline from the American College of Physicians and American Academy of Family Physicians. *Ann Intern Med*. 2020;173:739–748. doi: 10.7326/M19-3602.

2. Zeng C, Wei J, Persson MSM, et al. Relative efficacy and safety of topical non-steroidal anti-inflammatory drugs for osteoarthritis: A systematic review and network meta-analysis of randomised controlled trials and observational studies. *Br J Sports Med*. 2018;52(10):642–650.

3. Bally M, Dendukuri N, Rich B, et al. Risk of acute myocardial infarction with NSAIDs in real world use: Bayesian meta-analysis of individual patient data. *BMJ*. 2017;357:j1909.

4. Coxib and traditional NSAID Trialists' Collaboration. Vascular and upper gastrointestinal effects of non-steroidal anti-inflammatory drugs: Meta-analyses of individual participant data from randomised trials. *Lancet*. 2013;382(9894):769–779.

5. Olsen AS, Fosbøl EL, Lindhardsen J, et al. Duration of treatment with nonsteroidal anti-inflammatory drugs and impact on risk of death and recurrent myocardial infarction in patients with prior myocardial infarction. A Nationwide Cohort Study. *Circulation*. 2011;123:2226–2235.

6. Schmidt M, Christiansen CF, Mehnert F, et al. Non-steroidal anti-inflammatory drug use and risk of atrial fibrillation or flutter: Population based case–control study. *BMJ*. 2011;343:d3450.

7. Krijthe BP, Heeringa J, Hofman A, et al. Non-steroidal anti-inflammatory drugs and the risk of atrial fibrillation: A population-based follow-up study. *BMJ Open*. 2014;4(4):e004059.

8. Ungprasert P, Srivali N, Wijarnpreecha K, et al. Non-steroidal anti-inflammatory drugs and risk of venous thromboembolism: A systematic review and meta-analysis. *Rheumatology*. 2015;54(4):736–742.

9. Nourjah P, et al. Estimates of acetaminophen (Paracetamol)-associated overdoses in the United States. *Pharmacoepidemiol Drug Saf*. 2006;15:398–405.

10. Bower WA, et al. Population-based surveillance for acute liver failure. *Am J Gastroenterol*. 2007;102:2459–2463.

11. Mowry JB, Spyker DA, Brooks DE, et al. 2014 annual report of the American Association of Poison Control Centers' National Poison Data System (NPDS): 32nd annual report. *Clin Toxicol (Phila)*. 2015;53(10):962–1147.

12. Roberts E, Delgado Nunes V, Buckner S, et al. Paracetamol: Not as safe as we thought? A systematic literature review of observational studies. *Ann Rheum Dis*. 2016;75(3):552–559.

13. FDA Drug Safety Communication: FDA warns of rare but serious skin reactions with the pain reliever/fever reducer acetaminophen. Available at: http://www.fda.gov/Drugs/DrugSafety/ucm363041.htm. Accessed on December 29, 2013.

14. Toupin April K, Bisaillon J, Welch V, et al. Tramadol for osteoarthritis. *Cochrane Database Syst Rev*. 2019;(5):CD005522. doi: 10.1002/14651858.CD005522.pub3.

15. Riva JJ, Noor ST, Wang L, et al. Predictors of prolonged opioid use after initial prescription for acute musculoskeletal injuries in adults: A systematic review and meta-analysis of observational studies. *Ann Intern Med*. 2020;173:721–729. doi: 10.7326/M19-3600.

16. Els C, Jackson TD, Kunyk D, et al. Adverse events associated with medium- and long-term use of opioids for chronic non-cancer pain: An overview of Cochrane Reviews. *Cochrane Database Syst Rev*. 2017;10(10):CD012509.

17. Park K, Kim S, Ko YJ, et al. Duloxetine and cardiovascular adverse events: A systematic review and meta-analysis. *J Psychiatr Res*. 2020;124:109–114.

18. Ogata T, Ideno Y, Akai M, et al. Effects of glucosamine in patients with osteoarthritis of the knee: A systematic review and meta-analysis. *Clin Rheumatol*. 2018;37(9):2479–2487.

19. Allen KD, Choong PF, Davis AM, et al. Osteoarthritis: Models for appropriate care across the disease continuum. *Best Pract Res Clin Rheumatol*. 2016;30(3):503–535.

20. Patel IJ, Davidson JC, Nikolic B, et al. Standards of practice committee, with Cardiovascular and Interventional Radiological Society of Europe (CIRSE) endorsement. *J Vasc Interv Radiol*. 2012;23(6):727–736.

21. Thumboo J, O'Duffy JD. A prospective study of the safety of joint and soft tissue aspiration and injections in patients taking warfarin sodium. *Arthritis Rheum*. 1998;41(4):736–739.

22. Foremny GB, Pretell-Mazzini J, Jose J, et al. Risk of bleeding associated with interventional musculoskeletal radiology procedures. A comprehensive review of the literature. *Skeletal Radiol*. 2015;44(5):619–627.

23. Habib GS, Bashir M, Jabbour A. Increased blood glucose levels following intra-articular injection of methylprednisolone acetate in patients with controlled diabetes and symptomatic osteoarthritis of the knee. *Ann Rheum Dis*. 2008;67:1790–1791.

24. Habib G, Safi A. The effect of intra-articular injection of betamethasone acetate/betamethasone sodium phosphate on blood glucose levels in controlled diabetic patients with symptomatic osteoarthritis of the knee. *Clin Rheumatol*. 2009;28:85–87.

25. Habib GS, Abu-Ahmad R. Lack of effect of corticosteroid injection at the shoulder joint on blood glucose levels in diabetic patients. *Clin Rheumatol*. 2007;26:566–568.

26. Rogojan C, Hetland ML. Depigmentation: A rare side effect to intra-articular glucocorticoid treatment. *Clin Rheumatol*. 2004;23:373–375.

27. Lund IM, Donde R, Knudsen EA. Persistent local cutaneous atrophy following corticosteroid injection for tendinitis. *Rheumatol Rehabil*. 1979;18:91–93.
28. Shumaker PR, Rao J, Goldman MP. Treatment of local, persistent cutaneous atrophy following corticosteroid injection with normal saline infiltration. *Dermatol Surg*. 2005;31:1340–1343.
29. Clark SC, et al. Bilateral patellar tendon rupture secondary to repeated local steroid injections. *J Accid Emerg Med*. 1995;12:300–301.
30. Ford LT, DeBender J. Tendon rupture after local steroid injection. *South Med J*. 1979;72:827–830.
31. Chen SK, et al. Patellar tendon ruptures in weight lifters after local steroid injections. *Arch Orthop Trauma Surg*. 2009;129:369–372.
32. Scutt N, Rolf CG, Scutt A. Glucocorticoids inhibit tenocyte proliferation and tendon progenitor cell recruitment. *J Orthop Res*. 2006;24:173–182.
33. Paik NC, Seo JW. CT-guided needle aspiration of pneumothorax from a trigger point injection. *Pain Med*. 2011;12(5):837–841.
34. Jalul M, Humphrey AR. Radial artery injury caused by a sclerosant injected into a palmar wrist ganglion. *J Hand Surg Eur Vol*. 2009;34(5):698–699.
35. Fujita F, Moriyama T, Higashi T, et al. Methyl p-hydroxybenzoate causes pain sensation through activation of TRPA1 channels. *Br J Pharmacol*. 2007;151(1):153–160.
36. Epstein SP, Ahdoot M, Marcus E, et al. Comparative toxicity of preservatives on immortalized corneal and conjunctival epithelial cells. *J Ocul Pharmacol Ther*. 2009;25(2):113–119.
37. Dragoo JL, et al. The in vitro chondrotoxicity of single-dose local anesthetics. *Am J Sports Med*. 2012;40(4):794–799
38. Jacobs TF, et al. The effect of Lidocaine on the viability of cultivated mature human cartilage cells: An in vitro study. *Knee Surg Sports Traumatol Arthrosc*. 2011;19(7):1206–1213.
39. Wiater BP, et al. Risk factors for chondrolysis of the glenohumeral joint: A study of three hundred and seventy-five shoulder arthroscopic procedures in the practice of an individual community surgeon. *J Bone Joint Surg Am*. 2011;93(7):615–625.
40. Scheffel PT, et al. Glenohumeral chondrolysis: A systematic review of 100 cases from the English language literature. *J Shoulder Elbow Surg*. 2010;19(6):944–949.
41. Grishko V, et al. Apoptosis and mitochondrial dysfunction in human chondrocytes following exposure to lidocaine, bupivacaine, and ropivacaine. *J Bone Joint Surg Am*. 2010;92(3):609–618.
42. Dragoo JL, et al. Chondrotoxicity of low pH, epinephrine, and preservatives found in local anesthetics containing epinephrine. *Am J Sports Med*. 2010;38(6):1154–1159.
43. Miller RD, Pardo MC Jr. *Basics of Anesthesia*, 6th Ed. Philadelphia, PA: Elsevier Saunders, 2011:136.
44. Becker DE, Reed KL. Essentials of local anesthetic pharmacology. *Anesth Prog*. 2006;53(3):98–109.
45. Kreuz PC, Steinwachs M, Angele P. Single-dose local anesthetics exhibit a type-, dose-, and time-dependent chondrotoxic effect on chondrocytes and cartilage: A systematic review of the current literature. *Knee Surg Sports Traumatol Arthrosc*. 2018;26(3):819–830.
46. McAlindon TE, LaValley MP, Harvey WF, et al. Effect of intra-articular triamcinolone vs saline on knee cartilage volume and pain in patients with knee osteoarthritis: A randomized clinical trial. *JAMA*. 2017;317(19):1967–1975.
47. Rabih O, Darouiche MD, et al. Chlorhexidine-alcohol versus povidone-iodine for surgical-site antisepsis. *N Engl J Med*. 2010;362:18–26.
48. Wade RG, Burr NE, McCauley G, et al. The comparative efficacy of chlorhexidine gluconate and povidone-iodine antiseptics for the prevention of infection in clean surgery: A systematic review and network meta-analysis. *Ann Surg*. 2020. Sep 1. doi: 10.1097/SLA.0000000000004076. Epub ahead of print. PMID: 32773627.
49. Krobbuaban B, Diregpoke S, et al. Alcohol-based chlorhexidine vs. povidone iodine in reducing skin colonization prior to regional anesthesia procedures. *J Med Assoc Thai*. 2011;94(7):807–812.
50. Ostrander RV, Botte MJ, Brage ME. Efficacy of surgical preparation solutions in foot and ankle surgery. *J Bone Joint Surg Am*. 2005;87:980–985.
51. Bibbo C, Patel DV, Gehrmann RM, et al. Chlorhexidine provides superior skin decontamination in foot and ankle surgery: A prospective randomized study. *Clin Orthop Relat Res*. 2005;438:204–208.
52. Mangram, AJ, et al. CDC: Guideline for prevention of surgical site infection, 1999. *Infect Control Hosp Epidemiol*. 1999;20(4):250–266. Available at: http://www.cdc.gov/hicpac/pdf/guidelines/SSI_1999.pdf
53. Brown TR, et al. A clinical evaluation of chlorhexidine gluconate spray as compared with iodophor scrub for preoperative skin preparation. *Surg Gynecol Obstet*. 1984;158:363–366.
54. Denton GW. Chlorhexidine. In: Block SS, ed. *Disinfection, Sterilization, and Preservation*, 5th Ed. Philadelphia, PA: Lippincott Williams & Wilkins, 2001:321–336.
55. Berry PH, Dahl JD. The new JCAHO pain standards: Implications for pain management nurses. *Pain Manag Nurs*. 2000;1(1):3–12.
56. Zhu Y, Peng X, et al. Vapocoolant spray versus placebo spray/no treatment for reducing pain from intravenous cannulation: A meta-analysis of randomized controlled trials. *Am J Emerg Med*. 2018;36(11):2085–2092.
57. Gebauer's Pain Ease® Topical Anesthetic Skin Refrigerant Technical Data Document. Available at: http://www.gebauer.com/Portals/150313/docs/pe%20technical%20data%20document.pdf. Accessed on May 3, 2014.
58. Azar FM, Lake JE, Grace SP, et al. Ethyl chloride improves antiseptic effect of betadine skin preparation for office procedures. *J Surg Orthop Adv*. 2012;21(2):84–87.
59. Courtney P, Doherty M. Joint aspiration and injection and synovial fluid analysis. *Best Pract Res Clin Rheumatol*. 2013;27(2):137–169.

60. Pascual E, Sivera F, Andrés M. Synovial fluid analysis for crystals. *Curr Opin Rheumatol.* 2011;23(2):161–169.
61. Charalambous C, Paschalides C, Sadiq S, et al. Weight bearing following intra-articular steroid injection of the knee: Survey of current practice and review of the available evidence. *Rheumatol Int.* 2002;22(5): 185–187.
62. Chatham W, et al. Intraarticular corticosteroid injections: Should we rest the joints? *Arthritis Care Res.* 1989;2(2):70–74.
63. American Medical Association. CPT® 2021 Professional Edition, 2021:978. ISBN#: 978-1-64016-049-1.

3

Injectable Agents

James W. McNabb

LOCAL ANESTHETICS

Local anesthetics are membrane-stabilizing drugs. They act by inhibiting sodium influx through sodium-specific ion channels in the neuronal cell membrane. They reversibly decrease the rate of depolarization and repolarization of excitable membranes in nociceptors—thus interrupting pain impulses.

Local anesthetics are commonly injected either alone or with another compound, such as a corticosteroid when treating painful conditions. The injection of local anesthetic into joints or soft tissues serves several purposes. Administration of the local anesthetic provides short-term pain relief. This allows for patient feedback. It may provide a more comprehensive examination of the affected area without the limitation of pain. Although mixing steroids with local anesthetics is not recommended by the manufacturers of injectable corticosteroids, it is common clinical practice to mix a local anesthetic in the same syringe as the corticosteroid solution prior to injection. By convention, the clear liquid (local anesthetic) is drawn up in the syringe first, followed by the cloudy fluid (steroid). The added volume of the local anesthetic helps dilute the corticosteroid. This enables dispersion of steroid in a large joint space or bursa. Pain relief following injection confirms the proper placement of corticosteroid both to the clinician and to the patient. Although pain may return after the effect of the anesthetic wears off, the patient can be assured that the injected corticosteroid is properly placed and should begin to exert its clinical effect within 24 to 48 hours.

There are several commercially available choices of local anesthetics. Most commonly, the amide class of local anesthetics is used. The clinically significant characteristics of the amides are summarized in Table 3.1. Lidocaine (lignocaine, Xylocaine®) for local anesthetic injection is commercially available as 0.5%, 1%, and 2% concentrations with or without epinephrine. Duration of action for infiltration anesthesia without epinephrine is 30 to 120 minutes. For soft tissue injections, the author exclusively uses 1% lidocaine without epinephrine. This is commonly available in multiuse bottles containing the preservative, methylparaben. Lidocaine is also available in 2-mL single-use preservative-free vials. The 2% solution of lidocaine confers no clinically important advantages and increases the risk of toxicity following administration of large amounts of greater than 4.5 mg/kg. The inclusion of epinephrine likewise offers no clinical advantages with musculoskeletal injections/aspirations and is not used in these procedures to dilute the corticosteroid. In fact, lidocaine with epinephrine is acidic (pH = 4.5) and causes significant transient local burning pain upon injection.

Bupivacaine (Marcaine®, Sensorcaine®, Vivacaine®, Exparel®) is another commonly used local anesthetic. It has a longer onset of action but offers extended anesthetic effect. Duration of action for infiltration anesthesia without epinephrine is 120 to 240 minutes.

Characteristics of Common Local Anesthetics

Anesthetic	Onset of Action (min)	Duration Without Epinephrine (min)	Max. Dosage w/o Epinephrine (mg/kg)
Lidocaine	<1	30–120	4.5
Mepivacaine	3–20	30–120	6.0
Bupivacaine	2–10	120–240	2.5
Ropivacaine	3–15	120–240	2.5

Adapted from Kouba DJ, LoPiccolo MC, Alam M, et al. Guidelines for the use of local anesthesia in office-based dermatologic surgery. *J Am Acad Dermatol.* 2016;74:1201–1219; Park KK, Sharon VR. A review of local anesthetics: Minimizing risk and side effects in cutaneous surgery. *Dermatol Surg.* 2017;43:173–187.

Multidose vials also contain 1 mg of methylparaben as a preservative. Many clinicians prefer to mix 1% lidocaine with 0.25% bupivacaine in order to give the patient rapid onset of local anesthesia with an extended duration. However, there is no proven clinical benefit using this approach. Because of the additional steps required to draw up the separate anesthetics, preparation of this combination may increase the chance of contamination and needle stick injury. It may also give the patient a false sense of security since there is prolonged initial pain relief before the tissues have healed. Since the negative feedback from pain is absent for an extended period of time, the patient might suffer further injury such as tendon rupture through inadvertent use of the affected body area.

Mepivacaine (Carbocaine®) is a newer agent that is a shorter-acting homolog of bupivacaine. It is available as 1%, 2%, and 3% solutions for injection. It has a shorter onset of action and anesthetic effect. Duration of action for infiltration anesthesia without epinephrine is 30 to 120 minutes. This is available in multiuse bottles containing the preservative, methylparaben, and also as single-use preservative-free vials.

Ropivacaine (Naropin®) is a newer agent that is also a long-acting homolog of bupivacaine. It is available as a 0.5% solution for injection. It also has a longer onset of action and offers extended anesthetic effect. Duration of action for infiltration anesthesia without epinephrine is extended at 120 to 240 minutes. Ropivacaine is available in multiuse bottles containing the preservative, methylparaben, and also as single-use preservative-free vials.

Levobupivacaine (Chirocaine®) is the levo-enantiomer of bupivacaine. It is also a recently developed option for local anesthesia. Levobupivacaine is commercially available as 2.5, 5.0, and 7.5 mg/mL solutions. Both of these stereoisomers display less cardiovascular and central nervous system toxicity than does racemic bupivacaine.[1]

The pH of local anesthetics can be buffered to decrease local pain. The pH of 1% lidocaine without epinephrine is 6.5, while the pH of 1% lidocaine with epinephrine is 4.5. Bupivacaine is isotonic. Adding sterile 8.4% sodium bicarbonate to lidocaine with epinephrine at a ratio of 1:10 neutralizes the mixture and has been shown to provide significant pain relief. However, this is not a clinically important issue with joint injections because plain lidocaine is used and not lidocaine with epinephrine.

In general, the amount of local anesthetic injected is dependent on the injection site and disease process. The smallest volume of the lowest concentration of the anesthetic with the least side effect profile should be used. For instance, large volumes (5 to 10 mL) of lidocaine were commonly used in the past for treatment of large joints such as shoulders, SI joints, hips, and knees. More recently, the author has found equivalent anesthetic effect with much small volumes (0.5 to 1 mL) of mepivacaine or other anesthetics. This recommendation to limit anesthetic administration is made to decrease the possibility of local and systemic toxicity.

A discussion of chondrocyte toxicity of the amide class of local anesthetics is included in the Complications section of this chapter.

CORTICOSTEROIDS

Corticosteroids used for injection purposes are synthetic derivatives of hydrocortisone. The exact mechanism of action of corticosteroids is complex with various sites of action. They bind to glucocorticoid receptors regulating gene transcription. By altering the production of protein annexin-1, corticosteroids reduce cytokines and other inflammatory mediators.[2–4] They lead to down-regulation of immune function,[5] inhibition of cell-mediated immunity, and reduction in the number of macrophages and PMNs accumulating at inflammatory sites. There is also a vascular stabilizing effect by the inhibition of endothelial expression of adhesion molecules for neutrophils. Capillary dilation and vascular permeability are therefore reduced.[2,3] The end-effect is to reduce the amount of inflammation, thereby reducing swelling and pain.

Several corticosteroids are commercially available to use for joint and soft tissue injections (Table 3.2). These include triamcinolone acetonide (Kenalog®), triamcinolone diacetate (Aristocort®), triamcinolone hexacetonide (Aristospan®), methylprednisolone acetate (Depo-Medrol®), betamethasone acetate and sodium phosphate (Celestone Soluspan®), and dexamethasone acetate (Decadron-LA®). The agents differ with regard to their solubility, biological half-life, and potency as compared to hydrocortisone (Table 3.2). Different products have varying effects and solubility in the tissues. The solubility is inversely proportional to the biologic duration of effect of the agent. Hydrocortisone is almost never used because of its high solubility and very short duration of action. It also has significant mineralocorticoid activity that is not shared by the other agents.

TABLE 3.2

Properties of Injectable Corticosteroids

Corticosteroid	Relative Anti-inflammatory Potency	Solubility (%Wt/Vol)	Biologic Half-life (h)
Hydrocortisone acetate (Hydrocortone)	1	High 0.002	8–12
Triamcinolone acetonide (Kenalog®)	5	Intermediate 0.004	12–36
Triamcinolone hexacetonide (Aristospan®)	5	Intermediate 0.0002	12–36
Methylprednisolone acetate (Depo-Medrol®)	5	Intermediate 0.0014	12–36
Betamethasone acetate and sodium phosphate (Celestone Soluspan®)	25	Low/high	26–54
Dexamethasone acetate (Decadron-LA®)	25	Low	26–54

The common synthetic corticosteroids used in musculoskeletal procedures are derivatives of prednisolone. Corticosteroid preparations are either soluble or insoluble. Most corticosteroid preparations contain corticosteroid esters, which are highly insoluble in water and thus form microcrystalline suspensions.[6] The more insoluble, esterified corticosteroids remain at the injection sites far longer than do the soluble forms.

Dexamethasone preparations, however, are not esters and are freely soluble in water; hence, the preparation is clear (i.e., nonparticulate). The potential advantage of corticosteroid ester preparations is that they require hydrolysis by cellular esterases to release the active moiety and consequently should last longer in the joint than do nonester preparations.[7] On the other hand, freely water soluble preparations such as dexamethasone sodium phosphate and betamethasone sodium phosphate are taken up rapidly by cells and thus have a quicker onset of effect but with a concomitant reduced duration of action.[4]

Notably, the betamethasone formulation, Celestone Soluspan®, contains a combination of betamethasone salt and betamethasone ester and, therefore, may provide a dual action of quick onset and long duration of therapy. However, most studies have not shown a clinically significant difference between this product and other corticosteroid ester preparations in terms of onset or duration.[8,9]

Few studies have been conducted that directly compare the various agents in terms of their efficacy. A comparison of intra-articular administration of triamcinolone acetonide, triamcinolone hexacetonide, and a combination of betamethasone phosphate and acetate was conducted by Derendorf and colleagues. They demonstrated complete absorption of all corticosteroids from the site of injection over a period of 2 to 3 weeks. Because of its lower solubility, triamcinolone hexacetonide was absorbed more slowly than triamcinolone acetonide, thus maintaining synovial levels for a longer time and creating lower systemic corticoid levels. Endogenous hydrocortisone suppression correlated with exogenous steroid levels.[10] A systematic review of the relative efficacy of various corticosteroids was published by Garg in 2014. This included seven good quality trials that overall showed no difference in long-term efficacy between the medications that included triamcinolone acetate, triamcinolone hexacetonide, methylprednisolone, and betamethasone.[11] Similar results were reported by Cushman in 2018.[12] In a double blind study utilizing corticosteroid injections of knee joints in patients with rheumatoid arthritis, Hajialilo and colleagues found no difference in pain outcomes comparing triamcinolone hexacetonide and dexamethasone.[13] Another recent double-blind, randomized controlled trial including patients with rheumatoid arthritis or spondyloarthritis with an acutely swollen knee joint found no difference in pain at 24 weeks when injected with either triamcinolone acetonide or methylprednisolone acetate.[14]

No studies have been done that conclusively determine which corticosteroid is preferred for injection of joints versus soft tissues. Without good data, the selection of the particular corticosteroid agent is left to the preference of the individual clinician. Despite lack of literature support, some clinicians prefer to choose a relatively insoluble preparation for intra-articular use and a more soluble form for use in soft tissues and peritendinous injections. Considering medication availability, cost, and past clinical experience, the author prefers to use triamcinolone acetonide (40 mg/mL) for all injections, regardless of site. If another corticosteroid is chosen, then the equivalent dosage and volume of administration may be calculated from the comparison table (Table 3.3).

The dose of corticosteroid to be used generally depends on the injection site, disease process, and degree of inflammation. Unfortunately, there is no quality published medical literature to help in the determination of dosing. In general, the lowest possible dose should be used, at least with the initial injection of a structure. This recommendation is

TABLE 3.3

Equivalent Dosages of Injectable Corticosteroids

Corticosteroid Preparation	Trade Name	Equivalent Dose/Volume (mg/mL)
Triamcinolone acetonide	Kenalog®	40
Triamcinolone hexacetonide	Aristospan®	40
Methylprednisolone acetate	Depo-Medrol®	40
Dexamethasone acetate	Decadron-LA®	8
Betamethasone acetate and sodium phosphate	Celestone Soluspan®	6

made to balance the effectiveness of an injection with the desire to minimize the possibility of local and systemic toxicity. Suggested doses of corticosteroids are listed in each individual injection chapter. Table 3.3 presents equivalent dosages of corticosteroids used for injection. For the purposes of this book, all doses are expressed in milligrams of triamcinolone acetonide suspension (Kenalog). If the practitioner chooses to use another steroid, then the comparative dosage can be simply calculated from the table. For instance, if the chapter in this text indicates that 20 mg of triamcinolone is to be used for injection into the wrist joint, then one could use 20 mg of Kenalog®, 20 mg of Aristospan®, 20 mg of Depo-Medrol®, 4 mg of Decadron-LA®, or 3 mg of Celestone Soluspan®.

Information concerning the frequency of intra-articular corticosteroid injection appears to be primarily based upon professional opinion. An article published in 2014 reviewed this issue.[15] Hypothalamic–pituitary–adrenal axis (HPAA) suppression is the most common and dangerous, although often unrecognized and untreated, side effect of glucocorticoid administration. The risk and duration depend both on patient and treatment characteristics. Guaraldi and colleagues determined that a single 40-mg intrabursal injection of methylprednisolone acetate or triamcinolone acetate is sufficient to suppress the HPAA up to 45 days.[16] Although typically asymptomatic, patients should be instructed to recognize and report symptoms suggestive for hypocortisolism, to provide prompt diagnosis, and eventually, treatment, thus avoiding severe complications. The exact effect of repeated dosing and higher dosing is unknown. In general, most experts advocate that corticosteroid injections should be performed no more often than every 3 months. This non–evidence-based guide is an attempt to prevent potential steroid-related complications including HPAA suppression, osteoporosis, and local articular degradation.

The author typically uses only a small syringe when injecting solutions of anesthetic/corticosteroid. A 3-mL syringe is used at all joint and soft tissue injection sites. This accommodates up to 1 mL of local anesthetic (lidocaine or mepivacaine without epinephrine) and up to 1 mL of corticosteroid. Each syringe is prepared at the time of the procedure by drawing up the volume of local anesthetic first followed by corticosteroid. Prior to injecting a patient with the local anesthetic/corticosteroid mixture, a common observation is that the insoluble corticosteroid often precipitates along the dependent aspect of the syringe. Immediately before the local anesthetic/corticosteroid mixture is injected, 1 mL of air is aspirated into the syringe creating a "mixing bubble" (Fig. 3.1). The syringe is then rapidly rotated in order to disperse the corticosteroid evenly within the volume of local anesthetic. The needle of the syringe is then pointed upward and the small volume of air expelled before the needle is inserted into the skin at the target site.

FIGURE 3.1 ● Mixing bubble.

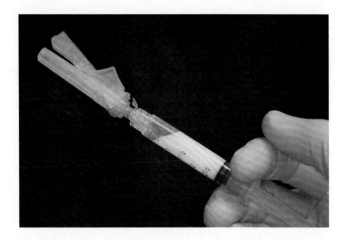

There is a common misconception that distributing the corticosteroid over a wide area enhances the effect from soft tissue injections. Practitioners frequently use a "fanning" or "peppering" technique to distribute the solution across the area of involvement. However, this practice is usually unnecessary. The volume of anesthetic/corticosteroid solution injected as a bolus will passively move along tendon sheaths and local fascia planes. Consideration might be given to "fanning" when injecting trochanteric pain syndrome because the involved area is frequently quite large.

VISCOSUPPLEMENTS

Hyaluronan (sodium hyaluronate) is a natural complex sugar of the glycosaminoglycan family. The concentration and size of endogenous hyaluronan are reduced in the joint fluid of patients with osteoarthritis. There are many commercially available products available for injection that can be used to supplement this substance in joint fluid. These agents are high molecular weight derivatives of hyaluronan, which are synthetically derived from rooster combs or produced by bacterial fermentation and extraction. Injection of exogenous, high molecular weight hyaluronic acid into the joint can interrupt the osteoarthritis cascade by down-regulating the production of the inflammatory cytokines and enzymes, restoring production of native hyaluronic acid, and slowing the progression of osteoarthritis. The exact mechanism of action of viscosupplements is unknown, but result in improved physical cushioning of the knee joint, restoration of favorable viscosity, stimulation of production of endogenous hyaluronan by synoviocytes, decreased inflammation, less pain, and improved knee joint function.

Viscosupplements serve an important role in the treatment of osteoarthritis of the knee. This condition is a chronic disease state that has a number of therapeutic options. Of these, weight reduction and physical therapy are the most effective measures. However, when pain persists, pharmacologic options may be utilized. Unfortunately, oral NSAIDs and acetaminophen are only modestly effective and possess significant toxicity. Opioids should not be used on a chronic basis in this condition. Corticosteroid injections are effective for short- to medium-term use, especially in patients experiencing an acute flare in pain and swelling. Viscosupplements occupy an important position in the mid- (3 months) to long-term (6 months) treatment of knee osteoarthritis. Their use may allow appropriate postponement of knee replacement surgery. They have a documented record of effectiveness and long-term safety. In addition, there may be specific advantages of viscosupplements in the treatment of patients who have brittle diabetes mellitus, those who have failed corticosteroid injections, patients who have received frequent corticosteroids and are in danger of the significant side effects from repeated administration, or those patients who have a rare allergy to corticosteroids.

Injectable hyaluronan products that are currently commercially available in the United States are listed in Table 3.4. They are classified by the U.S. Food and Drug Administration not as medications, but rather as medical devices. These agents are approved only for the treatment of pain in osteoarthritis of the knee joint in patients who have failed to respond adequately to conservative nonpharmacologic therapy and simple analgesics such as acetaminophen. Despite an increasing body of literature, the use of these viscosupplements in other joints besides the knee has not been approved to date by the FDA.

In a 2013 guideline based on consensus, the American Academy of Orthopaedic Surgeons deemed the use of intra-articular injections of hyaluronic acid as not an appropriate treatment modality.[17] On the other hand, the European-based Osteoarthritis Research Society International (OARSI) consensus guidelines published in 2019 now place hyaluronic acid injections as a Level 1B recommendation.[18] Evidence-based support in the medical literature for the use of hyaluronan derivatives is inconsistent, although there is an increasing body of literature documenting positive outcomes. The primary reason for the professional disagreement is due to differences in the studied hyaluronic acid products and especially the significant variations in the quality of trial designs and conduct.

TABLE 3.4

FDA-approved Viscosupplementation Products

Viscosupplementation products—synthetically derived from rooster combs
Gel-One® (Zimmer) http://gelone.zimmerbiomet.com/
    30 mg/mL—3-mL syringe given as a single injection
Synvisc® (Sanofi-Aventus) www.synvisc.com
    8 mg/mL—2-mL syringe given as three weekly injections
Synvisc-One® (Sanofi-Aventus) www.synviscone.com
    8 mg/mL—6-mL syringe given as a single injection
Hyalgan® (Fidia Pharma) www.hyalgan.com
    10 mg/mL—2-mL syringe given as three to five weekly injections
Supartz® (Bioventus) www.supartz.com
    10 mg/mL—2.5-mL syringe given as five weekly injections

Viscosupplementation products—produced by bacterial fermentation and extraction
Euflexxa® (Ferring) www.euflexxa.com
    10 mg/mL—2-mL syringe given as three weekly injections
Durolane® (Bioventus) www.durolane.com
    20 mg/mL—3-mL syringe given as a single injection
Gelsyn-3® (Bioventus) https://www.oakneepainrelief.com/gelsyn_3/
    16.8 mg/mL—2-mL syringe given as three weekly injections
Orthovisc® (Anika) https://www.anikatherapeutics.com/products/orthobiologics/orthovisc/
    15 mg/mL—2-mL syringe given as three to four weekly injections
Monovisc® (Anika) https://www.anikatherapeutics.com/products/orthobiologics/monovisc/
    22 mg/mL—4-mL syringe given as a single injection
Genvisc-850® (OrthogenRx) https://genvisc850.com/
    10 mg/mL—2.5-mL syringe given as five weekly injections
Hymovis (Fidia Pharma) https://hymovis.com/
    8 mg/mL—3-mL syringe given as two weekly injections

In an effort to address this, Xing and colleagues performed a PRISMA-compliant systematic review of overlapping meta-analyses that demonstrates hyaluronic acid injections are an effective intervention in treating knee osteoarthritis without increased risk of adverse events.[19] Furthermore, Altman showed that repeated courses of intra-articular injections of hyaluronic acid are an effective and safe treatment for knee osteoarthritis.[20]

Although these products are similar in many respects, there are significant differences in the physical properties of each one (Table 3.5). Some hyaluronate products are derived from processing of rooster combs. Others are extracted from bacteria that have been genetically engineered to produce exact copies of human hyaluronic acid. More important from a clinical standpoint is the molecular weight of the agent and cross-linking of the molecules. A higher molecular weight and the presence of cross-linking increase the residence time in the joint and generally predict a longer term response to treatment. Research suggests that there is an optimal molecular weight range that maximizes the ability of how hyaluronic acid interacts with cell surface receptors on synoviocytes, thereby maximizing the synthesis of native hyaluronic acid.[21] Optimal molecular weight molecules (between 500,000 and 4 million Daltons) bind strongly to cell surface receptors, maximizing the stimulation of native hyaluronic acid biosynthesis. In addition, the commercially available products also differ in their duration of effect (13 to 26 weeks) and in the number of injections needed for a treatment course (single injection vs. 3- to 5-weekly procedures). Single-injection hyaluronic acid injection therapies for the treatment of knee pain due to osteoarthritis offer similar efficacy to multi-injection regimens, reduce the exposure of patients to injection procedures, maximize the probability of treatment completion/compliance, decrease costs, and increase convenience for patients.[22] All of these preparations are prepackaged in sterile syringes. They are expensive, and provider knowledge of the reimbursement process is essential.

TABLE 3.5

FDA-approved Viscosupplements: Physical Properties

Product	Mol. Wt.	Elasticity	Viscosity	Cross-linked	Injections	Duration
Healthy young synovial fluid	6	117	45	No	N/A	
Osteoarthritic synovial fluid	1.1–1.9	1.9	1.4	No	N/A	
Euflexxa®	2.4–3.6	92	38	No	3	26 wk
Gel-One®	Unknown	Unknown	Unknown	Yes	1	13 wk
Hyalgan®	0.5–0.7	0.8	4	No	5	26 wk
Orthovisc®	1.0–2.9	60	46	No	3–4	22 wk
Hymovis®	0.5–0.7	Unknown	Unknown	No	2	26 wk
Supartz®	0.6–1.2	9	15	No	5	26 wk
Synvisc®	6	111	25	Yes	3	26 wk
Synvisc-One®	6	111	25	Yes	1	26 wk
Durolane®	Unknown	Unknown	Unknown	Yes	1	26 wk
Gelsyn-3®	1.1	Unknown	Unknown	Yes	3	26 wk
Genvisc-850®	0.62–1.2	Unknown	Unknown	No	5	30 wk
Monovisc®	1.0–2.9	Unknown	Unknown	Yes	1	26 wk

Administration is contraindicated in patients with known hypersensitivity to hyaluronan products or patients with current infections in or around the target knee. It is extremely important to ensure that injection of the viscosupplement is accurately placed within the knee joint. Thus, when performing an intra-articular knee injection of any viscosupplement, the operator must aspirate synovial fluid in order to document successful entry through the knee joint capsule. Ultrasound guidance of the aspiration and injection procedure is quite helpful in ensuring a successful procedure. Inadvertent injection extra-articularly, into the synovial tissues, into the fat pad, or intravascularly greatly increases the risk of adverse reactions. The most commonly reported adverse effects of the viscosupplements injections are transient local pain, arthralgia, joint stiffness, joint swelling, joint warmth, and gait disturbance. Use caution when injecting the rooster comb–derived products in patients allergic to avian proteins, feathers, or egg products.

BOTULINUM TOXIN

Botulinum neurotoxin is a group of seven related proteins produced by *Clostridium botulinum*. Of these, only type A and type B neurotoxins are approved for use in the United States. Botulinum toxin irreversibly binds to the presynaptic nerve membrane and blocks formation and transmission of acetylcholine at the neuromuscular junction. Botulinum toxin causes flaccid paralysis of the injected muscles. It effectively creates "medical splinting" of the target musculotendinous unit that prevents continued use. This functional forced rest of the target area for approximately 3 months allows the pathologic tissue an opportunity to heal.

Injections are performed using anatomic landmarks or with electromyographic guidance. Those affected muscles with highest clinical and EMG activity are injected. Therapeutic effect from the injection usually occurs in the first 7 days and the response lasts for an average of 12 weeks. Injections may be repeated every 3 to 4 months. Recovery occurs through proximal axonal sprouting and muscle reinnervation by formation of new neuromuscular junctions.

Effective treatment using botulinum toxin has been demonstrated in clinical studies to be effective in the treatment of various musculoskeletal disorders including cervical dystonias, cervicogenic headache, migraine headache, temporomandibular joint disorders associated with increased muscle activity, myofascial pain disorder, piriformis syndrome, limb dystonia (writer's cramp), lateral epicondylitis, and plantar fasciitis. A list of the botulinum toxin products currently approved for use in the United States is displayed in Table 3.6. At this time of publication, the use of botulinum neurotoxin for the

TABLE 3.6

Botulinum Neurotoxin

Botulinum neurotoxin type A products

Botox® (Allergan) http://www.allergan.com/products/eye_care/botox.htm
  100 units/vial

Dysport® (Ipsen) www.dysport.com
  500 units/vial

Botulinum neurotoxin type B product

MyoBloc® (Solstice Neurosciences) http://www.myobloc.com
  5,000 units/mL

treatment of musculoskeletal pain is approved by the U.S. Food and Drug Administration only for cervical dystonia in adult patients, for upper limb spasticity in adult patients, and for prophylaxis of headaches in adult patients with chronic migraine (≥15 days per month with headache lasting 4 hours a day or longer).[23] Use of botulinum toxin for other pain is considered off-label use. An individual practitioner however may consider it appropriate for use in patients with a condition that does not respond to, or is judged inappropriate for, other treatment options.

OTHER

Other investigational agents may earn a future role in the practice of medicine and be delivered via intra-articular injections. These include ketorolac (Toradol®),[24,25] and biologic agents such as etanercept (Enbrel®).[26] Sprifermin, an intra-articularly injected disease-modifying osteoarthritis drug, has shown promising results with increasing knee joint cartilage thickness.[27] An exciting future treatment may involve injecting appropriate viral vectors into joints to transfer genes into synoviocytes for the treatment of rheumatoid arthritis, psoriatic arthritis, other inflammatory arthritis, and osteoarthritis.[28,29]

REFERENCES

1. Miller RD, Pardo MC Jr. *Basics of Anesthesia*, 6th Ed. Philadelphia, PA: Elsevier Saunders; 2011: 140–141.
2. Schramm R, Thorlacius H. Neutrophil recruitment in mast cell-dependent inflammation: Inhibitory mechanisms of glucocorticoids. *Inflamm Res.* 2004;53:644–652.
3. Malemud CJ. Cytokines as therapeutic targets for osteoarthritis. *BioDrugs.* 2004;18:23–35.
4. Barnes PJ. Anti-inflammatory actions of glucocorticoids: Molecular mechanisms. *Clin Sci (Lond).* 1998;94:557–572.
5. Eymontt MJ, Gordon GV, Schumacher HR, et al. The effects on synovial permeability and synovial fluid leukocyte counts in symptomatic osteoarthritis after intraarticular corticosteroid administration. *J Rheumatol.* 1982;9:198–203.
6. MacMahon PJ, Eustace SJ, Kavanagh EC. Injectable corticosteroid and local anesthetic preparations: A review for radiologists. *Radiology.* 2009;252(3):647–661.
7. Wright JM, Cowper JJ, Page Thomas DP, et al. The hydrolysis of cortisol 21-esters by a homogenate of inflamed rabbit synovium and by rheumatoid synovial fluid. *Clin Exp Rheumatol.* 1983;1:137–141.
8. Blankenbaker DG, De Smet AA, Stanczak JD, et al. Lumbar radiculopathy: Treatment with selective lumbar nerve blocks—comparison of effectiveness of triamcinolone and betamethasone injectable suspensions. *Radiology.* 2005;237:738–741.
9. Stanczak J, Blankenbaker DG, De Smet AA, et al. Efficacy of epidural injections of Kenalog and Celestone in the treatment of lower back pain. *AJR Am J Roentgenol.* 2003;181:1255–1258.
10. Derendorf H, Möllmann H, Grüner A, et al. Pharmacokinetics and pharmacodynamics of glucocorticoid suspensions after intra-articular administration. *Clin Pharmacol Ther.* 1986;39(3):313–317.
11. Garg N, Perry L, Deodhar A. Intra-articular and soft tissue injections, a systematic review of relative efficacy of various corticosteroids. *Clin Rheumatol.* 2014;33(12):1695–1706.
12. Cushman DM, Bruno B, Christiansen J, et al. Efficacy of injected corticosteroid type, dose, and volume for pain in large joints: A narrative review. *PM R.* 2018;10(7):748–757.
13. Hajialilo M, Ghorbanihaghjo A, Valaee L, et al. A double-blind randomized comparative study of triamcinolone hexacetonide and dexamethasone intra-articular injection for the treatment of knee joint arthritis in rheumatoid arthritis. *Clin Rheumatol.* 2016;35(12):2887–2891.
14. Kumar A, Dhir V, Sharma S, et al. Efficacy of methylprednisolone acetate versus triamcinolone acetonide intra-articular knee injection in patients with chronic inflammatory arthritis: A 24-week randomized controlled trial. *Clin Ther.* 2017;39(1):150–158.
15. Johnston PC, Lansang MC, Chatterjee S, et al. Intra-articular glucocorticoid injections and their effect on hypothalamic-pituitary-adrenal (HPA)-axis function. *Endocrine.* 2015;48(2):410–416.
16. Guaraldi F, Gori D, Calderoni P, et al. Comparative assessment of hypothalamic-pituitary-adrenal axis suppression secondary to intrabursal injection of different glucocorticoids: A pilot study. *J Endocrinol Invest.* 2019;42(9):1117–1124.
17. Sanders JO, Murray J, Gross L. Non-arthroplasty treatment of osteoarthritis of the knee. *J Am Acad Orthop Surg.* 2014;22(4):256–260.
18. Bannuru RR, Osani MC, Vaysbrot EE, et al. OARSI guidelines for the non-surgical management of knee, hip, and polyarticular osteoarthritis. *Osteoarthritis Cartilage.* 2019;27(11):1578–1589.

19. Xing D, Wang B, Liu Q, et al. Intra-articular hyaluronic acid in treating knee osteoarthritis: A PRISMA-compliant systematic review of overlapping meta-analysis. *Sci Rep*. 2016;6:32790.

20. Altman R, Hackel J, Niazi F, et al. Efficacy and safety of repeated courses of hyaluronic acid injections for knee osteoarthritis: A systematic review. *Semin Arthritis Rheum*. 2018;48(2):168–175.

21. Smith MM, Ghosh P. The synthesis of hyaluronic acid by human synovial fibroblasts is influenced by the nature of the hyaluronate in the extracellular environment. *Rheumatol Int*. 1987;7(3):113–122.

22. McElheny K, Toresdahl B, Ling D, et al. Comparative effectiveness of alternative dosing regimens of hyaluronic acid injections for knee osteoarthritis: A systematic review. *Sports Health*. 2019;11(5):461–466.

23. Botox prescribing information. Available at: http://www.allergan.com/assets/pdf/botox_pi.pdf Accessed on August 2, 2020.

24. Min KS, St Pierre P, Ryan PM, et al. A double-blind randomized controlled trial comparing the effects of subacromial injection with corticosteroid versus NSAID in patients with shoulder impingement syndrome. *J Shoulder Elbow Surg*. 2013;22(5):595–601.

25. Lee SC, Rha DW, Chang WH. Rapid analgesic onset of intra-articular hyaluronic acid with ketorolac in osteoarthritis of the knee. *J Back Musculoskelet Rehabil*. 2011;24(1):31–38.

26. Roux CH, Breuil V, Valerio L, et al. Etanercept compared to intraarticular corticosteroid injection in rheumatoid arthritis: Double-blind, randomized pilot study. *J Rheumatol*. 2011;38(6):1009–1011.

27. Hochberg MC, Guermazi A, Guehring H, et al. Effect of intra-articular sprifermin vs placebo on femorotibial joint cartilage thickness in patients with osteoarthritis: The FORWARD randomized clinical trial. *JAMA*. 2019;322(14):1360–1370.

28. Evans CH, Ghivizzani SC, Robbins PD. Arthritis gene therapy and its tortuous path into the clinic. *Transl Res*. 2013;161(4):205–216.

29. Weber C, Armbruster N, Scheller C, et al. Foamy virus-adenovirus hybrid vectors for gene therapy of the arthritides. *J Gene Med*. 2013;15(3–4):155–167.

Orthobiologics

Francis G. O'Connor

4

REGENERATIVE MEDICINE

"Regenerative medicine" describes an emerging field of musculoskeletal medicine that employs the precise application of autologous, allogeneic, or proliferative injectable agents that focus on augmenting the body's endogenous repair capabilities at the specific injury site.[1] The growth of regenerative medicine has emerged from increasing evidence that has challenged the efficacy of conventional treatment options for the care of common musculoskeletal ailments. In 1999, Kraushaar and Nirschl, using electron microscopy of surgical sections from tennis elbow procedures, demonstrated the absence of inflammatory cells, questioning the role of inflammation, and paving the way for the identification of a degenerative pathway for overuse injuries by coining the term "angiofibroblastic tendinosis".[2] This identification of a degenerative process raised concern over the role of anti-inflammatory medication.[2] Traditionally, nonsteroidal anti-inflammatory medications have been prescribed by primary care providers for the management of these disorders, but with the increasing recognition of degenerative tendinopathy, their role has been called to question.[3] Corticosteroid injections, in particular, have been the subject of several systematic reviews that have identified that while in musculoskeletal soft tissue injuries they may provide short-term relief, there are concerns that these effects may in the long term be no better than placebo and, in some cases, harmful.[4] In the case of spine injections, including epidural steroid injections in the setting of subacute and chronic lumbar pain, an updated Cochrane review concluded that "there is currently insufficient evidence to support the use of [corticosteroid] injection therapy in subacute and chronic low-back pain".[5]

In addition to injectable agents for many joint and soft tissue disorders, conventional surgical procedures have also been challenged for their efficacy. Arthroscopic surgery for the repair of knee meniscal tears in patients over the age of 40 have been shown in a recent meta-analysis to be no better than sham surgery or conservative treatment,[6,7] while surgery for rotator cuff impingement has been challenged for failing to provide improved patient outcomes.[8] In the management of arthritis, joint replacement surgery has resulted in profound improvement in the quality of life for many patients, but these procedures are management techniques, and not without their own complications and risks.[9] These publications in the peer-reviewed medical literature have raised not only provider, but also patient, concern in the current approach to treating common musculoskeletal disorders, and focused consideration on other potential alternative treatments, to include the regenerative medicine model.

Mulvaney et al. have described the regenerative medicine treatment model as a paradigm shift from catabolism and tissue degeneration to anabolism and tissue repair.[1] In the setting of chronic injury, there are several postulated mechanisms for failed self tissue repair, as described by Mulvaney et al.:

1. "The body fails to recognize an injury and mounts an ineffective healing response.
2. The repair mechanism is overwhelmed by ongoing tissue insults such as chronic repetitive movements without adequate recovery, ligamentous laxity resulting in pathologic joint movement, and functional movement disorders resulting in pathologic movement.
3. The repair mechanisms are inhibited by a suboptimal healing milieu. Factors contributing to a catabolic, suboptimal healing milieu include, but are not limited to, exposure to toxins (including many pharmaceuticals), poor diet, obesity, lack of regular exercise, chronic systemic inflammation, chronic infection, poor sleep, hormonal deficiencies, and chronic stress."[10,11]

The aforementioned etiologies for a failure of self-repair are potential targets and opportunities for regenerative medicine and counseling. The objective of regenerative medicine treatment is to promote and augment native and natural processes.[1] While there is an abundance of regenerative therapies currently available to providers, this review focuses on the some of the more common therapies with the most robust evidence-based literature: prolotherapy; autologous blood; platelet-rich plasma therapy; and autologous stem cells.

PROLOTHERAPY

Prolotherapy, initially described by Hackett,[12] has been used as a treatment modality since the 1950s. The theory supporting prolotherapy as an intervention is that accumulated ligamentous laxity (through acute trauma or chronic microtrauma) allows the joints to move beyond their intended physiologic parameters. This disproportionate motion can then lead to pathologic responses including annular ligament tears resulting in vertebral disc bulges, or cartilage degradation resulting in osteoarthritis. Prolotherapy has generally been used as a regional modality, insofar as many ligaments work in concert to prevent abnormal joint motion. Prolotherapy is also used in the management of degenerative tendinopathies.[13]

The most studied "proliferant" solution is 15% dextrose, although other agents have been used (e.g., sodium morrhuate). When injected in or very proximal to a ligament or tendon, the hypertonic dextrose is thought to induce a mild cellular injury via a rapid osmotic shift of fluid, which in turn initiates an inflammatory response.[14] This focused initiation of the healing cascade is postulated to heal the previously unrecognized ligamentous injury and restore the damaged ligament to its ideal length and structure. By healing all or most of the major ligaments in a painful joint or section of spine, normal motion parameters will be restored, allowing the area to heal over time. Because the healing cascade is initiated by induction of inflammation, patients need to refrain from using anti-inflammatory medications for 7 days prior to treatment and in the posttreatment recovery period.

For years, the scientific evidence supporting the use of prolotherapy lagged behind its use in clinical practice. In the last decade, however, this lack of medical evidence has been effectively addressed by dedicated researchers. High-quality studies currently support the use of prolotherapy in many chronic injuries. One of the most significant of these studies was a multicenter RCT by Rabago and colleagues, in which the investigators followed 90 patients for 1 year and concluded that prolotherapy resulted in clinically meaningful improvement of pain, function, and stiffness scores for knee osteoarthritis (OA) when compared to saline injections or at-home exercise programs. The protocol used in the study targeted both intra-articular and ligament structures around the knee.[15] Hauser et al. published a systematic review of dextrose prolotherapy for chronic musculoskeletal pain. Their paper reviewed 14 RCTs and concluded the "use of dextrose prolotherapy is supported for treatment of tendinopathies, knee and finger Joint OA, and spinal/pelvic pain due to ligament dysfunction".[16] Dumais and colleagues conducted a randomized crossover study for the treatment of knee osteoarthritis and concluded "the use of prolotherapy is associated with a marked reduction in symptoms, which was sustained for over 24 weeks".[17] There are now many high-quality statistically significant studies supporting the use of prolotherapy in joint osteoarthritis, tendinopathies, and chronic spine pain.[13,18–22]

AUTOLOGOUS BLOOD

Autologous blood injections (ABI) contain platelets with growth factors that may help in the healing process of chronic injuries. Specifically identified in platelets are transforming growth factor-β, platelet-derived growth factor, insulin-like growth factor, vascular endothelial growth factor, and epidermal growth factor. These platelet growth factors stimulate the healing process and are thought to lead to repair of the damaged tissue. The hypothesis is that these growth factors stimulate angiogenesis and cell proliferation and increase tensile strength and the recruitment of repair cells.

The ABI procedure is easily performed in the clinical setting. A variable amount of blood is withdrawn from the patient by standard venipuncture; usually about 2 to 3 cc into a syringe with a variable amount of anesthetic. The combination of the blood and anesthetic is injected into and around the damaged tendon, usually with ultrasound guidance. A "peppering" technique is sometimes used to inject the autologous blood; this involves inserting the needle into the tendon, injecting some of the blood, withdrawing without emerging from the skin, slightly redirecting, and reinserting (see Chapter 6 on Advanced and Adjunctive Procedures that addresses fenestration). After the procedure, patients are usually advised to avoid strenuous or excessive use of the tendon for a few weeks, after which physical therapy is initiated. Although the procedure is minimally invasive, there are still potential side effects. These include a small risk of the area becoming infected and temporary pain at the injection site. ABI are advantageous over other procedures that involve the use of blood products, however, as due to the patient's own blood being injected, there is no risk of transfusion-transmitted infection or reactions.

The evidence is limited on the efficacy of ABI as a regenerative therapy. While ABI is utilized for a wide variety of tendinopathies, one of the common uses is for recalcitrant tennis elbow. In one study, 28 patients with lateral epicondylitis were injected with 2 mL of autologous blood under the extensor carpi radialis brevis. All patients had failed previous nonsurgical treatments including all or combinations of physical therapy, splinting, nonsteroidal anti-inflammatory medication, and prior steroid injections. After ABI therapy, 22 patients (79%) in whom nonsurgical modalities had failed were relieved completely of pain even during strenuous activity.[23] A subsequent meta-analysis by Chou et al. concluded that ABI is more effective than corticosteroid injection but not more effective than platelet-rich plasma (PRP) injection in treating lateral epicondylitis.[24] Finally, while ABI is promising, a systematic review by DeVos et al. commented that there are currently limited high-quality clinical studies. Future clinical studies should use a proper control group, randomization, blinding or validated disease-specific outcome measures to assess for pain and function. In addition, the authors note that a good experimental model for studying tendinopathy would be helpful for basic research.[25]

PLATELET-RICH PLASMA

PRP, defined as a concentration of platelets above baseline, has been in clinical use since the 1990s.[26] PRP is prepared from autologous blood by using centrifuge density separation with removal of the red blood cells and then further concentrating the platelet-rich fraction of the remaining plasma. Platelets activate (degranulate) when they contact air, broken fragments of collagen (such as at the site of damaged tissue) or sense another platelet in proximity undergoing degranulation. When platelets degranulate, they release alpha granules that contain the aforementioned growth factors that signal for inflammation and stimulate the body's endogenous repair mechanisms.

PRP has been shown to be an effective treatment modality in many well-done RCTs,[27–32] although some of the evidence had shown mixed results.[33] Laver et al. published a systematic review of the literature looking at 29 studies (11 RCTs) comparing PRP against hyaluronic acid (HA) for both knee and hip OA. They concluded that current clinical evidence supports the benefit of PRP treatment for knee and hip OA compared to several alternative treatments.[34] One issue that continues to confound the results of many RCTs comparing the tested substance to a saline-injected control is that there is reasonable evidence indicating that a saline injection is not a control but a treatment.[35] Another confounding issue in PRP research may be attributed to the fact that it is difficult to statistically account for, and to appropriately power studies for, variations in even similar types of injuries, posttreatment recovery regimes, method of injection, skill of the clinician, and concomitant pharmaceutical use (and many other factors). Also, there is not one homologous preparation of PRP that is being compared in the literature.[36] There are many commercially available systems and lab-based preparation protocols for the preparation of PRP. Furthermore, optimal platelet concentrations have not been established for musculoskeletal repair. The qualitative differences in PRP also is a confounding variable in research. The presence and concentrations of the various blood components—RBCs, WBCs, and platelets—all have been proposed to have either beneficial or deleterious effects. For example, there are some data to support that leukocyte-poor PRP is more beneficial than leukocyte-rich PRP for intra-articular applications, while leukocyte-rich PRP may be superior for intratendon applications.[37,38] Nonetheless, the clinical superiority of any one preparation has not been the subject of ongoing research.[39] Mautner et al. have described a comprehensive PRP nomenclature paper designed to define PRP based on the variable components to accurately and quickly describe the type of PRP being used in the prospective study.[36]

STEM CELLS

Autologous mesenchymal stems cells (MSCs) appear to facilitate musculoskeletal repair not so much by differentiating into the required target tissue but by binding to the injury site and acting in a paracrine fashion to facilitate tissue repair.[40] Autologous stem cell preparations can be created from adipose-derived MSCs and from bone marrow–derived MSCs. Currently, there is ongoing debate regarding which source is more optimal for musculoskeletal applications. Marrow-derived stem cells have been shown to have a higher osteogenic and chondrogenic potential with in vitro studies. But human studies investigating the use of adipose-derived stem cells for the treatment of osteoarthritis have shown comparable results to those for marrow-derived treatments. Furthermore, adipose has a significantly greater number of stem cells than bone marrow per equivalent unit of measurement. However, it remains to be seen whether any of these differences result in clinically meaningful differences in improved outcomes in human studies. All that being stated, the number of stem cells derived from both bone marrow and fat is exceedingly small; estimated at approximately 1 in 10,000. In addition, the number of viable cells that are actually delivered and survive with an injection is currently unknown.

Mulvaney et al. performed a review of the medical literature and found six RCTs using bone marrow and adipose-derived stem cells to treat knee arthritis, which concluded the following: there were no serious adverse events and there were superior radiological outcomes favoring stem cell injections.[1] Two trials reported improved histological outcomes, improved arthroscopically scored healing rates, and superior patient-reported outcomes. However, the level of evidence in some of the studies was reduced to level 3 due to perceived risk of bias.[41] Maddening et al. published a randomized, triple-blind, placebo-controlled trial using bone marrow aspirate concentrate (BMAC) for knee OA of 43 patients and concluded that BMAC was safe and provided clinically significant relief of pain for over 6 months versus placebo.[42] Centeno and colleagues published a study of 840 OA knees with long-term follow-up treated with bone marrow–derived stem cells and found this application to be both safe and efficacious.[43] Centeno and colleagues also published a prospective multisite study of 115 shoulder OA and rotator cuff tears treated with bone marrow–derived stem cells, which showed statistically significant improvement in DASH scores.[43] Hernigou et al. recently published their landmark RCT comparing total knee arthroplasty (TKA) with subchondral bone marrow injections for severe knee OA, with a 12-year follow-up. Both groups had similar favorable improvement. The cell therapy group showed improvement in both cartilage and bone marrow lesions. There were significantly greater medical and surgical complications following TKA compared to the cell injection group.[44] Although there is ongoing debate about which source of MSCs is superior for orthopedic regenerative applications, both need further high-quality RCT level evidence to support their clinical efficacy.

The Australasian College of Sports Physicians published a position statement in 2016 stating that autologous MSC stem cell therapy should have the same four phase trial safety testing as a new drug before being considered safe; their position statement was also covering potential use of culture expanded MSCs.[45] Regarding the safety of non–culture-expanded MSCs from either bone marrow or adipose tissue, current medical literature supports that both sources appear to be safe and reasonably efficacious for the treatment of knee and hip osteoarthritis and some tendinopathies and tendon tears; however, more high-quality research is needed.

SUMMARY

Regenerative medicine offers promising new approaches to musculoskeletal injuries. These therapies have been shown to be largely safe; however, there are limited evidence-based data to guide their utilization at this time. Importantly, a critical observation is that there is currently no evidence that current orthobiologic therapies available in the United States can lead to any tissue regeneration. It is critical that providers are honest with the data when discussing these approaches with patients and proceed with caution; more evidence and guidance will develop with time. The National Football League recently published guidance with key summary points that best addresses where we are currently with the routine utilization of orthobiologic therapies[46]:

- "Orthobiologic treatments, such as PRP and 'stem cells,' offer promise for pain relief and potentially improved healing of certain conditions affecting tendons, ligaments, and joints.

- The indications for use and the claims reporting tissue regeneration after PRP or stem cell therapy are not supported by the available evidence at this time.
- Indiscriminate use of orthobiologic treatments and/or lack of rigorous protocols for tissue processing and delivery can paradoxically put athlete health and safety at risk.
- Active research studies by scientists will help define the best indications and applications for biologic therapies that maximize both the benefit and safety for our athletes."

All that being stated, it is important to maintain perspective on the limited supporting medical evidence for many currently accepted treatments and surgeries. Regenerative options may be a safer and more physiologic treatment choice for many injuries and long-term patient health. Clinicians need to carefully and continuously assess the literature and do what they think is the best for their patient.

REFERENCES

1. Mulvaney SW, Tortland P, Shiple B, et al. Regenerative medicine options for chronic musculoskeletal conditions: A review of the literature. *Endurance Sports Med*. 2018;(Fall/Winter):6–15.
2. Kraushaar BS, Nirschl RP. Tendinosis of the elbow (tennis elbow). Clinical features and findings of histological, immunohistochemical, and electron microscopy studies. *J Bone Joint Surg Am*. 1999;81(2):259–278.
3. Kane SF, Olewinski LH, Tamminga KS. Management of chronic tendon injuries. *Am Fam Physician*. 2019;100(3):147–157.
4. Coombes BK, Bisset L, Vicenzino B. Efficacy and safety of corticosteroid injections and other injections for management of tendinopathy: A systematic review of randomised controlled trials. *Lancet*. 2010;376(9754):1751–1767.
5. Staal JB, de Bie RA, de Vet HC, et al. Injection therapy for subacute and chronic low back pain: An updated Cochrane review. *Spine (Phila Pa 1976)*. 2009;34(1):49–59.
6. Lee DY, Park YJ, Kim HJ, et al. Arthroscopic meniscal surgery versus conservative management in patients aged 40 years and older: A meta-analysis. *Arch Orthop Trauma Surg*. 2018;138(12):1731–1739.
7. Siemieniuk RAC, Harris IA, Agoritsas T, et al. Arthroscopic surgery for degenerative knee arthritis and meniscal tears: A clinical practice guideline. *BMJ*. 2017;357:j1982.
8. Khan M, Alolabi B, Horner N, et al. Surgery for shoulder impingement: A systematic review and meta-analysis of controlled clinical trials. *CMAJ Open*. 2019;7(1):E149–E158.
9. Skou ST, Roos EM, Laursen MB, et al. A randomized, controlled trial of total knee replacement. *N Engl J Med*. 2015;373(17):1597–1606.
10. Anderson K, Hamm RL. Factors that impair wound healing. *J Am Coll Clin Wound Spec*. 2012;4(4): 84–91.
11. Gosling CM, Forbes AB, Gabbe BJ. Health professionals' perceptions of musculoskeletal injury and injury risk factors in Australian triathletes: A factor analysis. *Phys Ther Sport*. 2013;14(4):207–212.
12. Hackett GS. Joint stabilization through induced ligament sclerosis. *Ohio State Med J*. 1953;49(10): 877–884.
13. Yelland MJ, Sweeting KR, Lyftogt JA, et al. Prolotherapy injections and eccentric loading exercises for painful Achilles tendinosis: A randomised trial. *Br J Sports Med*. 2011;45(5):421–428.
14. Jensen KT, Rabago DP, Best TM, et al Early inflammatory response of knee ligaments to prolotherapy in a rat model. *J Orthop Res*. 2008;26(6):816–823.
15. Rabago D, Patterson JJ, Mundt M, et al. Dextrose prolotherapy for knee osteoarthritis: A randomized controlled trial. *Ann Fam Med*. 2013;11(3):229–237.
16. Hauser RA, Lackner JB, Steilen-Matias D, et al. A systematic review of dextrose prolotherapy for chronic musculoskeletal pain. *Clin Med Insights Arthritis Musculoskelet Disord*. 2016;9:139–159.
17. Dumais R, Benoit C, Dumais A, et al. Effect of regenerative injection therapy on function and pain in patients with knee osteoarthritis: A randomized crossover study. *Pain Med*. 2012;13(8):990–999.
18. Smigel LR, Reeves KD, Lyftogt J, et al. Poster 385 caudal epidural dextrose injections (D5W) for chronic back pain with accompanying buttock or leg pain: A consecutive patient study with long-term follow-up. *PM R*. 2016;8(9S):S286–S287.
19. Dwivedi S, Sobel AD, DaSilva MF, et al. Utility of prolotherapy for upper extremity pathology. *J Hand Surg Am*. 2019;44(3):236–239.
20. Watson JD, Shay BL. Treatment of chronic low-back pain: A 1-year or greater follow-up. *J Altern Complement Med*. 2010;16(9):951–958.
21. Kim WM, Lee HG, Jeong CW, et al. A randomized controlled trial of intra-articular prolotherapy versus steroid injection for sacroiliac joint pain. *J Altern Complement Med*. 2010;16(12):1285–1290.
22. Ryan M, Wong A, Taunton J. Favorable outcomes after sonographically guided intratendinous injection of hyperosmolar dextrose for chronic insertional and midportion Achilles tendinosis. *AJR Am J Roentgenol*. 2010;194(4):1047–1053.

23. Calandruccio JH, Steiner MM. Autologous blood and platelet-rich plasma injections for treatment of lateral epicondylitis. *Orthop Clin North Am.* 2017;48(3):351–357.
24. Chou LC, Liou TH, Kuan YC, et al. Autologous blood injection for treatment of lateral epicondylosis: A meta-analysis of randomized controlled trials. *Phys Ther Sport.* 2016;18:68–73.
25. de Vos RJ, van Veldhoven PL, Moen MH, et al. Autologous growth factor injections in chronic tendinopathy: A systematic review. *Br Med Bull.* 2010;95:63–77.
26. Marx RE, Carlson ER, Eichstaedt RM, et al. Platelet-rich plasma: Growth factor enhancement for bone grafts. *Oral Surg Oral Med Oral Pathol Oral Radiol Endod.* 1998;85(6):638–646.
27. Smith PA. Intra-articular autologous conditioned plasma injections provide safe and efficacious treatment for knee osteoarthritis: An FDA-sanctioned, randomized, double-blind, placebo-controlled clinical trial. *Am J Sports Med.* 2016;44(4):884–891.
28. Dai WL, Zhou AG, Zhang H, et al. Efficacy of platelet-rich plasma in the treatment of knee osteoarthritis: A meta-analysis of randomized controlled trials. *Arthroscopy.* 2017;33(3):659–70.e1.
29. Peerbooms JC, Lodder P, den Oudsten BL, et al. Positive effect of platelet-rich plasma on pain in plantar fasciitis: A double-blind multicenter randomized controlled trial. *Am J Sports Med.* 2019;47(13): 3238–3246.
30. Gosens T, Peerbooms JC, van Laar W, et al. Ongoing positive effect of platelet-rich plasma versus corticosteroid injection in lateral epicondylitis: A double-blind randomized controlled trial with 2-year follow-up. *Am J Sports Med.* 2011;39(6):1200–1208.
31. Mishra AK, Skrepnik NV, Edwards SG, et al. Efficacy of platelet-rich plasma for chronic tennis elbow: A double-blind, prospective, multicenter, randomized controlled trial of 230 patients. *Am J Sports Med.* 2014;42(2):463–471.
32. Laudy AB, Bakker EW, Rekers M, et al. Efficacy of platelet-rich plasma injections in osteoarthritis of the knee: A systematic review and meta-analysis. *Br J Sports Med.* 2015;49(10):657–672.
33. Yerlikaya M, Talay Çaliş H, Tomruk Sütbeyaz S, et al. Comparison of effects of leukocyte-rich and leukocyte-poor platelet-rich plasma on pain and functionality in patients with lateral epicondylitis. *Arch Rheumatol.* 2018;33(1):73–79.
34. Laver L, Marom N, Dnyanesh L, et al. PRP for degenerative cartilage disease: A systematic review of clinical studies. *Cartilage.* 2017;8(4):341–364.
35. Bar-Or D, Rael LT, Brody EN. Use of saline as a placebo in intra-articular injections in osteoarthritis: Potential contributions to nociceptive pain relief. *Open Rheumatol J.* 2017;11:16–22.
36. Mautner K, Malanga GA, Smith J, et al. A call for a standard classification system for future biologic research: The rationale for new PRP nomenclature. *PM R.* 2015;7(4 Suppl):S53–S59.
37. Xu Z, Yin W, Zhang Y, et al. Comparative evaluation of leukocyte- and platelet-rich plasma and pure platelet-rich plasma for cartilage regeneration. *Sci Rep.* 2017;7:43301.
38. Zhou Y, Zhang J, Wu H, et al. The differential effects of leukocyte-containing and pure platelet-rich plasma (PRP) on tendon stem/progenitor cells—Implications of PRP application for the clinical treatment of tendon injuries. *Stem Cell Res Ther.* 2015;6(1):173.
39. Andia I, Martin JI, Maffulli N. Advances with platelet rich plasma therapies for tendon regeneration. *Expert Opin Biol Ther.* 2018;18(4):389–398.
40. Caplan AI. Why are MSCs therapeutic? New data: New insight. *J Pathol.* 2009;217(2):318–324.
41. Pas HI, Winters M, Haisma HJ, et al. Stem cell injections in knee osteoarthritis: A systematic review of the literature. *Br J Sports Med.* 2017;51(15):1125–1133.
42. Emadedin M, Labibzadeh N, Liastani MG, et al. Intra-articular implantation of autologous bone marrow-derived mesenchymal stromal cells to treat knee osteoarthritis: A randomized, triple-blind, placebo-controlled phase 1/2 clinical trial. *Cytotherapy.* 2018;20(10):1238–1246.
43. Centeno CJ, Al-Sayegh H, Bashir J, et al. A prospective multi-site registry study of a specific protocol of autologous bone marrow concentrate for the treatment of shoulder rotator cuff tears and osteoarthritis. *J Pain Res.* 2015;8:269–276.
44. Hernigou P, Auregan JC, Dubory A, et al. Subchondral stem cell therapy versus contralateral total knee arthroplasty for osteoarthritis following secondary osteonecrosis of the knee. *Int Orthop.* 2018;42(11):2563–2571.
45. Osborne H, Anderson L, Burt P, et al. Australasian College of Sports Physicians-position statement: The place of mesenchymal stem/stromal cell therapies in sport and exercise medicine. *Br J Sports Med.* 2016;50(20):1237–1244.
46. Rodeo S, Bedi A. 2019-2020 NFL and NFL physician society orthobiologics consensus statement. *Sports Health.* 2020;12(1):58–60.

5

Musculoskeletal Ultrasound

Francis G. O'Connor

INTRODUCTION

The utilization of ultrasound in musculoskeletal medicine has been transformative in the last decade; procedures previously exclusively done by interventional radiologists are now readily performed in the hands of the primary care provider at the point-of-care (see Fig. 5.1).[1,2] Interventional ultrasound is routinely taught in residency and fellowship education, and ultrasound is increasingly being integrated into anatomy instruction as a part of undergraduate medical education.[3] The American Medical Society for Sports Medicine (AMSSM) has recently published curricular guidelines for musculoskeletal ultrasound education.[4]

Evidence to support the "value added" of ultrasound guidance continues to accumulate.[1,2,5,6] Multiple publications have documented concerning variability in the accuracy of palpation-guided injections.[7,8] Eustace reported that only 29% of subacromial injections reached the intended target, while Blum et al. found that in a study of patients with knee osteoarthritis, 83% of palpation-guided injections were successful in finding the intra-articular space compared to 96% of ultrasound-guided injections (USGIs). Ultrasound needle guidance clearly has an advantage over palpation-guided injections in its real-time capability, and the ability to visualize soft targets helps the clinician avoid surrounding neurovascular structures. Publications continue to emerge supporting the observation that USGIs are more accurate, more efficacious, and potentially more cost effective. In 2015 the AMSSM published a consensus position stand on interventional musculoskeletal ultrasound. The document concluded: there is **strong** evidence that USGIs are more accurate; **moderate** evidence that USGIs are more efficacious; and finally, **preliminary** evidence USGIs are more cost effective.[5]

INDICATIONS

USGIs follow comparable guidance already discussed for palpation-guided injections; however, there are several other indications that favor the utilization of ultrasound (see Table 5.1). There are several technically challenging injections described in this fourth edition that warrant consideration for improved accuracy to facilitate either a more precise diagnosis or administer a medication in a specific location. An example of such an injection would be to the piriformis muscle, where a palpation-guided injection may be unable to delineate the location among multiple muscle groups in the deep posterior hip. A second clear indication is where local standard of care recommends that an injection be performed under fluoroscopic- or ultrasound guidance, for matters of either safety or accuracy. Examples where guidance may be required include intra-articular hip or facet joint injections (see Fig. 5.2).

Another common scenario for transitioning from a palpation-guided injection to an USGI is failure of the former injection to provide clinical improvement. An injection

FIGURE 5.1 ● Primary
care provider performing
office-based ultrasound-
guided suprapatellar knee
injection.

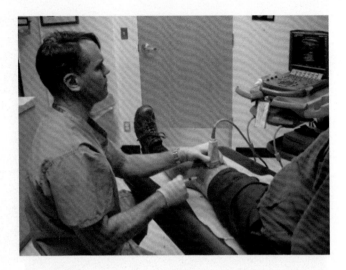

FIGURE 5.1 ● Primary
care provider performing
office-based ultrasound-
guided suprapatellar knee
injection.

failure is not uncommonly associated in a patient with comorbid obesity. Ultrasound-guidance may also be warranted for injection targets in close proximity to vulnerable neurovascular structures (e.g., femoral artery while performing an iliopsoas injection) or where a high-risk procedure in close proximity to a structure where needle puncture may be potentially harmful (e.g., lung with a complication of a pneumothorax).

CONTRAINDICATIONS

Contraindications for USGIs follow the identical precautions previously identified for palpation-guided injections. Importantly, however, it should be noted that using an ultrasound requires a three-dimensional recognition of anatomical relationships, and reasonable hand–eye coordination in order to successfully employ real-time needle guidance. It is critically important that the provider recognize his or her limitations, as the skillful use of ultrasound-guidance requires considerable investment in training and practice.

NORMAL ULTRASOUND ANATOMY SIGNALS

Musculoskeletal ultrasound is a remarkable tool that represents a dramatic innovation in the diagnosis and management of musculoskeletal disorders. This technology, however, is associated with a "significant" learning curve with new patterns to recognize and requires integrating knowledge of three-dimensional and cross-sectional anatomy with known palpation-evident superficial anatomical structures. A complete review of ultrasound anatomical signals is beyond the scope of this introduction, and the interested

TABLE 5.1

Ultrasound-Guided Injection Indications

Ultrasound Guidance Indication	Example
Accuracy	Piriformis
Recommended guidance	Intra-articular hip
Palpation-guided failure	Subacromial impingement (obesity)
Assess anatomy	Iliopsoas bursa—femoral artery
High-risk procedure	Proximity to the lung

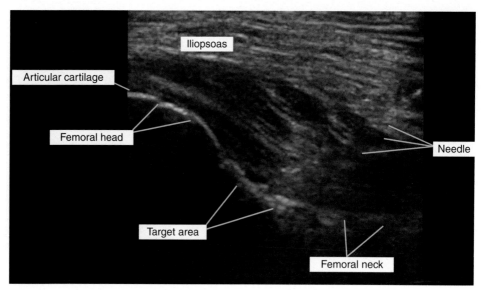

FIGURE 5.2 ● Needle approaching anterior hip capsule during intra-articular hip joint injection.

reader is referred to several excellent texts.[9,10] Basic anatomical structures, however, are introduced as well as the artifactual concepts of anisotropy and acoustic shadowing.

Ultrasound imaging produces three characteristic signals; hyperechoic, hypoechoic, and anechoic. "Hyperechoic" represents a strong reflection, with a bright echo-signal on B-mode (Brightness-mode) imaging. "Hypoechoic" is interpreted as a weak or lower-intensity (less bright) echo-signal, while "anechoic" represents a dark area, absent of echo-signal. These three terms are used to describe patterns characteristic of commonly encountered musculoskeletal structures (see Table 5.2): muscle (see Fig. 5.3); tendon (see Fig. 5.4); ligament (see Fig. 5.5); nerve (see Fig. 5.6); and bone (see Fig. 5.7).

TABLE 5.2

Ultrasound Signals for Common Anatomic Structures

Anatomical Structure	Ultrasound Signal
Muscle	• Hypoechoic with multiple hyperechoic lines, which represent fibro adipose septa or perimysium • Transverse—loosely arranged hyperechoic foci, resulting in a "starry night" appearance • Longitudinal—obliquely fascicular, "multipennate" appearance
Tendon	• Hyperechoic with anisotropy • Tightly arranged, bright lines longitudinally or bright dots transversely at right angles—compact fibrillary pattern
Nerve	• Linearly fascicular pattern with hypoechoic fascicles and hyperechoic connective tissue longitudinally • Transversely, clustered fascicles–"honeycomb," "cluster-of-grapes," or "speckled" appearance
Ligament	• Hyperechoic striated appearance that are more compact than tendons • Trilaminar appearance—central hypoechoic layer • Connect two osseous structures
Bone	• Intense hyperechoic appearance of cortical bone • Hyaline cartilage is hypoechoic or anechoic

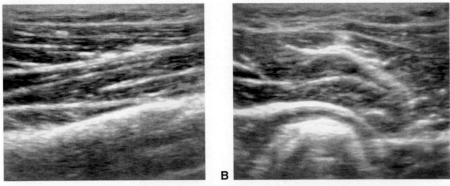

FIGURE 5.3 ● **A:** Muscle, long axis (multipennate). **B:** Muscle, short axis (starry night).

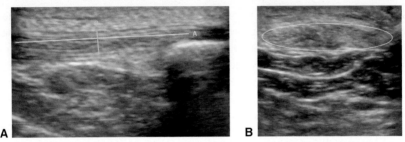

FIGURE 5.4 ● **A:** Tendon, long axis (Patellar tendon). *Lines* indicated by *A* and *B* illustrate borders of the patellar tendon. **B:** Tendon, short axis (Patellar tendon) (*yellow circle*).

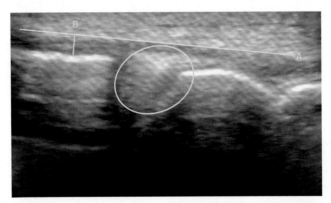

FIGURE 5.5 ● Ligament, long axis (medial collateral ligament). *Lines A* and *B* outline the width and length borders of the medial collateral ligament; the *circle* identifies the medial meniscus.

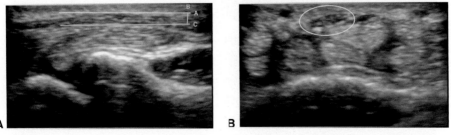

FIGURE 5.6 ● **A:** Nerve, long axis (median nerve). *Lines A, B,* and *C* outline the width and long axis borders of the median nerve. **B:** Nerve, short axis (median nerve), and tendons, short axis. The *yellow circle* outlines the median nerve in short axis.

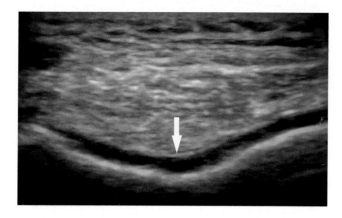

FIGURE 5.7 ● Bone and overlying articular cartilage (femoral sulcus). The *arrow* points directly to the femoral cartilage.

In addition to understanding normal ultrasound signaling, it is critical to understand sonographic artifacts in order to properly interpret an image. While there are many artifacts that affect musculoskeletal ultrasound imaging and needle guidance,[8,9] two warrant specific attention here: anisotropy and acoustic shadowing.

Anisotropy, a term commonly used in musculoskeletal ultrasound, is used to describe the artifact produced in certain tissues with tilting of the probe and resultant changes in observed echogenicity. Certain musculoskeletal structures, for example tendons, as a result of angular dependence, will demonstrate changes in echogenicity (hyperechoic to hypoechoic) with a change in the angle of the incident ultrasound beam (see Fig. 5.8). Recognition of this ultrasound artifact is critical as to not misinterpret this phenomenon as demonstrating pathology. Tendons are susceptible to anisotropy to a greater degree than nerves.

Acoustic shadowing is another commonly seen artifact key to understand for the provider utilizing musculoskeletal ultrasound. The ultrasound image relies on beam reflection for the production of an ultrasound image; when the beam encounters a highly reflective interface, for example bone or calcifications, there is no beam to further penetrate with resultant shadowing (see Fig. 5.9). This artifact may also occur when air or gas is in a tissue.

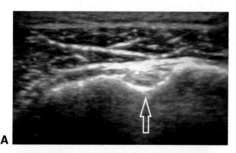

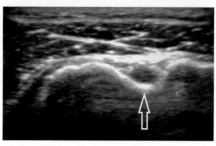

FIGURE 5.8 ● Short-axis view of biceps tendon demonstrating anisotropy. The *arrow* in **(A)** and **(B)** points directly to the biceps tendon in short axis. **(A)** illustrates hyperechoic signal with the probe perpendicular to the tendon. **(B)** illustrates anechoic signal when the probe is not directly perpendicular to the tendon.

FIGURE 5.9 ● Long-axis
view of an intra-articular hip
injection. *Arrow* illustrates
the acoustic shadowing deep
to the cortex of the femoral
neck.

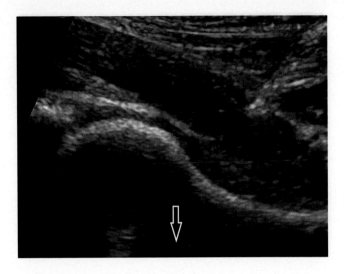

ULTRASOUND NEEDLE-GUIDANCE TERMINOLOGY

The performance of USGIs introduces specific terminology and definitions. Core to these definitions are understanding and describing the relationship of the transducer to the target and to the needle.[11] "Long-axis" ("longitudinal") images are where the long axis of the transducer is parallel to the anatomic target (see Fig. 5.10), while "short-axis" ("transverse") alignment is where the transducer is perpendicular to the target structure (see Fig. 5.11). "Out-of-plane" injections are where the transducer is perpendicular to the long-axis of the needle and only the hyperechoic needle tip or shaft can be visualized (see Fig. 5.12); whereas "in-plane" injections are where the transducer is parallel to the needle, and the entire segment of the needle shaft and tip are seen approaching the target (see Fig. 5.13). In-plane injections are preferred in clinical practice.

ULTRASOUND AND NEEDLE GUIDANCE

Performing an USGI successfully requires the integration of three factors: patient selection with appropriate indications, knowledge of ultrasound anatomy (sono-anatomy), and the ability to visualize and drive a needle to the intended target. The first two of

FIGURE 5.10 ● Long-axis
orientation, in-plane injection
(cubital tunnel).

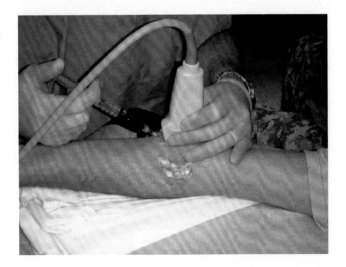

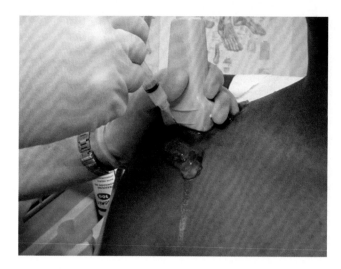

FIGURE 5.11 ● Short-axis orientation, out-of-plane injection (AC joint).

these factors are addressed with the cultivation of clinical acumen and knowledge. The third task requires practice aimed at both visuospatial and psychomotor development. Simultaneously controlling, visualizing and guiding a needle is a complex task, requiring hand–eye coordination with manual dexterity. The ultrasound probe can be manipulated in multiple directions to enhance both target and needle image acquisition. A useful pneumonic that identifies the various aspects of probe manipulation is "P.A.R.T."; pressure, alignment, rotation, and tilt (see Fig. 5.14).[12]

The pressure applied with the probe by the provider can considerably impact image quality, the echogenicity of the tissue, and can shorten the distance to the structure of interest. Pressure is generally applied evenly across the probe, but the provider may apply asymmetric pressure on one side in order to direct the US beam in the desired direction to facilitate a target or create more room for needle entrance. Axial relocation, or "translation," can be either in a long-axis or short-axis direction in relation to the transducer probe footprint. This axial motion has the principal goal of finding the structure of interest and positioning it optimally on the screen for needle advancement. Axial translation is also referred to as a "slide" in either the

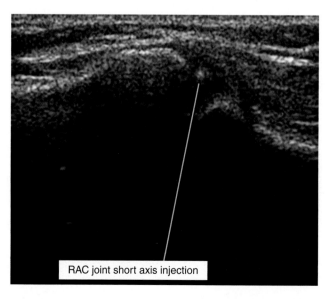

RAC joint short axis injection

FIGURE 5.12 ● Out-of-plane injection (AC joint).

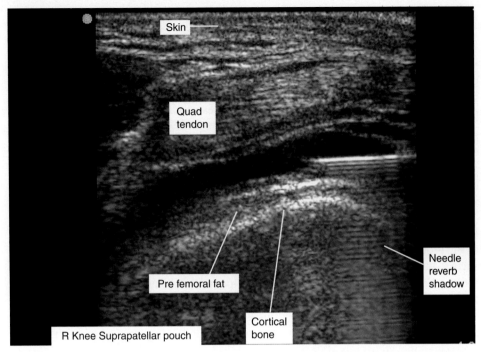

FIGURE 5.13 ● In-plane injection, short-axis (transverse) target image (suprapatellar recess).

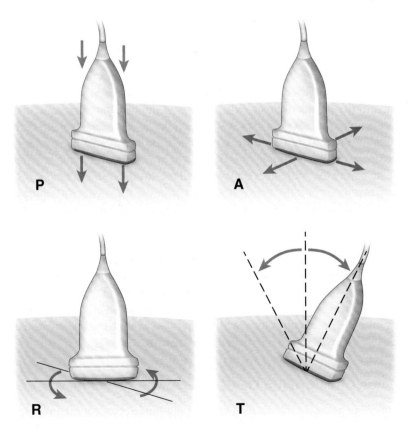

FIGURE 5.14 ● The PART pneumonic for probe motion: pressure, axial slide, rotation, and tilt.

TABLE 5.3

The STAR Technique for Needle Ultrasound Acquisition and Guidance

See	S	The participant is taught to look directly at the transducer and needle instead of the ultrasound screen, without moving the probe or needle.
Tilt	T	The participant tilts the transducer back and forth on a horizontal axis to achieve maximal brightness of the needle.
Align	A	The participant kept the same tilt and slide the transducer toward the needle (in the direction identified during "see") until the needle came into view.
Rotate	R	The participant turned the transducer on its long axis until full needle visualization was achieved.

long- or short-axis. "Rotation" is where the transducer is spun around the center axis of the probe; this facilitates an axial view of the target with its long axis parallel to the surface but not perpendicular to the current US plane. By continuous rotation of the probe to 90 degrees of the initial probe position, one can change the image of a structure from its short-axis to its long-axis view. Finally, "tilt" is where the transducer is angled in the plane of its short-axis; this is also described as "sweeping," "toggling," or "fanning" the probe. Tilting of the probe can facilitate a preview before the probe is engaged in a short-axis slide.

Learning to image the needle while performing real-time ultrasound guidance can be challenging and requires practiced hand–eye coordination with both the needle- and probe hands simultaneously. One group of educators developed the "**S.T.A.R.** Technique" (See, Tilt, Align, Rotate) to assist novice users in acquiring the necessary skills to perform USGIs (see Table 5.3 and Fig. 5.15).[13]

In addition to utilizing the STAR technique, a short-axis injection poses unique challenges, compared to a long-axis injection, as the needle is not seen the entire path during its approach to the intended target. When using an out-of-plane technique, the hyperechoic needle tip or shaft is only identified once it begins to cross the plane of the ultrasound beam. Accordingly, as the needle is advanced, the provider will be unable to image the needle tip until it has passed by this transducer plane. The technique required to see the needle tip during the entire injection is termed the "walk down" technique. This technique involves a series of transverse probe linear slides as the needle tip is progressively introduced, and followed by ultrasound imaging, more deeply into the soft tissue in the direction of the target. This out-of-plane technique can additionally be used to direct a needle deeper without moving the probe. The needle is introduced out-of-plane under the center of the probe in order to see the tip over the intended target, and then partially withdrawn to redirect deeper, and advanced again until the needle tip, deeper than before, is closer to the target. This is repeated until the needle tip arrives at the target. The repeated redirects are like taking steps as you walk the needle to the target. The critical observation is that once the needle tip comes in to view, it should not be advanced, as there is no reference as to where the needle tip is in the soft tissues.

ULTRASOUND GUIDANCE OF PROCEDURES

USGIs proceed in a comparable fashion to palpation-guided procedures with several distinct steps; these steps as originally described by Lento, with addition of adding documentation and several modifications, are listed in Table 5.4.[14]

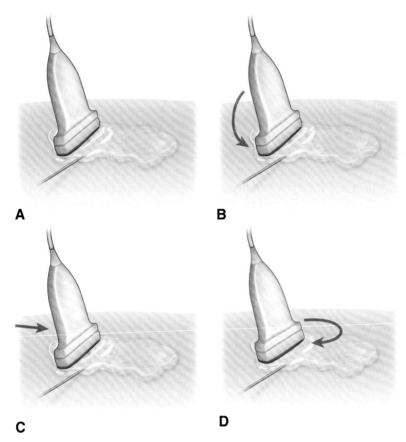

FIGURE 5.15 • The STAR technique for needle ultrasound acquisition and guidance. **A:** See. **B:** Tilt. **C:** Align. **D:** Rotate.

TABLE 5.4

Ultrasound-Guided Procedure Steps

Step	Procedure Action
1	History and physical
2	Obtain consent
3	Assemble equipment
4	Position patient and machine; enter patient ID
5	Preliminary scan
6	Demarcate skin
7	Don sterile gloves
8	Clean skin and drape as necessary
9	Draw up medications; local anesthesia as needed
10	Prepare probe, to include sterile cover as necessary
11	Attach syringe to needle
12	Place needle under probe and perform procedure
13	Documentation, reevaluate patient, clean equipment

Step 1: History and Physical

An ultrasound-guided injection's success depends upon a proper diagnosis; the history and physical examination, to include a review of diagnostic imaging tests, should be completed prior to commencing with an injection.

Step 2: Obtain Consent

As previously described, consent for all injections should be witnessed and documented in the medical record. Unique to an USGI, there should be a careful discussion of the role of the ultrasound as compared to a standard palpation-guided injection. Patients should additionally be asked if they would like to visualize the injection during the procedure. While the technology is of interest to most patients, some patients may become anxious and potentially vagal when witnessing a needle in their own body.

Step 3: Assemble Equipment

A sterile field should be considered to hold supplies for the injection. This step in the procedure is comparable to that discussed for palpation-guided injections.

Step 4: Position Patient and Machine

The ultrasound machine should be placed in-line, at eye level, and directly across from the injector, on the other side of the patient; this limits head motion and facilitates greater accuracy in needle placement and direction. The patient should be comfortable and relaxed, and if at all possible, in a supine position to limit the possibility of a vasovagal reaction. When holding the probe, the provider should learn to scan with the nondominant hand, as the dominant hand should be used to direct the needle. In addition, when holding the probe, the provider's fourth and fifth fingers should maintain skin contact to limit unintended motion and anchor the probe on the patient.

Step 5: Preliminary Scan

This preliminary scan confirms the diagnosis, identifies the target, and assists the provider in best determining whether an in-plane versus out-of-plane needle approach is optimal. The preliminary scan also assists the provider in determining appropriate needle length, as well as planning for modifications to the planned procedure (e.g., aspiration of a joint effusion prior to injection).

Step 6: Demarcate Skin

Marking the skin during the preliminary scan will assist in identifying the appropriate target and allowing facilitation of demarcating the location of the probe after the sterile preparation of the skin. The skin can be marked with an appropriate skin marking pen on either end of the probe, so that correct replacement can occur.

Step 7: Don Sterile Gloves

The appropriate gloves should be selected prior to performing the injection. Sterile gloves are only required if the provider intends to touch the location of the intended needle injection. The issue of sterile versus nonsterile gloves has previously been discussed in detail.

Step 8: Clean Skin

An appropriate skin cleaning agent (e.g., chlorhexidine gluconate) should be selected prior to performing the injection. Agents have been previously discussed, however, with ultrasound, a key variable will be ensuring compliance with the probe manufacturer's recommendations to avoid damage to the probe head.

Step 9: Draw Up Medications; Local Anesthesia as Needed

The procedure of drawing up medications and preparing the skin with local anesthesia prior to the injection are comparable to those utilized for palpation-guided injections.

Step 10: Prepare Probe

Preparation of the probe prior to performing an USGI is an area of active controversy and addressed by the American Institute of Ultrasound in Medicine (AIUM) Practice Parameter.[15] Most importantly, ultrasound-guided procedures should be performed in accordance with the provider's facility infection control guidelines. The patient's skin should appropriately be cleansed with an antiseptic cleanser. The ultrasound transducer also represents a potential source of contamination; accordingly, probes should be disinfected between each procedure according to manufacturer recommendations and facility-specific infection control guidelines.[15]

The use of sterile ultrasound gel, drapes, and probe covers/condoms may provide the best method to reduce the risk of contamination and infection. Alternatives include the use of a sterile glove covering the transducer combined with sterile gel, the use of a sterile condom covering the transducer combined with sterile gel, or the use of a sterile occlusive dressing, for example Tegaderm®, directly applied to the transducer face combined with sterile gel. Providers who use the "no-touch" technique, as previously described, place the transducer over the target region but away from the prepared skin entry site. The needle is passed through the prepared skin region and passes under the transducer within the body. This technique should only be used by experienced clinicians due to the risk of cross-contamination secondary to inadvertent transducer or needle movement.[15]

Step 11: Attach Syringe to Needle

Alternatively, the needle can be attached directly to extension tubing which is then attached to the syringe. This can be useful as the plunger can be more easily depressed without moving the needle tip.

Step 12: Place Needle Under Probe

Using the STAR technique, the actual needle (as opposed to the needle on the image screen) should be observed being introduced into the tissue deep to the probe. Once the actual needle is visualized as under the probe, the provider can then look to the screen and identify the needle on the ultrasound image. Short axis slides in an orthogonal plane are then utilized to maintain normal recognized anatomic relationships during the injection.

Step 13: Documentation

The AIUM Practice Parameter specifies clear guidance for proper procedure documentation.[15] "Adequate documentation is essential and should be permanently documented in the patient's medical record. Retention of the ultrasound examination should be consistent both with clinical needs and with relevant legal and local health care facility requirements. The procedure documentation should include the following: (a) Patient identification, (b) Facility identification, (c) Procedure date, (d) Requested procedure, including side of body, (e) Indication for the procedure, (f) Justification for ultrasound guidance, (g) Description of the target and relevant associated structures, both normal and abnormal, (h) Description of the use of ultrasound to localize the target and the essential elements of the procedure, including transducer position, approach to the target, and method of needle tracking (in plane or out of plane). Deviations from standard techniques are described and justified, (i) The type and amount of medication, if used, (j) Needle/device type and gauge, and (k) Specimens removed, if any, as well as their disposition."[15] The choice of aseptic technique used during the ultrasound-guided procedure should be documented in the report.

The AIUM Practice Parameter also provides guidance for proper image utilization and documentation.[15] "Preprocedural, intraprocedural, and post procedure still image(s) or videos: (a) Images should be labeled with the patient identification, facility identification, procedure date, and side (right or left) of the procedure site. (b) Inclusion of at least one image demonstrating the needle or device placed into the target region is required unless the indirect technique is used. (c) All images should be permanently archived and easily retrievable. (d) Variations from normal size or morphology should be recorded and accompanied by measurements."[15]

NEW ULTRASOUND TECHNOLOGY

Ultrasound technology continues to improve, with advancements in quality imaging in tools that have smaller interfaces and are more mobile in a variety of care settings. Integrated functions additionally make it easier for the user to produce high-caliber and clinically useful imaging. With continued improvements in high-resolution imaging, procedural interventions in and around finer structures (e.g., nerves), previously challenging in the best of hands, are becoming more common place. Finally, newer technologic advancements are moving ultrasound from station-based machines to hand-held portable devices. Handheld ultrasound systems can attach to a smart phone, provide excellent resolution and penetration, and conveniently drop into the end-user's lab coat. Accompanied by decreasing costs over time, these devices will provide primary care providers with wide accessibility to use musculoskeletal ultrasound and other point-of-care office and hospital applications.

REFERENCES

1. Sorensen B, Hunskaar S. Point-of-care ultrasound in primary care: A systematic review of generalist performed point-of-care ultrasound in unselected populations. *Ultrasound J*. 2019;11(1):31.
2. Sconfienza LM, Albano D, Allen G, et al. Clinical indications for musculoskeletal ultrasound updated in 2017 by European Society of Musculoskeletal Radiology (ESSR) consensus. *Eur Radiol*. 2018;28:5338–5351.
3. Berko NS, Goldberg-Stein S, Thornhill BA, et al. Survey of current trends in postgraduate musculoskeletal ultrasound education in the United States. *Skeletal Radiol*. 2016;45:475–482.
4. Finnoff JT, Berkoff DJ, Brennan F, et al. American Medical Society for Sports Medicine (AMSSM) recommended sports ultrasound curriculum for sports medicine fellowships. *Br J Sports Med*. 2015;49:145–150.
5. Finoff J, et al. American Medical Society for sports medicine position statement: Interventional musculoskeletal ultrasound in sports medicine. *Clin J Sports Med*. 2015;25:6–22.
6. Daniels EW, Cole D, Jacobs B, et al. Existing evidence on ultrasound-guided injections in sports medicine. *Orthop J Sports Med*. 2018;6(2):2325967118756576.

7. Bum Park Y, et al. Accuracy of blind versus ultrasound guided suprapatellar bursal injection. *J Clin Ultrasound.* 2012;40(1):20–25.

8. Eustace JA, et al. Comparison of accuracy of steroid placement with clinical outcomes in patients with shoulder symptoms. *Ann Rheum Dis.* 1995;38:59–63.

9. Jacobsen JA. *Fundamentals of Musculoskeletal Ultrasound*, 3rd Ed. Philadelphia, PA: Elsevier, 2018.

10. Bianchi S, Martionoli C, Abdelwahad IF, et al. *Ultrasound of the Musculoskeletal System.* New York: Springer-Verlag Berlin Heidelberg, 2008.

11. Visco CJ. Introduction to interventional ultrasound. In: Malanga G, Mautner K, eds. *Atlas of Ultrasound-Guided Musculoskeletal Injections.* New York: McGraw Hill, 2014.

12. Ihnatsenka B, Boezaart AP. Ultrasound: Basic understanding and learning the language. *Int J Shoulder Surg.* 2010;4(3):55–62.

13. Lam NC, Fishburn SJ, Hammer AR, et al. A randomized controlled trial evaluating the See, Tilt, Align, and Rotate (STAR) maneuver on skill acquisition for simulated ultrasound-guided interventional procedures. *J Ultrasound Med.* 2015;34(6):1019–1026.

14. Lento PH. Preparation and setup for musculoskeletal ultrasound-guided procedures. In: Malanga G, Mautner K, eds. *Atlas of Ultrasound-Guided Musculoskeletal Injections.* New York: McGraw Hill, 2014.

15. AIUM Practice Parameter for the Performance of Selected Ultrasound-Guided Procedures. Available at: https://www.aium.org/resources/guidelines/usGuidedProcedures.pdf. Last Assessed on December 22, 2019.

Advanced and Adjunctive Techniques

6

Francis G. O'Connor

Injections have empowered primary care providers to deliver a number of evidence-based therapies to directly treat soft tissue and articular disorders in musculoskeletal medicine.[1] The ability to precisely target injuries on-site has in turn aided in not only maximizing potential benefit but also limiting adverse systemic side effects. With the increased level of comfort and utilization of injections, importantly with the addition of ultrasound guidance, there has been a propagation of unique techniques and tools that can be utilized in musculoskeletal medicine.[2] The last decade has additionally added considerable evidence-based literature to support the "value added" of these interventions in improving cost-effective clinical outcomes when in the hands of point-of-care providers.[3] These advanced techniques can assist in achieving pain relief, affect mechanical change in soft tissue structures, and ultimately provide improved clinical care. The techniques discussed in this chapter include battlefield auricular acupuncture (pain management); barbotage (calcific tendinopathy); high-volume injection tendon brisement (tendinopathy/tenosynovitis); needle fenestration (tendinopathy); hydrodissection (nerve entrapment); hydrodilatation/hydroplasty (adhesive capsulitis); trigger point dry needling (myofascial pain); and percutaneous tenotomy with debridement (tendinopathy). While these techniques are reviewed and evidence is introduced to support their incorporation in clinical practice, it should be emphasized that these are considered advanced skills that require additional training and practice to employ skillfully.

Auricular Battlefield Acupuncture

Battlefield acupuncture (BFA) was developed by US Air Force physician Dr. Richard Niemtzow in 2001.[4] The technique was specifically developed to provide pain relief during a period when an opiate analgesic may not be typically utilized or appropriate, secondary to systemic effects that may interfere with mission completion. BFA is an extension of the longstanding technique of auriculotherapy and designed for the rapid relief of pain. Utilizing specific acupoints on the outer ear that are thought to interact with central nervous system pain processing, auricular BFA can provide a quick and convenient method to provide pain relief (see Fig. 6.1). The technique employs ASP (Aiguille Semi-Permanente) needles, which are semi-permanent, and have the characteristics of remaining in the ear acupoints for up to 3 to 4 days before being pushed out toward to the surface by the previous flattened epidermis. This pain relief has a variable duration from minutes to days, depending upon the individual and the pathology being addressed. While the technique was originally developed to assist in the management of wounded warfighters on the battlefield, BFA has widely grown in popularity and offers an alternative or adjunct to systemic analgesics.

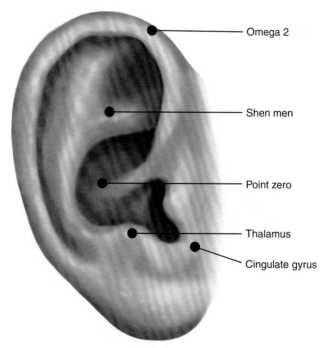

Omega 2

Shen men

Point zero

Thalamus

Cingulate gyrus

FIGURE 6.1 ● Auricular acupoints.

EVIDENCE

BFA has been utilized on the battlefield by medical acupuncturists and nonacupuncturists alike. While BFA has been increasingly employed, research has been limited in the field of auriculotherapy. A small randomized controlled trial ($n = 94$) of female patients with acute migraines demonstrated that auriculotherapy provided short-term pain relief when specific auricular acupoints were utilized.[5] Another pilot study of emergency room (ER) patients ($n = 87$) with a wide variety of pain complaints demonstrated a 23% reduction in pain for those receiving auriculotherapy before leaving the ER as compared to standard care, while both groups had the same level of pain reduction at 24 hours after the ER visit.[6] Finally, a recent meta-analysis was performed to assess the efficacy of auriculotherapy for pain relief in an emergency setting. The meta-analysis used data from several randomized studies and included 286 patients. There were no observed significant adverse effects and patient satisfaction was significantly improved. Results regarding if acupuncture reduced pain medication use, however, were equivocal. While study numbers were limited, ear acupuncture, either as a stand-alone or as an adjunctive technique, significantly reduced pain scores.[7] While current evidence is limited, BFA is becoming widely employed in the military and emergency medicine community and is proving to be a useful adjunct in managing acute pain.

CONTRAINDICATIONS

Active skin infection, needle phobia, and pregnancy are considered to be the only contraindications.

EQUIPMENT

- ASP or acupuncture needles (see Fig. 6.2)
- Alcohol pads

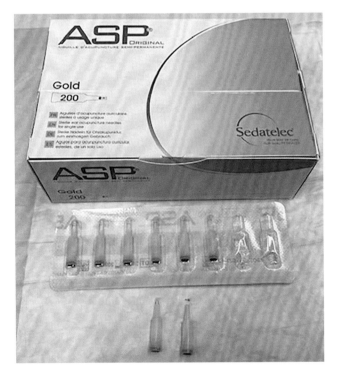

FIGURE 6.2 ● ASP needle. (ASP® from Sedatelec.)

PREPROCEDURAL INSTRUCTIONS

The patient should be informed that the indwelling needles or pins may be mildly uncomfortable but are generally well tolerated. The needles can be self-removed at any time; however, they will typically fall out in 2 to 10 days in most patients. Patients are additionally informed that pain relief may not be immediate and may take several days to achieve. Patients are instructed after initial placements that they should not engage in vigorous activity until they know the response they will get from the ASP needles.

ANESTHESIA

Typically no local anesthesia is required for BFA administration.

TECHNIQUE

The technique of BFA has been developed and described by Niemtzow.[4] The clinician performing the battlefield acupuncture "technique" first conducts an appropriate history and physical examination. The five acupoints are sequentially identified and needles are subsequently administered as indicated: cingulate gyrus, thalamic nuclei (anterior), omega 2, point zero, and shen men. This order of needle administration is commonly taught with acronym "CTOPS" or "CCTTOOPPSS" indicating the process of alternating between the ears.

1. Either the left or right ear is chosen for the placement of the needles; if the pain is not clearly lateralized, use the ear on the nondominant hand.
2. An ASP needle is first inserted into the cingulated gyrus.
3. The patient is allowed to ambulate for about 2 minutes to determine whether pain attenuation has occurred. If no pain attenuation has occurred, an ASP needle is inserted into the cingulate gyrus of the opposite ear and the patient ambulates to determine the new pain level.
4. If pain attenuation has been achieved via the cingulated gyrus, another ASP needle is placed in the anterior thalamic in the ear that has produced the most pain attenuation. The patient ambulates and the new pain level is determined.
5. Whichever ear insertion produces pain attenuation, ASP needles are placed in a similar sequential manner into omega 2, shen men, and point zero.
6. After the dominant ear has received ASP needles in all the "battlefield acupuncture" points, the pain level is evaluated. If the pain level is 0-1/10, the therapeutic goal is achieved. In the case where the pain level is above 1/10, the contralateral ear is needled in a similar manner.

AFTERCARE

The clinician should observe for ear irritation or infection; mild erythema after the procedure is to be expected. Typical postprocedure instructions include the following advice to patients:

• Do not be surprised if the pain increases over the first few days; this can be a normal reaction and should not be considered a failed treatment.
• The needles may be uncomfortable during sleep or when brushing against another object. If they are uncomfortable, they may be removed before failing out on their own, or one may use the Band-Aid that is provided in the BFA kit.

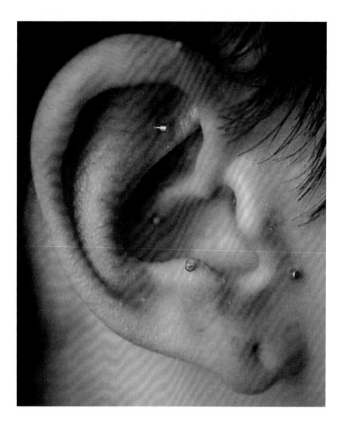

FIGURE 6.3 ● Auricular acupoints with ASP needles inserted.

- Watch for signs of infection, to include redness, discharge, or marked pain.
- Avoid excessive activity after the initial procedure and thereafter tailor activity based upon the initial response.
- Plan your activities to include some rest after the procedure; do not plan for a peak performance immediately after the procedure.
- Continue to take prescription medications as prescribed by one's regular physician.
- Keep written notes on the response to the procedure to be shared with the treating provider at follow-up visits.

CPT code:
- 97811—Acupuncture, one or more needles, without electrical stimulation

PEARLS

- BFA is a great adjunct to other treatments and also can be a guide to see if the patient will respond to more advanced acupuncture.
- BFA can be repeated at any interval but the usual protocol for an acute pain is as follows: initial, repeat in 3 to 6 days as efficacy wanes and then spread out time from there.
- For chronic pain, there will be a finite response, that is, every 1 to 2 weeks.
- If the pain is not clearly lateralized, use the ear on the nondominant hand; normal phone use may irritate ASP needles.
- If the pain has been significantly reduced, consider treating only one ear. This may facilitate the patient being able to achieve a comfortable sleeping position.

A video showing auricular battlefield acupuncture with insertion of ASP needles can be found in the companion eBook.

REFERENCES

1. Stephens MB, Beutler AI, O'Connor FG. Musculoskeletal injections: A review of the evidence. *Am Fam Physician.* 2008;78(8):971–976.
2. Finnoff JT, Hall MM, Adams E, et al. American Medical Society for Sports Medicine (AMSSM) position statement: Interventional musculoskeletal ultrasound in sports medicine. *PM & R.* 2015;7(2):151–168.e12.
3. Daniels EW, Cole D, Jacobs B, et al. Existing evidence on ultrasound-guided injections in sports medicine. *Orthop J Sports Med.* 2018;6(2):2325967118756576.
4. Niemtzow RC. Battlefield acupuncture: My story. *Med Acupunct.* 2018;30(2):57–58.
5. Allais G, Romoli M, Rolando S, et al. Ear acupuncture in the treatment of migraine attacks: A randomized trial on the efficacy of appropriate versus inappropriate acupoints. *Neurol Sci.* 2011;32(Suppl 1):S173–S175.
6. Goertz CMH, Niemtzow R, Burns SM, et al. Auricular acupuncture in the treatment of acute pain syndromes: A pilot study. *Mil Med.* 2006;171(10):1010–1014.
7. Jan AL, Aldridge ES, Rogers IR, et al. Does ear acupuncture have a role for pain relief in the emergency setting? A systematic review and meta-analysis. *Med Acupunct.* 2017;29(5):276–289.

Barbotage

Ultrasound-guided barbotage, a procedure of repeated injection and aspiration, is commonly used in the management of soft tissue calcific deposits.[1] Calcific tendinopathy has been identified and treated in a number of locations including the patellar and gluteal tendons but is most commonly identified in the tendons of rotator cuff about the shoulder. Rotator cuff calcific tendinopathy (RCCT), a common disease that occurs in up to 7.5% of asymptomatic adults and up to 20% of painful shoulders, is frequently diagnosed in women in their 40s and 50s. RCCT, which is not uncommonly disabling, can be treated conservatively with excellent results.[2]

The exact etiology of calcific tendinopathy is currently not understood but postulated to be the result of a local tissue degenerative cascade. The calcification process is specifically thought to be related to a cell-mediated disease in which metaplastic transformation of tenocytes into chondrocytes induces calcification inside the tendon.[3] Uhthoff describes the pathogenesis in three stages: (a) precalcific stage with fibrocartilaginous transformation within the tendon; (b) calcific stage with calcium deposition; and finally, the (c) postcalcific phase, in which self-healing and repair of the affected tendon occurs which can last several months.[4] In the calcific stage, a resorptive phase occurs, which is characterized by vascular invasion, edema, and increased intratendinous pressure with possible extravasation of calcium crystals in the subacromial bursa. This phase is usually associated with the development of acute pain that can be highly disabling and unresponsive to common analgesics.[2] The acute phase is generally associated with "softer" deposits with poorly defined borders, while the more chronic "harder" lesions tend to appear more granular with sharply defined borders.

EVIDENCE

Ultrasound-guided barbotage is a safe technique, with a high success rate and low complication rate.[5] There is currently no evidence assessing its effectiveness compared with other major treatment modalities including extracorporeal shock wave therapy, subacromial corticosteroid injections, dry needling, or arthroscopic calcific deposit excision. However, pending emerging evidence from ongoing clinical trials, a recent systematic review of 908 patients recommended ultrasound-guided barbotage.[6] Interestingly, de Witte et al. have two publications looking at 1-year and 5-year follow-up results of ultrasound-guided barbotage with a subacromial corticosteroid injection versus ultrasound-guided subacromial corticosteroid injection alone. While the results demonstrated a clear benefit at 1 year, there were no significant clinical or radiologic differences at the 5-year mark.[7,8]

As will be described, barbotage can be performed with both one- and two-needle techniques. There is one published study evaluating the efficacy of the one-needle technique versus the two-needle technique and found no significant difference in clinical outcomes at 1-year follow-up. However, the data suggested that a double-needle approach might be more appropriate to treat harder deposits, while one needle may be more useful in treating fluid, or softer calcifications.[9] In addition, recent evidence suggests that the utilization of warm saline has been shown both to reduce procedure duration and improve calcium deposit dissolution, particularly in cases of hard calcifications.[10] Finally, if ultrasound-guided barbotage is utilized, the evidence suggests that the procedure is optimally followed by a subacromial corticosteroid injection.[11]

CONTRAINDICATIONS

The barbotage procedure has comparable contraindications that apply to all bursal injections as previously described. In addition, ultrasound-guided barbotage is not indicated when patients are asymptomatic, the calcification is very small (≤5 mm), or the calcifications have migrated into the bursal space. There is additional evidence that patients with intraosseous migration of calcification experience worse results.[12]

EQUIPMENT

- One or two 18-guage needles (depending on the technique chosen: single or double needle)
- Two 25-guage needles for subacromial injections prior to and after the barbotage procedure
- Two syringes (20 mL and 3 mL)
- One 10-cm 18- or 20-guage spinal needle (optional)
- Bowl (to collect the washing fluid)
- Sterile saline solution (100 to 200 mL, warmed to 38°C to 40°C)
- Lidocaine 1% or mepivacaine (10 mL)
- Steroid (1 mL, 40 mg/mL)
- Ultrasound machine with high-frequency linear array transducer

PREPROCEDURAL INSTRUCTIONS

The patient should be placed in a supine position, to prevent patient movement during the procedure. The arm of the affected shoulder should lie completely extended along the body with a slight internal or external rotation, according to calcification location. The procedural guidance for utilization of ultrasound guidance, to include sterile technique, is detailed in the previous chapter of **Introduction to Ultrasound**.

ANESTHESIA

Using US guidance with an in-plane approach, inject up to 10-mL lidocaine or mepivacaine along the path of the needles into the subacromial bursa and around the calcification.

TECHNIQUE

US-guided barbotage is performed with patients in the supine position on a table; the two-needle and one-needle techniques are described by Sconfienza and Messina.[12] After sterile preparation of the skin and ultrasound probe as previously described, the target calcification is visualized with a high-frequency linear array transducer. Using a 25-guage needle, local anesthesia (up to 10 mL of lidocaine or mepivacaine) is injected in the subacromial bursa and around the calcification with an in-plane approach. When using the two-needle technique, the first needle is inserted into the lowest portion of the calcification with needle bevel open toward the probe. The second needle is then inserted into the calcification parallel and superficial to the first needle, with its bevel opposite to the first needle, 25 to 30 degrees of angulation, in order to create a correct washing circuit. The calcification is then filled with saline solution, applying a gentle intermittent pressure in order to dissolve its core and allowing the calcific fluid to exit through the second needle, until a complete internal emptying is visualized. As calcium fills the syringe, exchange is made with new syringes until no further calcium is expelled. Remaining observed calcification can be fenestrated with the needle. The procedure is then concluded with a subacromial steroid injection. The single-needle technique is comparable to the two-needle technique, with the caveat being that the calcification is punctured with one needle only. Washing is performed by pushing the syringe plunger to hydrate the deposit. Calcium then refluxes back together with the saline solution within the same syringe as the plunger is released.

The single-needle technique has been thought to have a lower risk of infection and bleeding. On the other hand, the use of two needles ensures an in–out flow of the saline solution outside the calcification, reducing the risk of calcification disruption and subsequent postprocedural bursitis.

AFTERCARE

There are currently no evidence-based guidelines for postprocedural care, however, Messina et al. have published their protocol.[9,12] They have suggested a short course of nonsteroidal anti-inflammatory drugs and relative rest (i.e., no elevation of the arm over the shoulder) for up to 2 weeks. This is followed by a short treatment of physical therapy. Imaging is not routinely used during follow-up. Patients are instructed to call if pain persists for more than a few days after treatment or in case of fever, or in case of pain recurrence after 2 months posttreatment.

CPT codes:
- 20551—Injection; single tendon origin/insertion
- 76942—Ultrasonic guidance for needle placement with imaging supervision and interpretation with permanent recording

PEARLS

- The initial subacromial injection should involve 5 to 10 mL of lidocaine to facilitate comfort for the patient during the procedure; corticosteroid into the subacromial space following the procedure decreases postprocedure pain.
- Warm saline to facilitate the barbotage has been demonstrated to reduce procedure duration and improve calcium deposit dissolution.
- Data suggest that that a double-needle approach might be more appropriate to treat harder deposits, while a one-needle approach may be more useful in treating fluid.
- Air infiltration into the soft tissues should be avoided as this may obscure visualization of the calcific deposit and surrounding sonoanatomy.
- Additional tips and tricks have been published and are available for the interested reader.[9]

 A video showing barbotage can be found in the companion eBook.

REFERENCES

1. Davidson J, Jayaraman S. Guided interventions in musculoskeletal ultrasound: What's the evidence? *Clin Radiol.* 2011;66(2):140–152.
2. Speed CA, Hazleman BL. Calcific tendinitis of the shoulder. *N Engl J Med.* 1999;340(20):1582–1584.
3. De Carli A, Pulcinelli F, Rose GD, et al. Calcific tendinitis of the shoulder. *Joints.* 2014;2(3):130–136.
4. Uhthoff HK, Sarkar K. Calcifying tendinitis. *Baillieres Clin Rheumatol.* 1989;3(3):567–581.
5. Lanza E, Banfi G, Serafini G, et al. Ultrasound-guided percutaneous irrigation in rotator cuff calcific tendinopathy: What is the evidence? A systematic review with proposals for future reporting. *Eur Radiol.* 2015;25(7):2176–2183.
6. Gatt DL, Charalambous CP. Ultrasound-guided barbotage for calcific tendonitis of the shoulder: A systematic review including 908 patients. *Arthroscopy.* 2014;30(9):1166–1172.
7. de Witte PB, Selten JW, Navas A, et al. Calcific tendinitis of the rotator cuff: A randomized controlled trial of ultrasound-guided needling and lavage versus subacromial corticosteroids. *Am J Sports Med.* 2013;41(7):1665–1673.
8. de Witte PB, Kolk A, Overes F, et al. Rotator cuff calcific tendinitis: Ultrasound-guided needling and lavage versus subacromial corticosteroids: Five-year outcomes of a randomized controlled trial. *Am J Sports Med.* 2017;45(14):3305–3314.
9. Sconfienza LM, Viganò S, Martini C, et al. Double-needle ultrasound-guided percutaneous treatment of rotator cuff calcific tendinitis: Tips & tricks. *Skeletal Radiol.* 2013;42(1):19–24.
10. Sconfienza LM, Bandirali M, Serafini G, et al. Rotator cuff calcific tendinitis: Does warm saline solution improve the short-term outcome of double-needle US-guided treatment? *Radiology.* 2012;262(2):560–566.
11. Arirachakaran A, Boonard M, Yamaphai S, et al. Extracorporeal shock wave therapy, ultrasound-guided percutaneous lavage, corticosteroid injection and combined treatment for the treatment of rotator cuff calcific tendinopathy: A network meta-analysis of RCTs. *Eur J Orthop Surg Traumatol.* 2017;27(3):381–390.
12. Messina C, Banfi G, Orlandi D, et al. Ultrasound-guided interventional procedures around the shoulder. *Br J Radiol.* 2016;89(1057):20150372.

Tendon Brisement/ High-Volume Injection

Tendon brisement—as opposed to fenestration and tenotomy, which directly approaches degenerative tendinopathy with intratendinous needling and debridement of abnormal angiofibroblastic tissue—focuses on disrupting adherent peritendinous neovessels and neonerves. Brisement was first described in 1997 and was initially meant to interrupt the degenerative cycle of the tendon proper by initiating a healing cascade, but in essence seems equivalent to currently described high-volume injections (HVIs).[1] Brisement specifically is the injection of fluid into the space between a tendon and its lining, peritenon, or peritendinous fat pad. While the exact mechanism of efficacy is unknown, this procedure is thought to potentially break up scar tissue, and disrupt associated neovessels and neonerves, and ultimately stimulate the healing of the tendon. Tendon brisement and HVI procedures essentially perform a hydrostatic decompression of soft tissues. Brisement procedures, or HVIs, are most commonly described with the Achilles tendon and patellar tendon but have also been described in other tendons with associated synovial sheaths, for example, the peroneal tendons.

EVIDENCE

There have been several manuscripts that have addressed HVI therapy. Ultrasound-guided HVI therapy for patellar tendinopathy was first described by Crisp and colleagues in 2008.[2] Nine patients with recalcitrant patellar tendinopathy, with associated neovascularity demonstrated by ultrasound, were treated with HVI between the patellar tendon and Hoffa's fat pad. The injection consisted of 10 mL of 0.5% bupivacaine, 25 mg of cortisone, and between 20 and 40 mL of normal saline, based upon the resistance encountered by the treating provider. Subjects reported significant improvement 2 weeks following the procedure.

A study by Chan et al. included 30 patients with refractory Achilles tendinopathy.[3] All patients underwent an HVI injection that included 10-mL 0.5% bupivacaine, 25-mg hydrocortisone, and 4 to 10 mL of normal saline that was administered between the anterior aspect of the Achilles tendon and Kager's fat pad. Vascularity was assessed with power Doppler and eccentric loading was subsequently prescribed. The results from visual pain scores showed a significant improvement in the short term (2 weeks), with a mean change of 50 mm, from a mean of 76 mm to a mean of 25 mm. There was also a statistically significant improvement in function with a mean gain of 50 mm, as well as a significant reduction demonstrated at a 30-week follow-up assessment.

In addition to the aforementioned studies, where HVI incorporated the utilization of a corticosteroid, there are a limited number of studies that employed fluid volume alone, generally a combination of lidocaine and normal saline (Wheeler[4], Mafulli[5]). While these studies demonstrated positive results, they involved limited numbers and lacked a control group for comparison. The HVI technique, while promising, and a potentially useful procedure in those who have otherwise failed conservative rehabilitative therapy, is limited by a lack of strong evidence at this time.

CONTRAINDICATIONS

The brisement/HVI procedure has comparable contraindications that apply to all bursal and peritendinous injections as previously described. The provider in particular should be cautious in an area where either a partial- or full-thickness tear in a tendon is evident, as either pain relief or an inappropriate intratendinous corticosteroid injection may propagate the tear.

EQUIPMENT

- One 21- to 22-guage needle
- Sterile saline solution (20 to 100)
- Lidocaine 1% (10 mL)
- Steroid (1 mL, 40 mg/mL) (optional)
- Ultrasound machine with high-frequency linear array transducer

PREPROCEDURAL INSTRUCTIONS

The patient should be placed in a supine position to prevent patient movement during the procedure. The limb of the affected extremity should lie completely extended along the body to facilitate optimal visualization. The procedural guidance for utilization of ultrasound guidance, to include sterile technique, is detailed in the previous chapter of **Introduction to Ultrasound**.

ANESTHESIA

Using US guidance with an in-plane approach, inject up to 10-mL lidocaine along the path of the needle's track through the skin and soft tissue proximal to the intended area of the brisement procedure.

TECHNIQUE

After the patient is placed in the appropriate position (e.g., prone for Achilles tendinopathy) and appropriately prepped and draped, the involved tendon is examined by ultrasound to identify the area of tendinopathy. The skin and subcutaneous tissue is anesthetized utilizing a 25-gauge needle. After the skin is anesthetized, a brisement or HVI can be performed, utilizing a 21- or 22-guage needle. The tendon is identified, or the tendon fat pad interface, using the linear probe being held perpendicular to the effected region. The needle then enters the area of interest, and a combination of lidocaine and normal saline is injected to tolerance and or resistance. The amount injected is variable, with the literature describing 5 to 100 mL. Some authors argue exceedingly large volumes may risk tendon rupture and/or compartment syndrome.

AFTERCARE

After tendon brisement or HVI, in particular for the Achilles or patellar tendon, the patient is asked to avoid excessive activity for several days. For the Achilles tendon, a walking boot is often used and, for the patellar tendon, a knee brace may be used. Such mechanical braces are not typically used for the upper extremity or greater trochanteric regions. The timing of stretching and physical therapy after tendon brisement is also variable in the literature.

CPT codes:
- 20550—Injection(s); single tendon sheath, or ligament, aponeurosis
  or
- 27899—Unlisted procedure, leg or ankle
- 76942—Ultrasonic guidance for needle placement with imaging supervision and interpretation with permanent recording

PEARLS

- Patients should be supine for the procedure to carefully observe for vasovagal syncope.
- Patients who have brisement or HVI near a weight-bearing tendon should have the limb protected for at least 48 to 72 hours.
- Physical therapy should commence after the procedure to facilitate optimal healing.

 A video showing tendon brisement can be found in the companion eBook.

REFERENCES

1. Johnston E, Scranton P Jr, Pfeffer GB. Chronic disorders of the Achilles tendon: Results of conservative and surgical treatments. *Foot Ankle Int*. 1997;18(9):570–574.
2. Crisp T, Khan F, Padhiar N, et al. High volume ultrasound guided injections at the interface between the patellar tendon and Hoffa's body are effective in chronic patellar tendinopathy: A pilot study. *Disabil Rehabil*. 2008;30(20–22):1625–1634.
3. Chan O, O'Dowd D, Padhiar N, et al. High volume image guided injections in chronic Achilles tendinopathy. *Disabil Rehabil*. 2008;30(20–22):1697–1708.
4. Wheeler PC, Tattersall C. Novel interventions for recalcitrant Achilles tendinopathy: Benefits seen following high-volume image-guided injection or extracorporeal shockwave therapy-a prospective cohort study. *Clin J Sport Med*. 2020;30(1):14–19.
5. Maffulli N, Del Buono A, Oliva F, Testa V, Capasso G, Maffulli G. High-volume image-guided injection for recalcitrant patellar tendinopathy in athletes. *Clin J Sport Med*. 2016;26(1):12–16.

Fenestration (Percutaneous Tenotomy)

The use of a needle to produce multiple punctate incisions or openings in a tendon for tendinopathy is termed tendon fenestration; the procedure is importantly distinguished by the absence of the use of an injectable agent.[1] Tenotomy, or percutaneous needle tenotomy, has also been used as a synonymous term in the literature and is often applied where the intervention results in tendon lengthening, release, or debridement. The theory behind this procedure is that repetitively passing the needle though the area of tendinosis disrupts the chronic degenerative process, causes bleeding and inflammation, and locally increases growth factors and other substances that promote healing. The primary goal of tendon fenestration is to convert a chronic tendon abnormality into an acute condition to facilitate improved healing. Needle fenestration is commonly utilized for tendinopathy in multiple structures including the patellar, elbow, gluteus medius, and Achilles tendons.

EVIDENCE

There have been multiple publications in the peer-reviewed literature to support the role of fenestration in treating common tendinopathies.[1-3] One of the first to report on the benefit of needle fenestration was McShane and colleagues.[4] In a study involving 52 patients, and a 22-month follow-up, they reported that 92% of subjects reporting good to excellent results. Krey et al. performed a recent systematic review of the literature on needle fenestration, finding only four manuscripts that met their inclusion criteria.[2] However, they did conclude that the current evidence suggests that tendon needling improves patient-reported outcome measures in patients with tendinopathy. They also concluded that there is a trend that shows that the addition of autologous blood products may further improve theses outcomes.

CONTRAINDICATIONS

There are several contraindications to consider when performing any ultrasound-guided percutaneous procedure. These include (a) patients with a bleeding disorder; (b) patients who are anticoagulated; and (c) the presence of local infection. The presence of an underlying tendon tear deserves discussion because the risk of tendon rupture as a complication of the procedure increases with the degree of a preexisting tendon tear. While there are no evidence-based guidelines, most authorities advocate fenestration with tendinosis, interstitial tearing, or partial-thickness tearing up to 50% of the tendon thickness, while avoiding fenestration if a tear is greater than 50% of the tendon thickness.[1-2]

EQUIPMENT

- 27-guage needle
- 22-guage needle
- 5- to 10-mL lidocaine 1%
- Ultrasound machine with high-frequency linear array transducer

PREPROCEDURAL INSTRUCTIONS

Prior to the fenestration procedure, the patient is instructed to avoid nonsteroidal anti-inflammatory medication for 2 weeks before and after the procedure. Avoidance of such medications theoretically may increase the chance of healing in that inflammation, growth factors, and the healing cascade will not be altered.

ANESTHESIA

Using US guidance with an in-plane approach, inject up to 10-mL lidocaine along the path of the needles into the peritendinous tissue of the intended needle fenestration procedure. Some patients have significant pain when the needle is at the surface of the tendon. Injection of an anesthetic agent at the tendon surface is often effective in significantly reducing symptoms. The amount of anesthetic agent should be minimized because it may potentially interfere with the healing process after fenestration.

TECHNIQUE

Ultrasound is first performed to confirm the presence of tendinosis and to plan the optimal approach to needle guidance. The area of tendinosis is targeted, which is usually near its enthesis or attachment to bone. The skin is then marked to indicate the proposed needle puncture site as well as the position of the transducer. This indicates the area that needs to be cleansed prior to the procedure, and additionally, it allows the transducer to be returned to the exact imaging plane. First, the skin is scrubbed with an appropriate cleansing agent and sterile drapes are placed around the puncture site. The ultrasound probe is then inserted into a sterile probe cover with gel, and sterile gel is used on the skin surface. Using a 27-gauge needle, the subcutaneous tissues are infiltrated with local anesthetic (Fig. 6.4). Regarding the size of the needle used for fenestration, we use

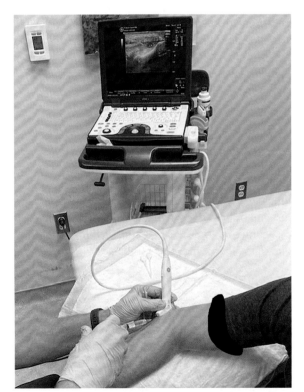

FIGURE 6.4 ● Needle fenestration of the tendon of the extensor carpi radialis brevis.

a 20-gauge needle for the shoulder, hip, and knee, and a 22-gauge needle for tendons about smaller joints. The length of the needle may be either 1.5 cm or 3 cm. The needle typically is inserted along the long-axis of the tendon, parallel to the transducer. Passing the needle in-plane, or parallel to the long-axis of the transducer, is often preferred for ultrasound guidance because the needle is visualized in its entirety. The needle can then be angle corrected during the procedure to provide real-time visualization of the fenestration.

A few technical aspects should be considered prior to entering the tendon to minimize any patient discomfort. First, the needle should be positioned in-plane, along the long axis of the transducer and tendon. Second, the needle should be placed at the proper angle while the needle is still at a very superficial level within the subcutaneous tissues. It is much easier to make changes in the needle trajectory while the needle is superficial. After entering deeper structures, such as muscle or tendon, the needle becomes more difficult to redirect. Once the needle is identified in-plane and the target visualized, the needle is advanced to the tendon abnormality. If the needle has a stylet, it should be removed prior to fenestration. The needle is then passed into the tendon, within the area of tendinosis, subsequently partially withdrawn and redirected, sequentially redirecting shallower or deeper to cover the area of tendinosis within the plane of the transducer. If the tendon abnormality is adjacent to bone, the needle is advanced to make contact with the bone. The transducer is turned 90 degrees to determine if the needle needs to be positioned or redirected medially or laterally relative to the short axis of the tendon. The needle is again partially retracted and then redirected and advanced medially or laterally, sequentially redirecting to cover the short-axis area of tendinosis. The transducer is then turned 90 degrees again, in-plane with the needle, and the fenestration continues in a similar manner, repeating until the target area has been satisfactorily fenestrated. If the patient is having symptoms, additional anesthetic agent may be injected into the tendon, although this should be minimized. The number of times the needle passes through the tendon varies but often ranges from 15 to 50 passes, depending on the size of the tendon abnormality. As the needle passes through the abnormal tendon, the tendon tends to soften. The procedure is terminated when the entire area of tendinosis is treated and feels soft during needle advancement.

AFTERCARE

After the tendon fenestration, the patient is asked to avoid nonsteroidal anti-inflammatory drugs for 2 weeks so as not to interfere with the healing process. For similar reasons, ice is avoided so as to not inhibit the induced inflammation, which is a precursor for tendon healing. For weight-bearing tendons, precautions should be considered to enhance healing and avoid the complication of tendon tear. For the Achilles tendon, a walking boot is often used and, for the patellar tendon, a knee brace is used. Such mechanical braces are not typically used for the upper extremity or greater trochanteric regions. The timing of stretching and physical therapy after tendon fenestration is also variable in the literature, although many authors advocate waiting 2 weeks after fenestration.

CPT codes:
- 20551—Injection; single tendon origin/insertion
- 76942 (optional)—Ultrasonic guidance for needle placement with imaging supervision and interpretation with permanent recording

PEARLS

- In addition to needle fenestration, it may be useful to consider the addition of either a prolotherapy injectant, autologous blood, or another regenerative agent.
- Advise the patient it may take up to 6 weeks postprocedure to see clinical benefits.
- NSAIDs should be avoided postprocedure as this negates the intent of inducing an inflammatory response.

 A video showing fenestration (percutaneous tenotomy) can be found in the companion eBook.

REFERENCES

1. Chiavaras MM, Jacobson JA. Ultrasound-guided tendon fenestration. *Semin Musculoskelet Radiol.* 2013;17(1):85–90.
2. Krey D, Borchers J, McCamey K. Tendon needling for treatment of tendinopathy: A systematic review. *Phys Sportsmed.* 2015;43(1):80–86.
3. Mattie R, Wong J, McCormick Z, et al. Percutaneous needle tenotomy for the treatment of lateral epicondylitis: A systematic review of the literature. *PM R.* 2017;9(6):603–611.
4. McShane JM, Shah VN, Nazarian LN. Sonographically guided percutaneous needle tenotomy for treatment of common extensor tendinosis in the elbow: Is a corticosteroid necessary? *J Ultrasound Med.* 2008;27(8):1137–1144.

Nerve Hydrodissection

Nerve hydrodissection, also identified as adhesiolysis neuroplasty, procedures have emerged in musculoskeletal medicine with the increasing utilization of ultrasound.[1,2] Nerve hydrodissection can be defined as the introduction of a solution under pressure between tissue planes to create separation and detach adhesions with the goal of releasing a potential soft tissue tethers or obstruction from an entrapped peripheral nerve.[1,3] Hydrodissection has been suggested as a safe and proven procedure for the blunt dissection of tissue planes. That being stated, guiding a needle along a small to medium size nerve in two axial planes is a high-skill level procedure.

While the use of hydrodissection in the treatment of peripheral nerve entrapment syndromes is a relatively new and emerging concept, the concept itself has been used for many years in a variety of settings. Hydrodissection has been used in urologic oncology to preserve the neurovascular bundle during radical prostatectomy and to prevent nerve damage during radiofrequency ablation of kidney tumors.[4,5] It has been used to preserve perforating arteries during breast reconstruction, as well as to define surgical planes during ophthalmologic procedures.[6,7] The most oft cited risk associated with peripheral nerve hydrodissection has been that of intraneural injection and resultant nerve damage. However, a study of 257 patients receiving peripheral nerve blocks before shoulder arthroscopy reported a 17% incidence of intraneural injection with zero patients experiencing postoperative neurologic complications.[8] A second study evaluated 72 cases of apparent intraneural injection, none of which resulted in any permanent nerve injury.[9] These findings suggest that while unintentional intraneural injections should be avoided, the complication of intraneural injection does not pose as ominous a risk as once thought.

EVIDENCE

Case reports have been published reporting successful treatment of peripheral neuropathies using hydrodissection techniques, such as a case of meralgia paresthetica as described by Mulvaney in 2011, and a case of foot drop as described by Tabor et al. in 2017.[10,11] However, these cases used local anesthetic or corticosteroid as part of the injectate solution. Improvement in radial nerve palsy signs and symptoms after ultrasound-guided perineural injection of D5W was noted in a single case report.[12] One recent study compared the use of corticosteroid injection versus D5W perineural injections of the median nerve in carpal tunnel syndrome patients. This study showed increased benefit in the D5W group compared with the corticosteroid group at 4 to 6 months of follow-up.[13]

CONTRAINDICATIONS

There are several contraindications to consider when performing any ultrasound-guided percutaneous procedure. These include (a) patients with a bleeding disorder; (b) patients who are anticoagulated; and (c) the presence of local infection. When approaching a nerve hydrodissection procedure, the provider should insure an accurate diagnosis of an entrapment neuropathy. In addition, patients with demonstrated distal evidence of atrophy or progressive weakness should be considered for surgical evaluation and consultation.

EQUIPMENT

- One 21- to 22-guage needle
- D5W solution (20 to 100)
- Lidocaine 1% (10 mL)
- Steroid (1 mL, 40 mg/mL) (optional)
- Ultrasound machine with high-frequency linear array transducer

PREPROCEDURAL INSTRUCTIONS

The patient should be placed in a supine position, to prevent patient movement during the procedure. The patient should be instructed to report any numbness or tingling during the procedure as this would warrant retraction and redirection of the needle. The procedural guidance for utilization of ultrasound guidance, to include sterile technique, is detailed in the previous chapter of **Introduction to Ultrasound**.

ANESTHESIA

The overlying skin is anesthetized using lidocaine 1% with epinephrine.

TECHNIQUE

Plan the procedure to hydrodissect the nerve in the direction of distal to proximal. The procedural area just proximal and distal to the site of entrapment is appropriately prepped by cleaning the skin overlying the path of the nerve with a single-use chlorhexidine sponge followed by application of sterile ultrasound gel. The transducer is cleansed with appropriate bactericidal wipes. The affected nerve is then visualized in the short axis where the nerve is most superficial and easy to visualize. Using a two-provider technique, the first provider uses ultrasound guidance to advance a 21- to 25-gauge ultrasound needle to a point just superficial and medial or lateral to the nerve in the surrounding connective tissue, dependent upon the related vascular anatomy (Fig. 6.3). Advance the needle initially in short axis (out-of-plane) to ensure you are over the correct nerve, then switch to long axis (in-plane) for precise depth control when approaching the nerve. The needle is attached to connector tubing, which is attached to a 10- to 20-mL syringe held by the second provider. The syringe is filled with 5% dextrose in water (D5W) solution as the sole injectate for this procedure. As the needle is approximated to the perineural connective tissue, the D5W is slowly injected to bluntly dissect the surrounding connective tissue from the nerve. Using fluid to maintain distance between the needle and the nerve, the needle is maneuvered superficially, deep, and circumferentially while injecting aliquots of fluid around the nerve until a complete hypoechoic ring (aka: halo) of fluid is visualized in both the short and long axes (Fig. 6.5). At this point, the nerve is visualized in long axis and further injectate is pushed through the syringe along the superficial aspect of the nerve, traveling along the length of the nerve segment and extending the area of hydrodissection through the site of entrapment.

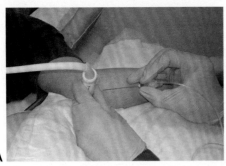
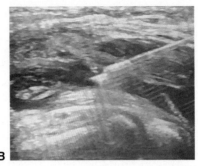

A   **B**

FIGURE 6.5 ● Nerve hydrodissection procedure. **A:** Needle out of plane approach for hydrodissection procedure of ulnar nerve in cubital tunnel. **B:** Needle in-plane long-axis approach for hydrodissection procedure of ulnar nerve in cubital tunnel.

If at any time during the procedure the nerve appears to be getting larger: STOP, as you are injecting intraneurally and high volumes may damage the nerve. If at any time during the procedure you see concentric rings of tissue expanding away from the nerve: STOP, you are injecting into the perineurium and high volumes may compress and damage the nerve.

AFTERCARE

Following the procedure, pressure should be applied as well as a surface bandage; a pressure dressing may increase friction and accentuate the tissues that caused the entrapment. Immediate physical therapy is recommended to reinforce physiologic nerve gliding.

CPT codes:
- Consider 20526—Injection, therapeutic, of carpal tunnel
- Consider 64450—Injection, nerve block, therapeutic, other peripheral nerve or branch
- Consider 64798 or 64704 for percutaneous neuroplasty. Coding should be discussed with a professional coder
- 76942—Ultrasonic guidance for needle placement with imaging supervision and interpretation with permanent recording

PEARLS

- Consider the utilization of buffered lidocaine; additionally, consider the use of 2% lidocaine if the patient is a known "slow metabolizer" of local anesthetics by history.
- Before starting the hydrodissection procedure, measure and document the nerve cross-sectional area and record comments on the appearance of the nerve (e.g., the nerve was 14 mm^2, and anechoic with the loss of the normal "bundle of grapes" appearance in cross section).
- A one-provider approach (hand on syringe approach) has the advantage of maintaining the sense of "injection pressure" during injection but requires greater skill, while the two-provider approach (hand on needle approach) affords greater precision in needle handling at the cost feeling injection pressure.
- 10- or 20-mL syringes are recommended for hydrodissection procedures. A larger syringe (e.g., 60 mL) is too large to have any sense of injection pressure with two providers and is too cumbersome to handle for one provider. Instead, have multiple full syringes available to support the planned procedure.
- Physical therapy and home exercise should emphasize nerve glide exercises.

A video showing a nerve hydrodissection procedure can be found in the companion eBook.

REFERENCES

1. Cass SP. Ultrasound-guided nerve hydrodissection: What is it? A review of the literature. *Curr Sports Med Rep*. 2016;15(1):20–22.
2. Norbury JW, Nazarian LN. Ultrasound-guided treatment of peripheral entrapment mononeuropathies. *Muscle Nerve*. 2019;60(3):222–231.
3. Bokey EL, Keating JP, Zelas P. Hydrodissection: An easy way to dissect anatomical planes and complex adhesions. *Aust N Z J Surg*. 1997;67(9):643–644.
4. Guru KA, Perlmutter AE, Butt ZM, et al. Hydrodissection for preservation of neurovascular bundle during robot-assisted radical prostatectomy. *Can J Urol*. 2008;15(2):4000–4003.
5. Lee SJ, Choyke LT, Locklin JK, et al. Use of hydrodissection to prevent nerve and muscular damage during radiofrequency ablation of kidney tumors. *J Vasc Interv Radiol*. 2006;17(12):1967–1969.
6. Ting J, Rozen WM, Morsi A. Improving the subfascial dissection of perforators during deep inferior epigastric artery perforator flap harvest: The hydrodissection technique. *Plast Reconstr Surg*. 2010;126(2):87e–89e.
7. Malavazzi GR, Nery RG. Visco-fracture technique for soft lens cataract removal. *J Cataract Refract Surg*. 2011;37(1):11–12.
8. Liu SS, YaDeau JT, Shaw PM, et al. Incidence of unintentional intraneural injection and postoperative neurological complications with ultrasound-guided interscalene and supraclavicular nerve blocks. *Anaesthesia*. 2011;66(3):168–174.
9. Bigeleisen PE. Nerve puncture and apparent intraneural injection during ultrasound-guided axillary block does not invariably result in neurologic injury. *Anesthesiology*. 2006;105(4):779–783.
10. Mulvaney SW. Ultrasound-guided percutaneous neuroplasty of the lateral femoral cutaneous nerve for the treatment of meralgia paresthetica: A case report and description of a new ultrasound-guided technique. *Curr Sports Med Rep*. 2011;10(2):99–104.
11. Tabor M, Emerson B, Drucker R, et al. High-stepping cross-country athlete: A unique case of foot drop and a novel treatment approach. *Curr Sports Med Rep*. 2017;16(5):314–316.
12. Chen S-R, Shen Y-P, Ho T-Y, et al. Ultrasound-guided perineural injection with dextrose for treatment of radial nerve palsy: A case report. *Medicine (Baltimore)*. 2018;97(23):e10978.
13. Wu Y-T, Ke M-J, Ho T-Y, et al. Randomized double-blinded clinical trial of 5% dextrose versus triamcinolone injection for carpal tunnel syndrome patients. *Ann Neurol*. 2018;84(4):601–610.

Capsular Hydrodilatation/ Hydroplasty

Capsular hydrodilatation, also known as hydroplasty, is a nonsurgical intervention used in the management of adhesive capsulitis, also known as frozen shoulder.[1] Adhesive capsulitis is a common disorder encountered by primary care providers with an estimated prevalence of 2% to 5% of the general population. Most patients diagnosed with adhesive capsulitis are women between 40 and 60 years of age, with the disorder commonly associated with both diabetes mellitus and hypothyroidism. Adhesive capsulitis is defined as a pathologic process in which contracture of the glenohumeral capsule is a hallmark, where there is restriction of both active and passive range of motion. Clinically, it presents as pain, stiffness, and dysfunction of the affected shoulder; the natural history of frozen shoulder has been described as a progression through three phases: painful, stiffness, and recovery, also known as freezing, frozen, and thawing. Adhesive capsulitis is generally considered self-limited; however, it can persist for years with some patients never regaining full function of their shoulder.[2]

EVIDENCE

Hydrodilatation (capsular distension) is a nonoperative treatment that involves an injection of local anesthetic into the shoulder capsule at high pressure to distend, stretch, or rupture the joint capsule. Although therapeutic regimens will differ between units, common to most is the instillation of a large volume of saline containing steroid, local anesthetic, and contrast material into the glenohumeral joint under imaging guidance, typically around 30 mL. A randomized controlled study of 46 patients compared hydrodilatation with placebo and demonstrated statistically and clinically significant improvement in functional outcome scores at 6 weeks following intervention.[3] One study comparing hydrodilatation, to glenohumeral and subacromial injections, found that while there was no significant difference at 6 months, that hydrodilatation provided faster relief.[4] Finally, a Cochrane review found that there is "silver" level evidence that capsular distension with saline and steroid provides short-term benefits in pain, range of movement, and function in adhesive capsulitis; however, it is uncertain whether this is better than alternative interventions.[5]

CONTRAINDICATIONS

- Anticoagulation/coagulopathy
- Systemic sepsis
- Allergies to contrast, steroid or local anesthetic
- Acute trauma

EQUIPMENT

- One 22-guage needle for the hydrodilatation procedure
- One 25-guage needle for soft tissue injection prior to the hydrodilatation procedure

- Four syringes ((2)20 mL and (2)3 mL)
- Surgical tubing and three way stop cock (optional)
- Bowl (to collect the washing fluid)
- Sterile saline solution (100 to 200 mL)
- Lidocaine 1% or mepivacaine (10 mL)
- Steroid (1 mL, 40 mg/mL)
- High-frequency linear array transducer

PREPROCEDURAL INSTRUCTIONS

For the preferred, posterior approach (see below), the patient should be placed in a lateral decubitus position, with the target shoulder up and non–weight bearing. The arm of the affected shoulder should lie in a neutral-adducted position. The procedural guidance for utilization of ultrasound guidance, to include sterile technique, is detailed in the previous chapter of **Introduction to Ultrasound**.

ANESTHESIA

Using US guidance with an in-plane approach, inject up to 10-mL lidocaine along the path of the needles into the glenohumeral joint.

TECHNIQUE

Hydrodilatation, also known as hydroplasty, can be performed from an anterior or a posterior approach. The posterior approach is our preferred approach and is accomplished with the following steps:

1. The patient is positioned in a side lying position with the affected shoulder up. The forearm should be internally rotated to facilitate opening the posterior glenohumeral joint.
2. A high-frequency linear or curvilinear probe can then be used to identify the infraspinatus and posterior glenohumeral joint.
3. After a sterile site preparation, an in-plane injection proceeds with the 25-guage needle, providing track local anesthesia.
4. The injection then proceeds with a 22-guage spinal needle along the previous identified track, until the joint capsule is penetrated (Fig. 6.6). At this point, local anesthetic and corticosteroid is injected into the joint. The syringe is then changed to a 20-cc syringe of normal saline; optionally, an extension tubing with a three way stop cock can be attached.
5. Normal saline 0.9% is then introduced into the joint (10 to 40 mL) to produce a hydraulic distention of the joint.

AFTERCARE

Following the procedure, pressure should be applied as well as a bandage. Immediate physical therapy is recommended to reinforce capsular range of motion.

CPT codes:
- 20610—Arthrocentesis, aspiration and/or injection, major joint or bursa; without ultrasound guidance
- 20611—With ultrasound guidance, with permanent recording and reporting

FIGURE 6.6 • Hydrodilatation procedure of the posterior glenohumeral joint.

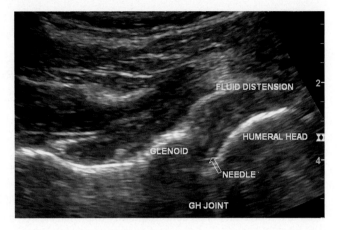

PEARLS

- Patients should be supine following the procedure to carefully observe for vasovagal syncope.
- A suprascapular nerve block can be considered prior to the procedure to facilitate patient comfort.
- Physical therapy immediately after the procedure is highly recommended to optimally leverage the hydrodilatation procedure.

 A video showing capsular hydrodilatation/hydroplasty can be found in the companion eBook.

REFERENCES

1. Halverson L, Maas R. Shoulder joint capsule distension (hydroplasty): A case series of patients with "frozen shoulders" treated in a primary care office. *J Fam Pract*. 2002;51(1):61–63.
2. Ramirez J. Adhesive capsulitis: Diagnosis and management. *Am Fam Physician*. 2019;99(5):297–300.
3. Buchbinder RGS, Forbes A, Hall S, et al. Arthrographic joint distension with saline and steroid improves function and reduces pain in patients with painful stiff shoulder: Results of a randomised, double blind, placebo controlled trial. *Ann Rheum Dis*. 2004;63(3):302–309.
4. Yoon JP, Chung SW, Kim J-E, et al. Intra-articular injection, subacromial injection, and hydrodilatation for primary frozen shoulder: A randomized clinical trial. *J Shoulder Elbow Surg*. 2016;25(3):376–383.
5. Buchbinder R, Green S, Youd JM, et al. Arthrographic distension for adhesive capsulitis (frozen shoulder). *Cochrane Database Syst Rev*. 2008;(1):CD007005.

Myofascial Trigger Point Dry Needling

Myofascial pain syndrome is a common condition that arises from muscles or related fascia and is associated with painful myofascial trigger points (MTrPs). Each trigger point is a highly localized, hyperirritable focal area in a palpable, taut band of skeletal muscle fibers. Patients present frequently to primary care physicians with this condition. Although the trigger points may be injected with corticosteroids or local anesthetics, the nodules are also commonly treated with multiple needle piercings without the introduction of an injectant. This practice of "dry needling" is attributed to Travell and Simons who empirically developed techniques involving the passage of needles into isolated trigger points for the treatment of myofascial pain syndrome.[1] This therapeutic modality, also known as intramuscular stimulation, is based on theories similar, but not exclusive, to traditional acupuncture. However, dry needling targets discrete trigger points, which are the direct and palpable source of pain, rather than traditional meridians.

Dry needling is an invasive procedure in which a standard hollow hypodermic needle or a solid core acupuncture needle is inserted through the skin and directly into a MTrP (Fig. 6.7). Proper dry needling of a MTrP will elicit both referred pain and a "local twitch response." This is an involuntary spinal cord reflex in which the muscle fibers in the taut band quickly contract. The local twitch response indicates the proper placement of the needle in a trigger point. At the site of an active trigger point, there are elevated levels of inflammatory mediators, known to be associated with persistent pain states and myofascial tenderness. This local milieu positively changes with the occurrence of a local twitch response.[2] Lewit demonstrated that the therapeutic effect from passage of a needle is distinct from that of the injected substance.[3]

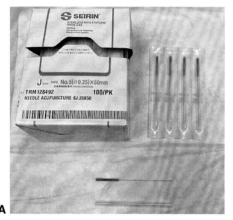
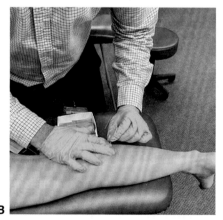

A **B**

FIGURE 6.7 ● Myofascial trigger point dry needling procedure. **A:** Dry needles. (Lhasa OMS.) **B:** Dry needling technique to lateral gastrocnemius.

EVIDENCE

An examination of the peer-reviewed literature regarding the benefit of dry needling is inconclusive. There are randomized clinical trials indicating both positive effects and no difference.[4-7] The use of ultrasound may improve the accuracy, clinical response, and safety of the procedure.[8] A recent systematic review, however, indicated no difference in outcomes in patients treated with dry needling for the treatment of myofascial pain syndrome.[9] Another comprehensive review yielded insufficient evidence to make any recommendations about acupuncture or dry needling for acute low back pain.[10] For chronic low back pain, however, results show that acupuncture is more effective for pain relief and improving function than no treatment or sham treatment in the short term. The technique has a small incremental effect when added to other conventional therapies but is not more effective than are other conventional and "alternative" treatments.

Most reported studies suffer from significant methodologic limitations and may not be generalizable.[10,11] Furthermore, rigorous evidence regarding the potential physiologic mechanisms of actions and effects of this modality is sparse and incomplete. Studies performed in an acupuncture setting do not necessarily apply to dry needling.[12] Since it appears that significant symptomatic improvement occurs in some patients who are treated with injection of MTrPs, further high-quality research is required to determine the proper place of this intervention in the treatment of myofascial pain syndrome. Areas that need to be addressed include proper study design that include blinding, randomization, use of controls, and sufficient numbers of patients.

Several adverse effects associated specifically with dry needling have been reported. These include pain, hematoma, syncopal episodes, and pneumothorax.[13] Overall, the rate of complications is low, and dry needling/acupuncture provided by experienced physicians is considered a safe treatment.[14]

CONTRAINDICATIONS

There are few contraindications to dry needling; however, there are some concerns that would preclude dry needling. Patients with either a needle phobia, a belief the technique will not help, or an unwillingness to participate in the procedure, or consent, present clear contraindications. Dry needling should not be performed over an area with either evidence of cellulitis or lymphedema as both may potentially worsen with needle intervention. Relative contraindications include, but are not limited to, abnormal bleeding tendencies, a severely compromised immune system (e.g., cancer, HIV, hepatitis, etc.), vascular disease, diabetes mellitus, pregnancy, frail patients, epilepsy, allergy to metals or latex, children, and individuals taking certain prescriptive medications (e.g., significant mood-altering medication, blood thinning agents, etc.). Additional relative contraindications include an altered psychological status, anatomic considerations (extreme caution must be taken over the pleura and lungs, blood vessels, nerves, organs, joints, prosthetic implants, implantable electrical devices, etc.), needling near a surgical site within 4 months of the surgical procedure, and a decreased ability to tolerate the procedure.

Indications	ICD-10 Code
Fibromyalgia/fibromyositis	M79.7
Spinal enthesopathy	M46.0
Cervicalgia	M54.2
Tension headache	G44.2

PREPROCEDURAL INSTRUCTIONS

The patient should be placed in a comfortable position, to prevent patient movement during the procedure. The patient should be instructed to report any numbness or tingling during the procedure as this would warrant retraction and redirection of the needle. The procedural guidance for percutaneous injections, to include sterile technique, is detailed in the previous chapter of **Introduction to Ultrasound**.

EQUIPMENT

- 3-mL syringe
- Needle choices:
  - 25-gauge, 1- to 2-in. needle (standard hollow hypodermic needle)
  - A 0.30 × 50-mm solid core acupuncture needle. The 0.30 corresponds to the gauge, or diameter, of the needle, and the 50 corresponds to length
- (Optional) 0.5 to 1 mL of 1% lidocaine without epinephrine per trigger point
- One alcohol prep pad
- Two povidone–iodine prep pads
- Sterile gauze pads
- Sterile adhesive bandage

ANESTHESIA

Skin distraction or local anesthesia of the skin using topical vapocoolant spray.

TECHNIQUE

Standard Hollow Hypodermic Needle

1. The needle entry point is located directly over the nodule(s).
2. At that site, press firmly on the skin with the retracted tip of a ballpoint pen. This indention represents the entry point for the needle.
3. After the landmarks are identified, the patient should not move.
4. Prep the insertion site with alcohol. Current standards of care in the United States recommend preparing the skin with 70% isopropyl alcohol prior to needling, as well the practitioner utilizing gloves during the intervention.[15]
5. Achieve good local anesthesia by using topical vapocoolant spray.
6. With the nondominant hand, firmly press on either side of the nodule with the index and long fingers in order to "fix" the position of the muscular nodule.
7. Position the needle and syringe at a 30- to 45-degree angle to the skin with the tip of the needle directed toward the trigger point.
8. Using the no-touch technique, introduce the needle at the insertion site.
9. Advance the needle carefully into the nodule until the needle tip is located in the center of the trigger point. Successful entry into the nodule will be accompanied by a quick muscle contraction known as the local twitch response. There may also be increased pain at the site of the trigger point or referred pain. Leave the needle in place until the muscle twitch (spasm) relaxes.
10. If performing dry needling, partially withdraw the needle from the nodule and back to the subcutaneous fat before advancing again into the trigger point. Repeat the process 5 to 10 times or until the twitch response is extinguished.

11. If desired, 0.5 to 1 mL of 1% lidocaine without epinephrine may be injected slowly into the nodule during the final entry of the needle—though it should be noted that this would constitute a trigger point injection, rather than dry needling alone.
12. Finally, withdraw the needle through the skin.
13. Apply a sterile adhesive bandage.
14. Massage and stretch each of the injection sites.
15. Reexamine the area of involvement in 5 minutes to confirm pain relief and observe for any complications.

Solid Core Acupuncture Needle

In addition to the hollow needle technique, solid core acupuncture needles can be utilized, with some modifications to the aforementioned technique. The trigger point is identified using palpation methods previously described. A pincer grip technique is employed to gently lift the skin. Additionally, flat palpation can be utilized to take up the slack of the skin. A high-quality, sterile, disposable, solid filament needle is then inserted directly through the skin, or using a guide tube that is then removed.[16] The depth of needle penetration must be sufficient to engage the MTrP. Once the needle has penetrated the skin and is inserted into the muscle, techniques vary: the practitioner may utilize a slow, steady, lancing, or pistoning motion in and out of the muscle (termed, "dynamic needling"); he or she may leave the needle in situ (termed, "static needling"); or the needle may be rotated several revolutions in order to draw the fascia or soft tissues.[16] Baldry[17] recommends leaving the needle in situ for 30 to 60 seconds for "average responders," or up to 2 to 3 minutes in "weak responders." While there is no consensus as to which technique is ideal using a solid core needle, it is the opinion of the author that dynamic needle is superior to static needling (without intramuscular electrical stimulation) in most cases.

AFTERCARE

- Ice, heat, stretching, and/or physical therapy as indicated.
- Treatment of the underlying condition.
- Consider follow-up examination in 2 weeks.

CPT codes:
- 20552—Injection of single or multiple trigger point(s) without imaging guidance
- 20553—Injection of trigger point(s) in three+ muscle groups without imaging
- 20560—Needle insertion(s) without injection(s); 1 or 2 muscle(s)
- 20561—Needle insertion(s) without injection(s); 3 or more muscles

These codes are used only once in each session, regardless of the number of injections performed.

PEARLS

- The key objective with this procedure is to elicit the local twitch response when directing a needle into a MTrP.
- Avoid advancing the needle so deeply as to risk complications including pneumothorax.

 A video showing a myofascial trigger point injection can be found in the companion eBook.

REFERENCES

1. Simons DG, Travell JG, Simons LS. *Travell and Simons' Myofascial Pain and Dysfunction: The Trigger Point Manual*, 2nd Ed. Philadelphia. PA: Lippincott Williams & Wilkins, 1999.
2. Vulfsons S, Ratmansky M, Kalichman L. Trigger point needling: Techniques and outcome. *Curr Pain Headache Rep*. 2012;16(5):407–412.
3. Lewit K. The needle effect in the relief of myofascial pain. *Pain*. 1979;6(1):83–90.
4. Tekin L, Akarsu S, Durmuş O, et al. The effect of dry needling in the treatment of myofascial pain syndrome: A randomized double-blinded placebo-controlled trial. *Clin Rheumatol*. 2013;32(3):309–315.
5. Ga H, Choi J-H, Park C-H, et al. Acupuncture needling versus lidocaine injection of trigger points in myofascial pain syndrome in elderly patients—A randomised trial. *Acupunct Med*. 2007;25(4):130–136.
6. Barbagli P, Bollettin R, Ceccherelli F. Acupuncture (dry needle) versus neural therapy (local anesthesia) in the treatment of benign back pain. Immediate and long-term results. *Minerva Med*. 2003;94(4 Suppl 1): 17–25.
7. Hong CZ. Lidocaine injection versus dry needling to myofascial trigger point. The importance of the local twitch response. *Am J Phys Med Rehabil*. 1994;73(4):256–263.
8. Chiavaras MM, Jacobson JA. Ultrasound-guided tendon fenestration. *Semin Musculoskelet Radiol*. 2013;17(1):85–90.
9. Cummings TM, White AR. Needling therapies in the management of myofascial trigger point pain: A systematic review. *Arch Phys Med Rehabil*. 2001;82(7):986–992.
10. Furlan AD, van Tulder MW, Cherkin DC, et al. Acupuncture and dry-needling for low back pain. *Cochrane Database Syst Rev*. 2005;(1):CD001351.
11. Tough EA, White AR, Cummings TM, et al. Acupuncture and dry needling in the management of myofascial trigger point pain: A systematic review and meta-analysis of randomised controlled trials. *Eur J Pain*. 2009;13(1):3–10.
12. Cagnie B, Dewitte V, Barbe T, et al. Physiologic effects of dry needling. *Curr Pain Headache Rep*. 2013;17(8):348.
13. Witt CM, Pach D, Brinkhaus B, et al. Safety of acupuncture: Results of a prospective observational study with 229,230 patients and introduction of a medical information and consent form. *Forsch Komplementmed*. 2009;16(2):91–97.
14. White A, Hayhoe S, Hart A, et al. Adverse events following acupuncture: Prospective survey of 32,000 consultations with doctors and physiotherapists. *BMJ*. 2001;323(7311):485–486.
15. Stephens MB, Beutler AI, O'Connor FG. Musculoskeletal injections: A review of the evidence. *Am Fam Physician*. 2008;78(8):971–976.
16. Finnoff JT, Hall MM, Adams E, et al. American Medical Society for Sports Medicine (AMSSM) position statement: Interventional musculoskeletal ultrasound in sports medicine. *PM & R*. 2015;7(2):151–168.e12.
17. Baldry P. Superficial versus deep dry needling. *Acupunct Med*. 2002;20(2-3):78–81.

Tenotomy With Debridement

Ultrasound-guided percutaneous tenotomy with debridement is a recently FDA-approved procedure that is indicated for recalcitrant tendinopathy. Current specific indications include extensor and flexor tendinopathy at the elbow; patellar and Achilles tendinopathy; and plantar fasciopathy. One technique (Tenex™) relies on the concept of "phaco-emulsification," which is a technique utilized during cataract surgery. In this technique, an ultrasonic vibrating needle tip emulsifies the area of tendinopathy, while a second lumen in the needle system suctions the debrided tissue. The system requires real-time ultrasound guidance, and a handheld instrument that utilizes an 18-gauge double-lumen needle.[1] A second technique (TenJet™) involves a pressurized, high-velocity stream of saline and suction, which offers an alternative to ultrasonic debridement.

EVIDENCE

There are several published studies that have looked at the role and efficacy of percutaneous ultrasonic tenotomy with debridement (PUT). Barnes et al. prospectively studied 19 patients, aged 38 to 67 years, in whom greater than 6 months of conservative management for medial (7) or lateral (12) elbow tendinopathy had failed.[2] They demonstrated that PUT appeared to be a safe and effective treatment option for chronic, refractory lateral, or medial elbow tendinopathy up to 1 year after the procedure. This study, however, like other published studies to date, are limited to case series; accordingly, the efficacy of PUT compared to other treatment options is unknown at this time. While this is a promising new technology, that offers yet another alternative to surgical intervention, further study is warranted to assess the role of this intervention.

CONTRAINDICATIONS

There are several contraindications to consider when performing any ultrasound-guided percutaneous procedure. These include (a) patients with a bleeding disorder; (b) patients who are anticoagulated; and (c) the presence of local infection. The presence of underlying tendon tear deserves discussion because the risk of tendon rupture as a complication of the procedure increases with the degree of a preexisting tendon tear.

EQUIPMENT

- 27-guage needle
- 22-guage needle
- 5- to 10-mL lidocaine 1% or mepivacaine
- Handheld device with equipment kit (depends on system used)
- High-frequency linear array transducer

PREPROCEDURAL INSTRUCTIONS

The patient should be placed in a supine position, to prevent patient movement during the procedure. The limb of the affected extremity should lie completely extended along the body to facilitate optimal visualization. The procedural guidance for utilization of ultrasound guidance, to include sterile technique, is detailed in the previous chapter of **Introduction to Ultrasound**.

ANESTHESIA

Using US guidance with an in-plane approach, inject up to 10-mL lidocaine along the path of the needle's track through the skin and soft tissue proximal to the intended area of the brisement procedure.

TECHNIQUE

Ultrasound is first performed to confirm the presence of tendinosis and to plan the optimal approach to needle guidance. The area of tendinosis is targeted, which is usually near its enthesis or attachment to bone. The needle typically is inserted along the long axis of the tendon, parallel to the transducer. Passing the needle in-plane, or long axis to the transducer, is the preferred method for ultrasound guidance because the needle is visualized in its entirety. The needle can then be angle corrected during the procedure to provide real-time visualization of the debridement. The skin is then marked to indicate the proposed needle puncture site as well as the position of the transducer. This indicates the area that needs to be cleansed prior to the procedure, and additionally, it allows the transducer to be returned to the exact imaging plane. First, the skin is scrubbed with an appropriate cleansing agent and sterile drapes are placed around the puncture site. The ultrasound probe is then inserted into a sterile probe cover with gel, and sterile gel is used on the skin surface. Using a 27-gauge needle, the subcutaneous tissues are infiltrated local anesthetic (Fig. 6.8).

A no. 11-blade scalpel is then utilized to make a stab incision to permit entry of the PUT device. The PUT device is then introduced to the area of tendinopathy, where it can be activated with the use of a foot pedal. The PUT device is redirected over the area of tendinopathic tissue comparable to a needle fenestration procedure (see above). When the procedure is concluded, wound closure is accomplished with a sterile adhesive dressing.

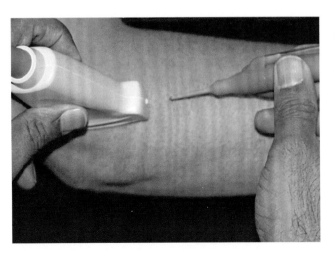

FIGURE 6.8 ● Equipment and location for ultrasound guided elbow percutaneous tenotomy with ultrasonic debridement procedure.

AFTERCARE

Postprocedure care and rehabilitation is highly variable dependent upon the area and degree of clinical debridement. Comparable to the fenestration procedure, the patient is asked to avoid nonsteroidal anti-inflammatory drugs for 2 weeks so as not to interfere with the healing process. For similar reasons, ice is avoided so as to not inhibit the induced inflammation, which is a precursor for tendon healing. For weight-bearing tendons, precautions should be considered to enhance healing and avoid the complication of tendon tear. For the Achilles tendon, a walking boot is often used and, for the patellar tendon, a knee brace is used. Such mechanical braces are not typically used for the upper extremity or greater trochanteric regions. The timing of stretching and physical therapy after tendon debridement is also variable in the literature, although many authors advocate waiting 2 weeks after debridement.

CPT codes:
- Shoulder: 23405 (tenotomy single tendon), or if appropriate 23406 (multiple tendons through same incision), also potentially use 23000 (removal of subdeltoid calcareous deposits, open)
- Achilles: 27605 (tenotomy percutaneous, Achilles tendon local anesthesia)
- Hip: 27006 (tenotomy abductors and/or extensor of hip open), 27000 (tenotomy, adductor of hip, percutaneous), 27062 (excision of trochanteric bursa or calcification), and 27060 (excision of ischial bursa)
- Foot: 28008 (fasciotomy, foot and or toe)
- Knee: 27306 (tenotomy, percutaneous, adductor or hamstring single tendon)
- Elbow: 24357 (tenotomy, elbow, lateral or medial: percutaneous)

PEARLS

- Advise the patient it may take up to 6 weeks postprocedure to see clinical benefits.
- NSAIDs should be avoided postprocedure as this negates the intent of inducing an inflammatory response.

 A video showing tenotomy with debridement can be found in the companion eBook.

REFERENCES

1. Peck E, Jelsing E, Onishi K. Advanced ultrasound-guided interventions for tendinopathy. *Phys Med Rehabil Clin N Am*. 2016;27(3):733–748.
2. Barnes DE, Beckley JM, Smith J. Percutaneous ultrasonic tenotomy for chronic elbow tendinosis: A prospective study. *J Shoulder Elbow Surg*. 2015;24(1):67–73.

7

Direct Local Injection

James W. McNabb

Direct injection by infiltration of a local anesthetic into the skin is a valuable method to provide precise anesthesia. This injection is done in a discrete area so that a minor skin procedure may be performed painlessly. Generally, 1% lidocaine with epinephrine at 1:100,000 (5 mg/mL) is the anesthetic choice for most skin procedures—whereas 1% lidocaine without epinephrine or 1% mepivacaine without epinephrine is used for musculoskeletal injections. If anesthesia is required for more than 60 min, bupivacaine 0.25% with or without epinephrine used alone, or mixed with lidocaine may be considered. The addition of epinephrine to the local anesthetic provides certain advantages, including prolongation of anesthetic duration of action and vasoconstriction to provide some hemostasis. Due to dermal vasoconstriction, there is blanching of the skin in the affected area. This affords the advantage of allowing visual estimation of the area of anesthesia—thus decreasing the possibility of cutting skin that is not anesthetized. The epinephrine-induced vasoconstriction also delays absorption of lidocaine. The prolongation in the rate of absorption decreases the risk of toxicity and increases the maximum recommended dose of lidocaine from 4 to 7 mg/kg.[1] The addition of epinephrine permits the use of larger volumes of the local anesthetic, if needed.

Several methods may be used to reduce the pain of injection caused by insertion of the needle and infiltration of the anesthetic into the skin. Ideally, the smallest needle, usually 30 gauge, should be used. Adjunctive techniques include use of topical vapocoolant spray or physical skin distraction to decrease the pain associated with needle insertion. Quick insertion of the needle into the skin, warming the injection fluid,[2] and injecting the anesthetic solution slowly[3] all decrease pain. If clinically indicated, injecting into the subcutaneous tissue is less painful than is infiltrating directly into the dermis. However, placement subcutaneously without concomitant intradermal injection increases the time to full-skin anesthesia to approximately 5 min.

The pH of lidocaine with epinephrine is 4.5. Thus, it is acidic and causes intense burning pain upon injection. As an option, lidocaine/epinephrine buffered with sodium bicarbonate to achieve a neutral pH above 6.8[4] significantly decreases the injection pain.[5,6] Buffering of the solution is particularly useful in circumstances where the pain of local anesthetic injection is not tolerated such as in large areas of infiltration, in sensitive areas such as the face or genitalia, and in children.[7] To buffer the anesthetic, mix one part of 8.4% sodium bicarbonate to nine parts of 1% lidocaine with epinephrine immediately prior to the procedure. Mixing of the solutions may be done within the syringe that is to be used for the injection. Simply, draw up both solutions, add 0.5 mL of air, and rotate the syringe to mix. Then, invert the syringe and expel the air bubble before proceeding. Raising the pH reduces the pain of injection without affecting the onset or efficacy of local anesthesia.

PATIENT POSITION

- Any, but generally recumbent on the examination/procedure table with the area of concern presented to the clinician.

ANESTHESIA

- Use topical vapocoolant spray to decrease the pain associated with injection. Alternatively, skin distraction methods may be employed.

EQUIPMENT

- Topical vapocoolant spray
- 3-mL syringe
- 30-gauge, 1/2-in. needle
- 1% lidocaine with epinephrine
- 8.4% sodium bicarbonate (optional)
- One alcohol prep pad
- Sterile gauze pads

TECHNIQUE

1. Draw up 2 to 3 mL of 1% lidocaine/epinephrine in a 3-mL syringe.
2. If desired, mix a nine-part volume of 1% lidocaine/epinephrine with a one-part volume of 8.4% sodium bicarbonate within the syringe.
3. Prep the insertion site with the alcohol pad.
4. Use topical vapocoolant spray or manual skin distraction to achieve transient local anesthesia.
5. Using the no-touch technique, insert the needle through the skin by a single, quick needle stick (Fig. 7.1).
6. Advance the needle at an angle below the center of the lesion in the subdermal tissue. Withdraw the syringe plunger to ensure that there is no blood return in the syringe to suggest intravascular needle placement. Inject approximately 1 to 2 mL of the anesthetic solution.

FIGURE 7.1 ● Direct local injection.

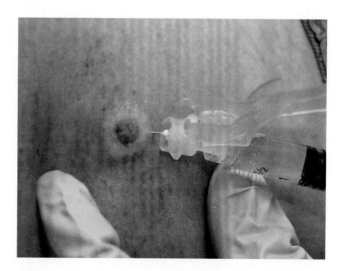

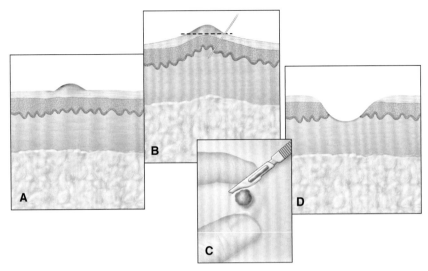

FIGURE 7.2 ● Steps in direct local injection.

7. Then, withdraw the needle slightly while keeping it in the skin and then readvance the needle to a point in the deep dermis that is directly under the center of the skin lesion. Inject approximately 1 mL of the anesthetic solution. This intradermal injection produces a wheal directly underneath the lesion.
8. The lesion is thus "floated" upward. This adds to procedure safety by increasing tissue depth and separating subcutaneous structures (vessels, nerves, tendons) from the surgical instrument (Fig. 7.2).
9. Remove the needle and apply direct pressure with the gauze pad.
10. Proceed with the skin procedure only after complete anesthesia is ensured in the target area.

AFTERCARE

• None needed

CPT code:
• None (injected local anesthesia is considered part of the skin procedure CPT code.)

 A video showing a direct local anesthetic injection can be found in the companion eBook.

REFERENCES

1. Tetzlaff JE. The pharmacology of local anesthetics. *Anesthesiol Clin North Am.* 2000;18:217–233.
2. Hogan ME, vanderVaart S, Perampaladas K, et al. Systematic review and meta-analysis of the effect of warming local anesthetics on injection pain. *Emerg Med.* 2011;58(1):86–98.
3. Hamelin ND, St-Amand H, Lalonde DH, et al. Decreasing the pain of finger block injection: Level II evidence. *Hand (N Y).* 2013;8:67–70.
4. Bancroft JW, et al. Neutralized lidocaine: Use in pain reduction in local anesthesia. *J Vasc Interv Radiol.* 1992;3(1):107–109.
5. Masters JE. Randomised control trial of pH buffered lignocaine with adrenaline in outpatient operations. *Br J Plast Surg.* 1998;51(5):385–387.
6. Hanna MN, et al. Efficacy of bicarbonate in decreasing pain on intradermal injection of local anesthetics: A meta-analysis. *Reg Anesth Pain Med.* 2009;34(2):122–125.
7. Davies RJ. Buffering the pain of local anaesthetics: A systematic review. *Emerg Med (Fremantle).* 2003;15(1):81–88.

Field Block Injection

The injection of local anesthetic into skin around an area of a planned surgical procedure is termed a field block. This procedure is a useful method to provide anesthesia to a larger area than that achieved with direct local injection. It is commonly used to provide anesthesia immediately prior to surgical excision of a skin lesion. It is also used when direct injection into, or distortion of, the surgical site is not desired. Use of a field block allows a smaller volume of anesthetic to affect a larger area. In this procedure, the local anesthetic is injected circumferentially into the dermis around the surgical site using only two points of needle entry. Infiltration of the anesthetic creates a diamond-shaped virtual "fence" that prevents the nerve impulses from leaving the targeted field of skin. For the reasons noted in "Direct Local Injection," 1% lidocaine with epinephrine (optionally buffered with sodium bicarbonate) is the anesthetic choice for this skin procedure. If anesthesia is required for more than 60 min, bupivacaine 0.25% with or without epinephrine used alone, or mixed with lidocaine may be considered.

Instead of inserting the needle oriented perpendicular to the skin, this procedure is performed in a horizontal plane to the skin surface. The operator identifies the area of excision that requires anesthesia, which includes the lesion and surrounding surgical margins. Excisions are usually performed using a fusiform shape. The insertion sites of the needle are located just beyond the corners of the fusiform outline. A longer needle (usually a 1-in. 30-gauge needle for use on the face or a 2-in. 25-gauge needle for other areas) is inserted into the skin and advanced within the dermis (without injection) to a point that is outside of the margin of the excision and just past the midpoint of the lesion. The local anesthetic solution is then injected into the dermis as the needle is slowly withdrawn. Before the needle is removed from the skin, the tip is redirected and advanced to the other side of the planned excision. After the local anesthetic is injected, the needle is withdrawn and the process repeated on the opposite side of the lesion.

PATIENT POSITION

- Any, but generally recumbent on the examination/procedure table with the area of concern presented to the clinician.

ANESTHESIA

- Use topical vapocoolant spray to decrease the pain associated with injection. Alternatively, skin distraction methods may be employed.

EQUIPMENT

- Topical vapocoolant spray
- 5- or 10-mL syringe
- 1-in. 30-gauge needle for face or a 2-in. 25-gauge needle for other areas

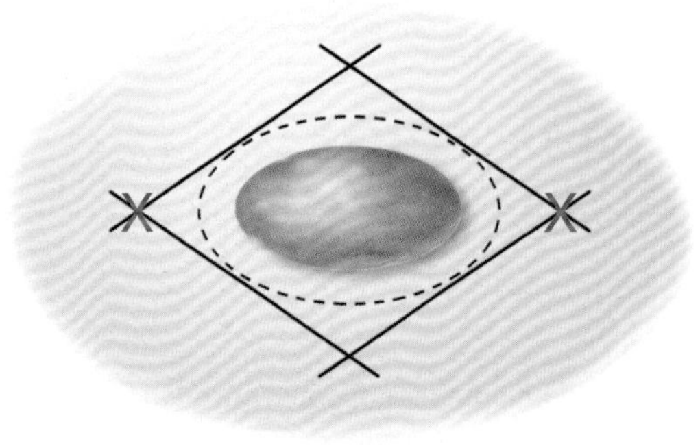

FIGURE 7.3 ● Location for field-block local anesthesia injection.

- 1% lidocaine with epinephrine
- 8.4% sodium bicarbonate (optional, but recommended)
- Alcohol prep pad(s)
- Sterile gauze pads

TECHNIQUE

1. Draw up 5 to 10 mL of 1% lidocaine/epinephrine in a 5- or 10-mL syringe.
2. If desired, mix a nine-part volume of 1% lidocaine/epinephrine with a one-part volume of 8.4% sodium bicarbonate within the syringe.
3. Identify the needle insertion sites located just beyond the points of the fusiform outline (Fig. 7.3).
4. Prep the insertion sites with the alcohol pad(s).
5. Use topical vapocoolant spray or manual skin distraction to achieve transient local anesthesia.
6. Using the no-touch technique, insert a long needle (usually a 1-in. 30-gauge needle for use on the face or a 2-in. 25-gauge needle for other areas), oriented in a horizontal plane, through the skin using a single, quick needle stick.
7. Advance the long needle within the dermis (without injection) to a point that is outside of the margin of the excision and just past the midpoint of the lesion. The location of the needle tip can be observed as it is advanced.
8. The local anesthetic is injected and infused into the dermis as the needle is slowly withdrawn. The intradermal injection produces a wheal along the needle tract (Fig. 7.4).

FIGURE 7.4 ● Field block.

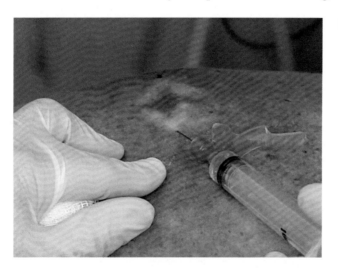

9. Before the needle is removed from the skin, the tip is redirected and advanced to the other side of the width of the excision.
10. After the local anesthetic is injected, the needle is withdrawn completely and the process repeated on the opposite side of the lesion.
11. After the intradermal anesthetic infusion has been completed, remove the needle and apply direct pressure with the gauze pad.
12. Proceed with the skin procedure only after complete anesthesia is ensured in the target area.

AFTERCARE

• None needed

CPT code:
• None (injected local anesthesia is considered part of the skin procedure CPT code.)

 A video showing a field-block injection can be found in the companion eBook.

Digital Nerve Block

Injection of local anesthetic around the digital nerves is a useful procedure to provide anesthesia of the thumbs, fingers, and toes so that surgical procedures may be conducted on those digits. The addition of epinephrine in the local anesthetic is desirable to extend the time of action of the anesthetic and to decrease bleeding in the operative field. For many years, conventional teaching was that epinephrine should be avoided in acral areas that contain end-arterioles such as the fingers, toes, penis, tip of nose, and earlobes, or skin flaps with marginal viability. However, there is a growing body of considerable evidence that withholding epinephrine in patients with normal vascular flow is not necessary and is in fact a "medical myth."

The idea that epinephrine should never be injected into fingers originated between 1920 and 1940, when procaine was used with and without epinephrine, with resulting reports of finger necrosis. Nearly all of the 48 reported cases of finger necrosis attributable to procaine local anesthesia occurred before 1950, with most implicating procaine injected without epinephrine.[1] Procaine is very acidic, with a pH of 3.6, and it further acidifies to a pH as low as 1 with prolonged storage. This acidity, not the addition of epinephrine, is likely responsible for the historical reports of finger necrosis.[2]

An extensive review of the literature from 1880 to 2000, a prospective series in 3,110 patients[3] retrospective reviews of 1,111 cases[4] and 1,334 cases,[5] as well as another review of 4,953 cases involving surgery of the nose, ears, extensive flaps, and skin grafts,[6] have definitively documented that it is safe to use lidocaine with epinephrine in acral areas and digits. Remarkably, there were no instances of vascular complications associated with the use of epinephrine reported in any of these published articles. Ultimately, the decision whether or not to use lidocaine with epinephrine rests with the medical provider. This may be particularly important in patients with medical conditions that lead to vascular compromise, including Raynaud's phenomenon, connective tissue disease, advanced diabetes, peripheral vascular disease, and Buerger's disease (thromboangiitis obliterans).

The thumbs, fingers and toes are innervated by two sets of nerves that course in the medial and lateral aspect of each digit. There are pairs of dorsal and palmar/plantar nerves. Each nerve is associated with a corresponding artery. The objective of a digital nerve block is to bathe each of the four nerves in local anesthetic with epinephrine to achieve operative anesthesia while avoiding injury to the vascular structures and digit. Traditionally this procedure has been performed utilizing a two-injection dorsal technique and more recently a web space two-injection technique. However, there is a growing body of evidence that demonstrates preference, and at least equivalent efficacy, for a single-injection technique into the volar subcutaneous tissues at the proximal digit.[7-11]

Lidocaine (1%) with epinephrine has a similar onset of action, but is significantly less painful and has a shorter duration of action than bupivacaine (0.5%).[12-14] Therefore, the current preferred method to perform a digital nerve block is a single injection of 2 mL of 1% lidocaine with epinephrine (1:100,000) into the volar subcutaneous tissue at the proximal digit to create a firm, turgid feel to the tissue. This technique is referred to as the

SIMPLE block (single, subcutaneous, injection, at the middle, proximal phalanx, using lidocaine, with epinephrine).[1]

Relevant Anatomy: (Fig. 7.5)

PATIENT POSITION

- Recumbent on the examination/procedure table with the hand or foot extended to the clinician.

ANESTHESIA

- Use topical vapocoolant spray to decrease the pain associated with injection. Alternatively, skin distraction methods may be employed.

EQUIPMENT

- Topical vapocoolant spray
- 3-mL syringe
- 30-gauge, 1/2-in. needle
- 2 mL of 1% lidocaine with epinephrine
- One alcohol prep pad
- Sterile gauze pads

TECHNIQUE

1. Locate the needle insertion site over the palmar/plantar crease at the junction of the digit and the palm or sole of the foot.[15]
2. Prep the insertion site with the alcohol pad.
3. Use topical vapocoolant spray or manual skin distraction to achieve transient local anesthesia.[4]

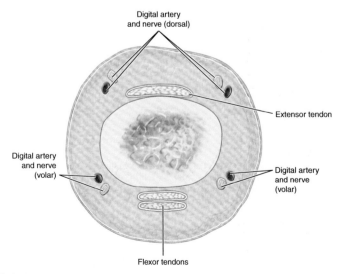

Digital artery and nerve (dorsal)

Extensor tendon

Digital artery and nerve (volar)

Digital artery and nerve (volar)

Flexor tendons

FIGURE 7.5 ● Digital anatomy.

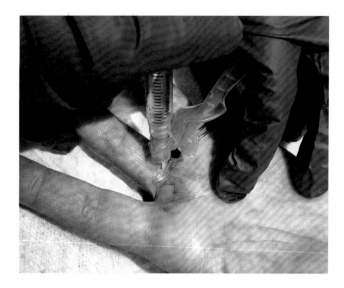

FIGURE 7.6 ● Digital nerve block.

4. Using the no-touch technique, insert the 30-gauge 1/2-in. needle perpendicularly through the skin using a single, quick needle stick. Advance the needle in a few millimeters through the skin into the subcutaneous tissue (Fig. 7.6).
5. Withdraw the plunger of the syringe to ensure that there is no blood return.
6. Inject 2 mL of lidocaine with epinephrine as a bolus in the subcutaneous tissue.
7. Remove the needle and apply direct pressure with a gauze pad—spreading the local anesthetic up to the digital nerves.
8. Allow at least 5 to 10 min for the anesthesia to take effect.
9. Repeat the procedure if necessary.
10. Proceed with the procedure only after complete anesthesia is ensured in the digit.

AFTERCARE

• None needed

CPT code:

• None (injected local anesthesia is considered part of the skin procedure CPT code.)

 A video showing a digital nerve block injection can be found in the companion eBook.

REFERENCES

1. Denkler K. A comprehensive review of epinephrine in the finger: To do or not to do. *Plast Reconstr Surg.* 2001;108(1):114–124.
2. Thomson CJ, Lalonde DH, Denkler KA, et al. A critical look at the evidence for and against elective epinephrine use in the finger. *Plast Reconstr Surg.* 2007;119(1):260–266.
3. Lalonde D, Bell M, Benoit P, et al. A multicenter prospective study of 3,110 consecutive cases of elective epinephrine use in the fingers and hand: The Dalhousie Project clinical phase. *J Hand Surg Am.* 2005;30(5):1061–1067.
4. Chowdhry S, Seidenstricker L, Cooney DS, et al. Do not use epinephrine in digital blocks: Myth or truth? Part II. A retrospective review of 1111 cases. *Plast Reconstr Surg.* 2010;126(6):2031–2034.
5. Chapeskie H, Juliao A, Payne S, et al. Evaluation of the safety of epinephrine in digital nerve blockade: Retrospective case series analysis of 1334 toe surgeries. *Can Fam Physician.* 2016;62(6):e334–e339.
6. Häfner HM, Röcken M, Breuninger H. Epinephrine-supplemented local anesthetics for ear and nose surgery: Clinical use without complications in more than 10,000 surgical procedures. *J Dtsch Dermatol Ges.* 2005;3(3):195–199.

7. Hung VS, Bodavula VK, Dubin NH. Digital anaesthesia: Comparison of the efficacy and pain associated with three digital nerve block techniques. *J Hand Surg Br*. 2005;30(6):581–584.
8. Williams JG, Lalonde DH. Randomized comparison of the single-injection volar subcutaneous block and the two-injection dorsal block for digital anesthesia. *Plast Reconstr Surg*. 2006;118(5):1195–1200.
9. Bashir MM, Khan FA, Afzal S, et al. Comparison of traditional two injections dorsal digital block with volar block. *J Coll Physicians Surg Pak*. 2008;18(12):768–770.
10. Tzeng YS, Chen SG. Tumescent technique in digits: A subcutaneous single-injection digital block. *Am J Emerg Med*. 2012;30(4):592–596.
11. Martin SP, Chu KH, Mahmoud I, et al. Double-dorsal versus single-volar digital subcutaneous anaesthetic injection for finger injuries in the emergency department: A randomised controlled trial. *Emerg Med Australas*. 2016;28(2):193–198.
12. Schnabl SM, Unglaub F, Leitz Z, et al. Skin perfusion and pain evaluation with different local anaesthetics in a double blind randomized study following digital nerve block anaesthesia. *Clin Hemorheol Microcirc*. 2013;55(2):241–253.
13. Alhelail M, Al-Salamah M, Al-Mulhim M, et al. Comparison of bupivacaine and lidocaine with epinephrine for digital nerve blocks. *Emerg Med J*. 2009;26(5):347–350.
14. Thomson CJ, Lalonde DH. Randomized double-blind comparison of duration of anesthesia among three commonly used agents in digital nerve block. *Plast Reconstr Surg*. 2006;118(2):429–432.
15. Bancroft JW, et al. Neutralized lidocaine: Use in pain reduction in local anesthesia. *J Vasc Interv Radiol*. 1992;3(1):107–109.

Facial Nerve Blocks

Facial nerve blocks are utilized to achieve anesthesia of various regions of the face. The technique is used when direct injection into the surgical field or distortion of the surgical site is not desired. In this case, a small volume of the local anesthetic is injected around the specific nerve that innervates a defined area of skin. Therefore, a small volume affects a much larger area than would otherwise be possible using local injections. This decreases excessive pain and bruising associated with multiple injections. It also reduces the total amount of local anesthetic required, thus minimizing the potential for medication toxicity. There are three classic nerve blocks that are commonly performed to provide anesthesia to most of the face. These are the supraorbital/supratrochlear, infraorbital, and mental nerve blocks. Each of these nerves is a terminal sensory branch of the fifth cranial nerve, and each has its own discrete foramen to exit the bony structures. Once the foramen is located, a small amount of anesthetic (0.5 to 1 mL) can be injected at that site to provide the desired effect. As shown in Figure 7.7, all of the three facial foramina are located along a line drawn in a vertical (sagittal) orientation from the center of the patient's pupil.

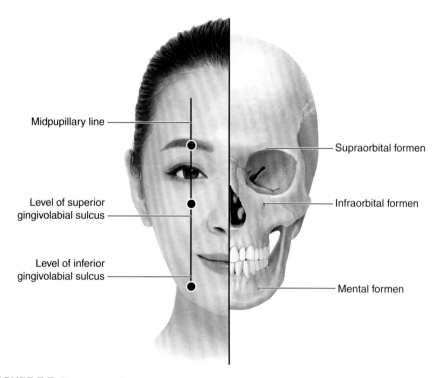

FIGURE 7.7 ● Foramina for nerve blocks.

The supraorbital foramen is the easiest to identify. It is located superior to the center of the pupil and palpated as a subtle depression in the supraorbital ridge underneath the eyebrow. The supratrochlear nerve is commonly injected along with the supraorbital nerve to extend the anesthetic effect to the midline of the forehead. The nerve is located at the supraorbital ridge immediately superior to the inner canthus of the eye. In most people, this is located at the medial aspect of the eyebrow.

The infraorbital foramen may be found in the maxilla about 1.5 cm inferior to the infraorbital rim—and in line with the pupil. A depression in the maxilla cannot be palpated.

Finally, the mental nerve is located along the same line drawn in a vertical (sagittal) orientation from the center of the patient's pupil. It is positioned at the midpoint of the height of the mandible. A discrete depression is also not palpable.

To confirm the correct location, firm palpation directly over each of the foramen elicits a sensation of intense, dull pain, not found in adjacent areas. From a coding standpoint, all injections to establish local anesthesia for a surgical procedure are considered part of that procedure. As such, they are included in the CPT procedural code and not billed separately.

Supraorbital and Supratrochlear Nerve Blocks

The supraorbital and supratrochlear nerves are perhaps the easiest of the facial nerve blocks to perform. These nerves are terminal sensory branches of the ophthalmic trunk of the fifth cranial nerve. The blocks are used to administer reversible local anesthesia to the forehead. Various procedures including laceration repair, skin lesion removal, photodynamic therapy, or laser facial skin resurfacing of the forehead may be performed utilizing these blocks. Headache disorders including cluster, tension, and migraine headaches may also be treated in part by performing these blocks.[1,2]

Relevant Anatomy: (Fig. 7.8)

PATIENT POSITION

- With the patient supine on the examination table and the patient's head rotated toward the clinician, the clinician stands lateral to the side of the face that is being injected.

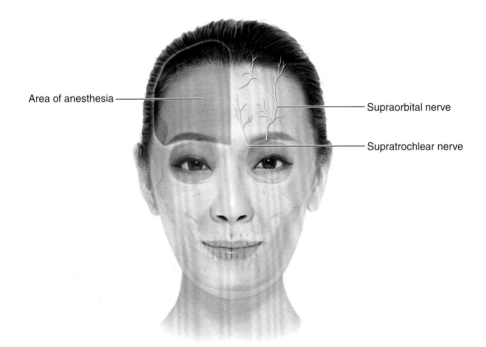

FIGURE 7.8 ● Supraorbital and supratrochlear nerves and innervated areas.

LANDMARKS

1. The supraorbital foramen is located superior (sagittal) to the center of the pupil and is palpated as a subtle depression in the supraorbital ridge underneath the eyebrow.
2. In an anatomic study of skulls, supraorbital foramina were found to be approximately 25 mm lateral to the midline, 30 mm medial to the temporal crest of the frontal bone, and 2 to 3 mm superior to the supraorbital rim. Additional exits for branches of the supraorbital nerve were present in 14% of skulls.[3]
3. The supratrochlear nerve is located at the supraorbital ridge superior (sagittal) to the inner canthus of the eye. In most people, this is located at the medial aspect of the eyebrow.
4. At sites located immediately superior to the eyebrow over each nerve location, press firmly on the skin with the retracted tip of a ballpoint pen. This indention represents the entry point for the needle.

ANESTHESIA

- Preinjection use of topical vapocoolant spray is not advised due to the close proximity to the eyes. However, skin distraction techniques may be employed.

EQUIPMENT

- Topical vapocoolant spray
- 3-mL syringe
- 30-gauge, 1/2-in. needle
- 1 mL of 1% lidocaine with or without epinephrine (depending on anticipated procedure time)
- One alcohol prep pad
- Sterile gauze pad

TECHNIQUE

1. Prep the insertion site with the alcohol pad.
2. Firmly place the tip of the nondominant hand index finger over the edge of the orbital rim just below the location of the supraorbital foramen. This prevents accidental passage of the needle below the rim and helps to keep the anesthetic up in proper position.
3. Position the needle at a 90-degree angle to the skin just above the eyebrow with the tip of the needle directed toward the supraorbital foramen.
4. In order to provide topical anesthesia, spray PainEase mist onto a sterile cotton swab until saturated. Then, apply the swab over the point of injection.
5. Using the no-touch technique, quickly introduce the needle at the insertion site.
6. Advance the needle directly over the supraorbital foramen, touch the bone, and withdraw about 1 mm.
7. Withdraw the plunger of the syringe to ensure that there is no blood return.
8. Inject 1 mL of 1% lidocaine with or without epinephrine directly over the supraorbital foramen.
9. Following injection, withdraw the needle.

10. Repeat the process for the supratrochlear nerve with the needle positioned over the supraorbital ridge immediately superior to the inner canthus of the eye.
11. Proceed with the skin procedure only after complete anesthesia is ensured in the target area.

AFTERCARE

• None needed

CPT code:
• None (injected local anesthesia is considered part of the skin procedure CPT code.)
• 64400—Injection, anesthetic agent; trigeminal nerve, any division or branch

 A video showing supraorbital/supratrochlear nerve block injections can be found in the companion eBook.

REFERENCES

1. Blumenfeld A, Ashkenazi A, Napchan U, et al. Expert consensus recommendations for the performance of peripheral nerve blocks for headaches—A narrative review. *Headache.* 2013;53(3):437–446.
2. Ilhan Alp S, Alp R. Supraorbital and infraorbital nerve blockade in migraine patients: Results of 6-month clinical follow-up. *Eur Rev Med Pharmacol Sci.* 2013;17(13):1778–1781.
3. Gupta T. Localization of important facial foramina encountered in maxillo-facial surgery. *Clin Anat.* 2008;21(7):633–640.

Infraorbital Nerve Block

The infraorbital nerve is a terminal sensory branch of the maxillary trunk of the fifth cranial nerve. This block is used to administer reversible local anesthesia to the medial midface excluding the central nose. Various procedures including skin and upper lip laceration repair, photodynamic therapy, laser facial skin resurfacing of the midface/upper lip, skin and upper lip filler placement, or skin lesion removal may be performed following this block.

Relevant Anatomy: (Fig. 7.9)

PATIENT POSITION

- With the patient supine on the examination table and the patient's head rotated toward the clinician, the clinician stands lateral to the side of the face that is being injected.

LANDMARKS

1. In an anatomic study of skulls, infraorbital foramina were found to be 28.5 mm lateral to the midline and approximately 7 mm inferior to the inferior orbital rim and along

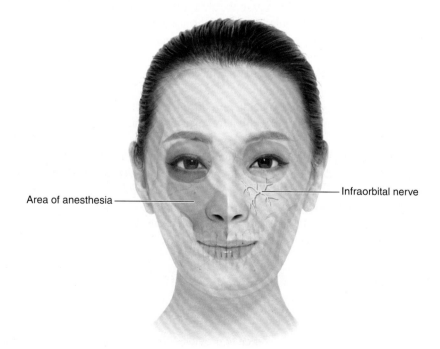

Area of anesthesia —————————————— Infraorbital nerve

FIGURE 7.9 ● Infraorbital nerve and innervated area.

a line drawn in a vertical (sagittal) orientation from the center of the patient's pupil.[1] A depression in the maxilla at the site of the foramen is not palpable. To confirm the location, firm pressure directly over the foramen elicits the sensation of intense, dull pain, not found in adjacent areas.

2. At that site, press firmly on the skin with the retracted tip of a ballpoint pen. This indention represents the entry point for the needle when using the transdermal approach.

ANESTHESIA

- Preinjection use of topical vapocoolant spray is not advised due to the close proximity to the eyes. However, skin distraction techniques may be employed.

EQUIPMENT

- Headlamp or other light source (for intraoral approach)
- Topical vapocoolant spray (optional)
- 3-mL syringe
- 30-gauge, 1/2-in. needle for transdermal approach or a 25-gauge 1½-in. needle for intraoral approach
- 1 mL of 1% lidocaine with or without epinephrine (depending on anticipated procedure time)
- One alcohol prep pad (for transdermal approach)
- Sterile gauze pad

TECHNIQUE (TRANSDERMAL)

1. Prep the insertion site with the alcohol pad.
2. Position the needle perpendicularly to the skin at the location over the maxilla identified above. The tip of the needle is directed toward the infraorbital foramen.
3. Provide skin distraction by pinching, stretching, and/or rubbing adjacent skin at the same time that the needle is being inserted into the skin. Or, in order to provide topical anesthesia, spray PainEase mist onto a sterile cotton swab until saturated. Then, apply the swab over the point of injection.
4. Using the no-touch technique, quickly introduce the needle at the insertion site.
5. Advance the needle over the infraorbital foramen, touch the bone, and withdraw about 1 mm.
6. Withdraw the plunger of the syringe to ensure that there is no blood return.
7. Inject 1 mL of 1% lidocaine with or without epinephrine directly over the infraorbital foramen.
8. Following injection, withdraw the needle.
9. Proceed with the skin procedure only after complete anesthesia is ensured in the target area.

TECHNIQUE (INTRAORAL)

1. Patient position is the same as described above, but with the patient's neck extended in order to tilt the head back.
2. Use a headlamp or other light source to provide good illumination for the procedure.
3. Grasp the upper lip with gauze and elevate it superiorly.

4. Identify the maxillary third to fourth tooth from midline (canine/first premolar). The infraorbital foramen is located just superior to the apex of the gingivolabial mucosal reflection between these teeth.
5. A 1½-in. 25-gauge needle is positioned in the sagittal plane, directed toward the ipsilateral pupil.
6. The needle is quickly inserted at this point and advanced approximately 0.5 cm to a position over the infraorbital foramen.
7. Withdraw the plunger of the syringe to ensure that there is no blood return.
8. Inject 1 mL of 1% lidocaine with or without epinephrine directly over the infraorbital foramen.
9. Following injection, withdraw the needle.
10. Proceed with the skin procedure only after complete anesthesia is ensured in the target area.

AFTERCARE

• None needed

CPT code:
• None (injected local anesthesia is considered part of the skin procedure CPT code.)

 Videos showing transdermal and intraoral infraorbital nerve block injections can be found in the companion eBook.

REFERENCE

1. Gupta T. Localization of important facial foramina encountered in maxillo-facial surgery. *Clin Anat.* 2008;21(7):633–640.

External Nasal Nerve Block

Infraorbital nerve blocks provide reversible anesthesia to the lateral nasal skin but not to the central portion of the nose. Blocks of the external nasal nerves supplement nasal anesthesia by providing anesthesia of the skin over the cartilaginous nasal dorsum and the tip of the nose.

The external nasal nerve is a terminal sensory branch of the anterior ethmoidal nerve from the trunk of the fifth cranial nerve. It emerges 5 to 10 mm lateral to the nasal midline at the osseous junction of the distal edge of the nasal bones.

Various procedures including skin laceration repair, photodynamic therapy, laser facial skin resurfacing of the nose, or skin lesion removal may be performed following this block.

Relevant Anatomy: (Fig. 7.10)

PATIENT POSITION

- With the patient supine on the examination table and the patient's head rotated toward the clinician, the clinician stands lateral to the side of the face that is being injected.

LANDMARKS

1. Palpate the distal rim of the nasal bone at the osseous cartilaginous junction. Select and mark an injection site 7.5 mm lateral to the midline.[1]

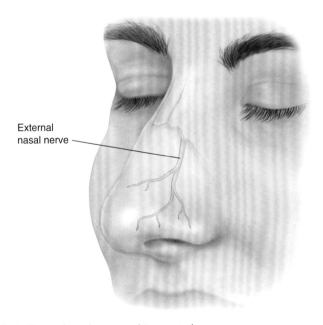

External nasal nerve

FIGURE 7.10 ● External nasal nerve and innervated area.

2. At that site, press firmly on the skin with the retracted tip of a ballpoint pen. This indention represents the entry point for the needle.

ANESTHESIA

- Preinjection use of topical vapocoolant spray is not advised due to the close proximity to the eyes. However, skin distraction techniques may be employed.

EQUIPMENT

- Topical vapocoolant spray
- 3-mL syringe
- 30-gauge, 1/2-in. needle
- 1 mL of 1% lidocaine with or without epinephrine (depending on anticipated procedure time)
- One alcohol prep pad
- Sterile gauze pad

TECHNIQUE

1. Prep the insertion site with the alcohol pad.
2. Position the needle perpendicularly to the skin over the lateral nose at the osseous cartilaginous junction as identified above.
3. Provide skin distraction by pinching, stretching, and/or rubbing adjacent skin at the same time that the needle is being inserted into the skin. Or, in order to provide topical anesthesia, spray PainEase mist onto a sterile cotton swab until saturated. Then, apply the swab over the point of injection.
4. Using the no-touch technique, quickly introduce the needle at the insertion site.
5. Advance the needle only into the deep dermis. (When attempting to advance the needle into the subcutaneous tissue, it is very easy to advance the needle too far and enter the nasal cavity.)
6. Withdraw the plunger of the syringe to ensure that there is no blood return.
7. Slowly inject 1 mL of 1% lidocaine with or without epinephrine into the tissue.
8. Following injection, withdraw the needle.
9. Proceed with the skin procedure only after complete anesthesia is ensured in the target area.

AFTERCARE

- None needed

CPT code:
- None (injected local anesthesia is considered part of the skin procedure CPT code.)

 A video showing the external nasal nerve block injection can be found in the companion eBook.

REFERENCE

1. Moskovitz JB, Sabatino F. Regional nerve blocks of the face. *Emerg Med Clin North Am.* 2013;31(2):517–527.

Mental Nerve Block

The mental nerve is a terminal sensory branch of the mandibular trunk of the fifth cranial nerve. This block is used to administer reversible local anesthesia to the lower midface. Various procedures including skin and lower lip laceration repair, photodynamic therapy, laser facial skin resurfacing of the midface/lower lip, skin and lower lip filler placement, or skin lesion removal may be performed following this block.

Relevant Anatomy: (Fig. 7.11)

PATIENT POSITION

- With the patient supine on the examination table and the patient's head rotated toward the clinician, the clinician stands lateral to the side of the face that is being injected.

LANDMARKS

1. In an anatomic study of skulls, mental foramina were on average, 25.8 mm lateral to the midline and about 13 mm superior to the inferior mandibular margin and along a line drawn in a vertical (sagittal) orientation from the center of the patient's pupil.[1] A depression in the mandible at the site of the foramen is difficult to palpate. To confirm

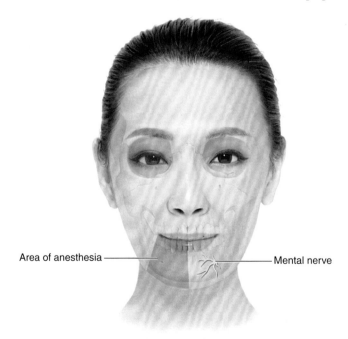

Area of anesthesia —————— —————— Mental nerve

FIGURE 7.11 ● Mental nerve and innervated area.

the location, firm pressure directly over the foramen elicits the sensation of intense, dull pain, not found in adjacent areas.
2. At that site, press firmly on the skin with the retracted tip of a ballpoint pen. This indention represents the entry point for the needle when using the transdermal approach.

ANESTHESIA

- Use topical vapocoolant spray to decrease the pain associated with injection. Alternatively, skin distraction methods may be employed.

EQUIPMENT

- Headlamp or other light source (for intraoral approach)
- 3-mL syringe
- 30-gauge, 1/2-in. needle for transdermal approach or a 25-gauge 1½-in. needle for intraoral approach
- 1 mL of 1% lidocaine with or without epinephrine (depending on anticipated procedure time)
- One alcohol prep pad (for transdermal approach)
- Sterile gauze pad

TECHNIQUE (TRANSDERMAL)

1. Prep the insertion site with the alcohol pad.
2. Position the needle perpendicularly to the skin at the location over the mandible identified above. The tip of the needle is directed toward the mental foramen.
3. Use topical vapocoolant spray to decrease the pain associated with injection. Alternatively, provide skin distraction by pinching, stretching, and/or rubbing adjacent skin at the same time that the needle is being inserted into the skin.
4. Using the no-touch technique, quickly introduce the needle at the insertion site.
5. Advance the needle over the mental foramen, touch the bone, and withdraw about 1 mm.
6. Withdraw the plunger of the syringe to ensure that there is no blood return.
7. Inject 1 mL of 1% lidocaine with or without epinephrine directly over the mental foramen.
8. Following injection, withdraw the needle.
9. Proceed with the skin procedure only after complete anesthesia is ensured in the target area.

TECHNIQUE (INTRAORAL)

1. Use a headlamp or other light source to provide good illumination for the procedure.
2. Grasp the lower lip with gauze and retract it inferiorly.
3. Identify the mandibular third to fourth tooth from midline (canine/first premolar). The infraorbital foramen is located just inferior to the apex of the gingivolabial mucosal reflection between these teeth.
4. A 1½-in. 25-gauge needle is positioned in the sagittal plane, directed inferiorly toward the mental foramen.

5. The needle is quickly inserted at this point and advanced approximately 0.5 cm to a position over the mental foramen.
6. Withdraw the plunger of the syringe to ensure that there is no blood return.
7. Inject 1 mL of 1% lidocaine with or without epinephrine directly over the mental foramen.
8. Following injection, withdraw the needle.
9. Proceed with the skin procedure only after complete anesthesia is ensured in the target area.

AFTERCARE

• None needed

CPT code:
• None (injected local anesthesia is considered part of the skin procedure CPT code.)

 Videos showing transdermal and intraoral mental nerve block injections can be found in the companion eBook.

REFERENCE

1. Gupta T. Localization of important facial foramina encountered in maxillo-facial surgery. *Clin Anat.* 2008;21(7):633–640.

External Ear Field Block

The external ear has complex innervation with four nerves contributing to sensory input. As illustrated in Fig. 7.12A, the auriculotemporal nerve innervates the superior aspect of the external ear, the lesser occipital nerve is responsible for the mid posterior external ear, and the great auricular nerve innervates the inferior aspect of the ear. Importantly, the auricular branch of the vagus nerve provides sensory input for the external ear canal and the central aspect of the external ear.

The injection of local anesthetic into skin around an area of a planned surgical procedure is termed a field block. This technique allows a small volume of anesthetic to affect a larger area. In this case, the points of needle entry are located immediately superior and inferior to the ear. Intradermal infiltration of the anesthetic creates a diamond-shaped virtual "fence" of anesthesia circumferentially around the ear. The local anesthetic of choice for this procedure is 1% lidocaine with epinephrine (optionally buffered with sodium bicarbonate).

If the external ear canal or the central aspect of the external ear will be involved in the surgical procedure, then direct local injection into the affected area will be required

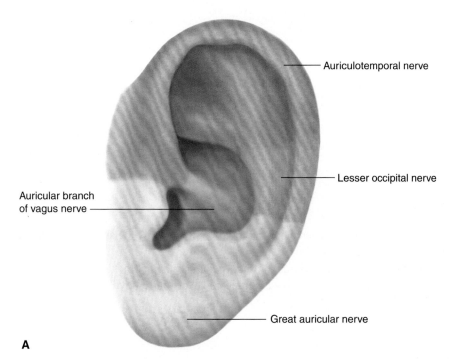

Auriculotemporal nerve

Lesser occipital nerve

Auricular branch of vagus nerve

Great auricular nerve

A

FIGURE 7.12 ● **A:** The auriculotemporal nerve innervates the superior aspect of the external ear, the lesser occipital nerve is responsible for the mid posterior external ear, and the great auricular nerve innervates the inferior aspect of the ear.

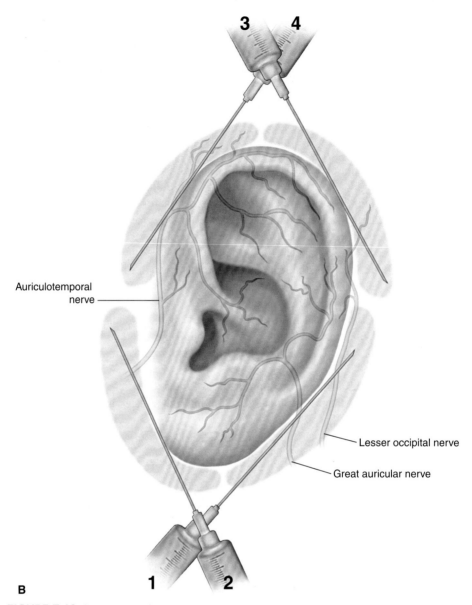

FIGURE 7.12 ● (*Continued*) **B:** Identify the needle insertion sites located immediately superior and also just inferior to the external.

to provide supplementary anesthesia to the skin innervated by the auricular branch of the vagus nerve.

The most common procedures for this type of anesthetic block involve ear laceration repair, hematoma evacuation, and ear skin lesion excision/removal.

Relevant Anatomy: (Fig. 7.12A and B)

PATIENT POSITION

• Supine on the examination table with the head of the bed slightly elevated

ANESTHESIA

- Use topical vapocoolant spray to decrease the pain associated with injection. Alternatively, skin distraction methods may be employed.

EQUIPMENT

- Topical vapocoolant spray
- 10-mL syringe
- 1 ½-in. or a 2-in. 25-gauge needle
- 1% lidocaine with epinephrine
- 8.4% sodium bicarbonate
- Alcohol prep pad(s)
- Sterile gauze pads

TECHNIQUE

1. Draw up and mix 9 mL of 1% lidocaine/epinephrine with 1 mL of 8.4% sodium bicarbonate (if desired) within the syringe.
2. Identify the needle insertion sites located immediately superior and also just inferior to the external ear (Fig. 7.12B).
3. Prep the insertion sites with alcohol pad(s).
4. Use topical vapocoolant spray to decrease the pain associated with injection. Alternatively, provide skin distraction by pinching, stretching, and/or rubbing adjacent skin at the same time that the needle is being inserted into the skin.
5. Start with the superior injection site. Using the no-touch technique, insert a 1 ½-in. or a 2-in. 25-gauge needle through the skin with a single, quick needle stick.
6. Advance the long needle in a horizontal plane within the dermis to points anterior and posterior to the ear. The location of the needle tip can be observed as it is advanced.
7. Withdraw the plunger of the syringe to ensure that there is no blood return.
8. The local anesthetic is injected and infused into the dermis as the needle is slowly withdrawn. The intradermal injection produces a wheal along the needle tract.
9. Before the needle is removed from the skin, the tip is redirected and advanced to the other side of the ear.
10. Again, withdraw the plunger of the syringe to ensure that there is no blood return.
11. After the local anesthetic is injected, the needle is withdrawn and the process repeated at the inferior aspect of the ear.
12. After the intradermal anesthetic infusion has been completed, remove the needle and apply direct pressure to the injection sites with the gauze pad.
13. Proceed with the skin procedure only after complete anesthesia of the ear is ensured in the target area.

AFTERCARE

- None needed

CPT code:
- None (injected local anesthesia is considered part of the skin procedure CPT code.)

 A video showing an external ear field-block injection can be found in the companion eBook.

Greater Occipital Nerve Block

Patients occasionally present to the primary care office for the treatment of headaches caused by greater occipital neuralgia. The greater occipital nerve, which is composed of C2 sensory fibers, can become entrapped as it passes through the aponeurotic attachments of the trapezius and semispinalis capitis muscles to the occipital bone. Typically, the pain of occipital neuralgia begins in the neck and then spreads to the vertex, ear, frontal area, and even the eyes. The International Classification of Headache Disorders 3rd edition describes occipital neuralgia as unilateral or bilateral paroxysmal, shooting or stabbing pain in the posterior part of the scalp, in the distribution(s) of the greater, lesser and/or third occipital nerves, sometimes accompanied by diminished sensation or dysesthesia in the affected area and commonly associated with tenderness over the involved nerve(s); and pain is eased temporarily by local anesthetic block of the nerve.[1] The pain of occipital neuralgia may reach the fronto-orbital area through trigeminocervical interneuronal connections in the trigeminal spinal nuclei.

There is an increasing body of evidence that greater occipital nerve injections are a safe and effective technique to treat headache pain. Suboccipital steroid injections of the greater occipital nerve for the treatment of cluster headaches received a Level A recommendation in the 2016 American Headache Society Evidence-Based Guidelines.[2] In a population of 159 childhood and adolescent patients with disabling headaches of various diagnoses, unilateral injections of the greater occipital nerve were shown to be an effective treatment with rapid onset, and with minimal side effects.[3] In a 5-year retrospective study of 562 patients, greater occipital nerve blocks effectively reduced pain in the acute treatment of patients with migraine headaches.[4] Also, in a single-center retrospective study of 190 adult patients with migraine headaches, occipital nerve blocks used as adjunctive therapy showed safety and efficacy measured by the reduction in pain.[5] Furthermore, ultrasound guidance has been demonstrated to increase the effectiveness of the greater occipital nerve injection procedure.[6]

Indications	ICD-10 Code
Headache	R51
Occipital neuralgia	M54.81
Cervicogenic headache	R51
Cluster headache	C44.009
Migraine headache	G43.909

Relevant Anatomy: (Fig. 7.13)

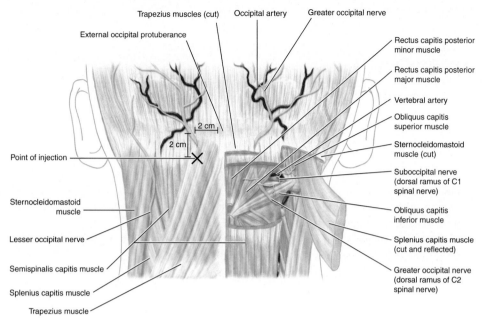

Trapezius muscles (cut) Occipital artery Greater occipital nerve

External occipital protuberance

Rectus capitis posterior minor muscle

Rectus capitis posterior major muscle

Vertebral artery

Obliquus capitis superior muscle

Sternocleidomastoid muscle (cut)

Suboccipital nerve (dorsal ramus of C1 spinal nerve)

Obliquus capitis inferior muscle

Splenius capitis muscle (cut and reflected)

Greater occipital nerve (dorsal ramus of C2 spinal nerve)

2 cm

2 cm

Point of injection

Sternocleidomastoid muscle

Lesser occipital nerve

Semispinalis capitis muscle

Splenius capitis muscle

Trapezius muscle

FIGURE 7.13 ● Suboccipital region. (From Gest TR. *Lippincott Atlas of Anatomy*, 2nd Ed. Philadelphia, PA: Wolters Kluwer, 2019.)

PATIENT POSITION

- The patient sitting on an exam stool with neck flexed and leaning forward with the forehead resting on the patient's crossed arms, which are resting on the pullout foot tray of the exam table. The clinician stands behind the patient and slightly lateral on the side of treatment.

LANDMARKS

1. Find the inion of the external occipital protuberance at the midline of the occipital bone.
2. The point of injection of the greater occipital nerve is 2 cm lateral to the external occipital protuberance along the superior nuchal line and then 2 cm inferior (caudal).[7]
3. At the point where the greater occipital nerve courses over the occipital bone, pressure over the nerve will elicit pain. Mark that spot with an ink pen.
4. At that site, press firmly on the skin with the retracted tip of a ballpoint pen. This indention represents the entry point for the needle.
5. After the landmarks are identified, the patient should not move the neck.

ANESTHESIA

- Transient topical anesthesia using vapocoolant spray is difficult over the posterior occiput, especially in patients who have thick hair. However, skin distraction techniques may be employed.

EQUIPMENT (FOR A SINGLE UNILATERAL INJECTION)

- 3-mL syringe
- 25-gauge, 1-in. needle

- 1 mL of 1% lidocaine without epinephrine
- 1 mL of 0.5% bupivacaine without epinephrine
- 1 mL of the steroid solution (40 mg of triamcinolone acetonide)
- One alcohol prep pad
- Two povidone–iodine prep pads
- Sterile gauze pads

TECHNIQUE

1. Part the hair and prep the insertion site with alcohol followed by the povidone–iodine pads.
2. Position the needle and syringe perpendicular to the skin with the tip of the needle directed anteriorly toward the inferior nuchal line of the occiput.
3. Provide skin distraction by pinching, stretching, and/or rubbing adjacent skin at the same time that the needle is being inserted into the skin.
4. Using the no-touch technique, introduce the needle at the insertion site (Fig. 7.14).
5. Advance the needle toward the location of the greater occipital nerve until the needle tip contacts the occiput at the inferior nuchal line. Back up the needle 1 to 2 mm.
6. Withdraw the plunger of the syringe to ensure that there is no blood return.
7. Inject the anesthetic/steroid solution as a bolus around the greater occipital nerve. The injected solution should flow smoothly into the tissues. If increased resistance is encountered, advance or withdraw the needle slightly before attempting further injection.
8. Following injection, withdraw the needle and apply direct pressure with a gauze pad until all bleeding has stopped.
9. Reexamine the greater occipital nerve in 1 to 5 min to assess pain relief.

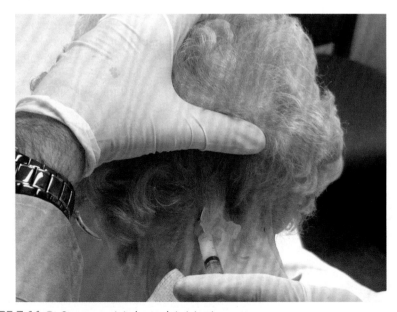

FIGURE 7.14 ● Greater occipital neuralgia injection.

AFTERCARE

- Analgesics, muscle relaxants, ice, physical therapy, musculoskeletal manipulation, and/or other modalities as indicated.
- Consider follow-up examination in 2 weeks.

CPT code:
- 64405—Injection, anesthetic agent; greater occipital nerve

PEARLS

- Occipital neuralgia must be distinguished from occipital referral of pain from the atlantoaxial or upper zygapophyseal joints or from tender trigger points in neck muscles or their insertions.[8]

 A video showing a greater occipital nerve block injection can be found in the companion eBook.

REFERENCES

1. https://ichd-3.org/13-painful-cranial-neuropathies-and-other-facial-pains/13-4-occipital-neuralgia/. Accessed on August 23, 2020.
2. Robbins MS, Starling AJ, Pringsheim TM, et al. Treatment of cluster headache: The American Headache Society Evidence-Based Guidelines. *Headache*. 2016;56(7):1093–1106.
3. Puledda F, Goadsby PJ, Prabhakar P. Treatment of disabling headache with greater occipital nerve injections in a large population of childhood and adolescent patients: A service evaluation. *J Headache Pain*. 2018;19(1):5.
4. Allen SM, Mookadam F, Cha SS, et al. Greater occipital nerve block for acute treatment of migraine headache. *J Am Board Fam Med*. 2018;31(2):211–218.
5. Ebied AM, Nguyen DT, Dang T. Evaluation of occipital nerve blocks for acute pain relief of migraines. *J Clin Pharmacol*. 2020;60(3):378–383.
6. Palamar D Uluduz D Saip S, et al. Ultrasound-guided greater occipital nerve block: an efficient technique in chronic refractory migraine without aura? *Pain Physician*. 2015;18(2):153-162.
7. Loukas M, El-Sedfy A, Tubbs RS, et al. Identification of greater occipital nerve landmarks for the treatment of occipital neuralgia. *Folia Morphol (Warsz)*. 2006;65(4):337–342.
8. Tetzlaff JE. The pharmacology of local anesthetics. *Anesthesiol Clin North Am*. 2000;18:217–233.

Headache Nerve Blocks

Headache peripheral nerve blocks are useful procedures that may be done to relieve the pain of various headaches[1] including muscular tension, cervicogenic,[2] migraine,[3–5] cluster,[6–8] chronic daily headache, paroxysmal hemicrania, and hemicrania continua.[9] They may be used in patients who have failed home medications and may help patients with medication overuse headaches to wean off of acute therapy.[10] Nerve blocks also may be appropriate for children[11,12] and pregnant patients.[13]

These injection techniques are used to provide reversible local anesthesia in order to achieve effective blockade of any or all of the bilateral greater occipital, lesser occipital, auriculotemporal, zygomaticotemporal, supraorbital, and supratrochlear nerves. Selection of the single nerve or multiple nerves to be injected is clinically determined on the basis of local pain or pain radiation when the nerve of interest is compressed. Multiple cranial nerve blocks may provide an efficacious, well tolerated, and reproducible transitional treatment for chronic headache disorders when greater occipital nerve blocks have been unsuccessful.[14] Corticosteroids may be added to the greater occipital nerve injections to provide longer term symptomatic relief. In fact, suboccipital steroid injections of the greater occipital nerve for the treatment of cluster headaches received a Level A recommendation in the 2016 American Headache Society Evidence-Based Guidelines.[15] On the other hand, several small studies are inconclusive regarding the efficacy of adding steroids to local anesthetics for the treatment of migraine headache.[16]

Pain relief from the headache nerve block injections commonly lasts longer than the usual expected anesthetic effect of the lidocaine and bupivacaine. Almost all patients experience pain relief after receiving anesthetic nerve blocks, but there is no way to predict which patients will experience long-term pain relief.

Contraindications to peripheral nerve blocks include a known allergy to a local anesthetic, open skull defect, and an overlying skin infection. Pregnancy is a relative contraindication.

Indications	ICD-10 Code
Muscular tension headache	G44.209
Migraine headache	G43.909
Cluster headache	C44.009
Occipital neuralgia	M54.81
Cervicogenic headache	R51
Chronic daily headache	R51
Paroxysmal hemicrania	G44.039
Hemicrania continua	G43.909

Relevant Anatomy: (Fig. 7.15)

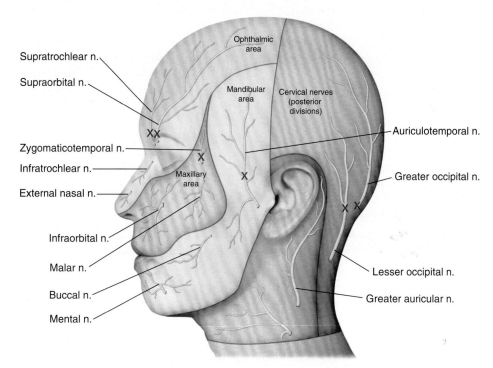

FIGURE 7.15 Scalp nerves and their innervated areas. The *red X* indicates the injection sites for each nerve.

PATIENT POSITION

- For the greater occipital and lesser occipital nerve injections, the patient is positioned sitting on an exam stool with neck flexed and leaning forward with the forehead resting on the patient's crossed arms, which are resting on the pullout foot tray of the exam table. The clinician stands behind the patient and slightly lateral on the side of treatment.
- For the auriculotemporal and zygomaticotemporal nerve injections, the patient is positioned lying supine on the examination table with the head of the bed slightly elevated. The clinician stands lateral to the side of the face that is being injected.
- For the supraorbital and supratrochlear nerve injections, the patient is positioned lying supine on the examination table with the patient's head rotated toward the clinician. The clinician stands lateral to the side of the face that is being injected.

LANDMARKS

1. Refer to the Greater Occipital Nerve Chapter for the location of this nerve.
2. The point of injection of the lesser occipital nerve is over the medial border of the sternocleidomastoid muscle. The position of the injection is 1 cm inferior and over the lateral third of a line between the external occipital protuberance and the mastoid process. Pressure over the nerve will often elicit pain.
3. The point of injection of the auriculotemporal nerve is 1.5 cm anterior to the ear at the level of the tragus.
4. The point of injection of the zygomaticotemporal nerve is 1.5 cm posterior to the lateral orbital rim above the zygomatic arch.
5. Refer to the Supraorbital and Supratrochlear Nerve Injection Chapter for location of these nerves.

ANESTHESIA

- Transient topical anesthesia of the skin using a vapocoolant spray is not advised for use with the supratrochlear, supraorbital, and zygomaticotemporal nerves due to the close proximity of the injection sites to the eyes. Transient topical anesthesia using vapocoolant spray is difficult over the posterior occiput, especially in patients who have thick hair. However, skin distraction techniques may be employed.

EQUIPMENT (IF ALL SITES WILL BE INJECTED BILATERALLY)

- One 5-mL syringe
- Two 10-mL syringes
- Two 30-gauge, 1/2-in. needles and one 25-gauge, 1-in. needle
- 10 mL of 1% lidocaine without epinephrine
- 10 mL of 0.5% bupivacaine without epinephrine
- 2 mL of the steroid solution (40 mg/mL of triamcinolone acetonide)
- Alcohol prep pads
- Sterile gauze pads

TECHNIQUE

1. Over each of the nerve block injection sites, press firmly on the skin with the retracted tip of a ballpoint pen. These indentions represent the entry points for the needles.
2. Prep each of the insertion sites with alcohol pads.
3.
   - One 10-mL syringe is used for the bilateral greater occipital and lesser occipital nerve injections. Fill the 10-mL syringe with 4 mL of 1% lidocaine without epinephrine, 4 mL of 0.5% bupivacaine without epinephrine, and 2 mL of the steroid solution (triamcinolone acetonide 40 mg/mL). Mix the contents of each syringe. Attach a 25-gauge, 1-in. needle.
   - One 10-mL syringe is used for bilateral auriculotemporal and zygomaticotemporal nerve injections. Fill the 10-mL syringe with 4 mL of 1% lidocaine without epinephrine and 4 mL of 0.5% bupivacaine without epinephrine. Mix the two anesthetics in each syringe. Attach a 30-gauge, 1/2-in. needle.
   - One 5-mL syringe is used for the bilateral supraorbital and supratrochlear nerve injections. Fill the 5-mL syringe with 2 mL of 1% lidocaine without epinephrine and 2 mL of 0.5% bupivacaine without epinephrine. Mix the two anesthetics in each syringe. Attach a 30-gauge, 1/2-in. needle.
4. Provide skin distraction by pinching, stretching, and/or rubbing adjacent skin at the same time that the needle is being inserted into the skin.
5. Using the no-touch technique, quickly introduce the needles at each insertion site.
6.
   - For the greater occipital nerve headache injections, follow the technique described in the dedicated chapter and infuse 2.5 mL of the lidocaine/steroid mixture at the site of each greater occipital nerve.
   - For the lesser occipital nerve headache injections, position the 25-gauge, 1-in. needle perpendicular to the skin at the identified point of entry. Advance the needle toward the location of that nerve until the needle tip contacts the occiput at the superior nuchal line. Back up the needle 1 to 2 mm. Withdraw the plunger of the syringe to ensure that there is no blood return. Inject 2.5 mL of the anesthetic/steroid mixture over each lesser occipital nerve site.
   - For the auriculotemporal and zygomaticotemporal nerve headache injections, position the 30-gauge, 1/2-in. needle perpendicular to the skin at each of the injection

sites described above. Advance it into the subcutaneous tissue under the injection site. Withdraw the plunger to ensure that there is not intravascular placement. Inject 2 mL of the anesthetic mixture at the site of each nerve.

- For the supraorbital and supratrochlear nerve headache injections, follow the technique described in the dedicated chapter and infuse 1 mL of the anesthetic mixture around each supraorbital and supratrochlear nerve.

7. Following the injections, withdraw the needles and apply direct pressure. For supraorbital and supratrochlear injections, press and push the anesthetic up the forehead and away from the eyes.

8. Reexamine the patient in 1 to 5 min to assess pain relief.

AFTERCARE

- None needed

CPT codes:

- 64400—Injection, anesthetic agent; trigeminal nerve, any division or branch
- 64402—Injection, anesthetic agent; facial nerve
- 64405—Injection, anesthetic agent; greater occipital nerve
- 64450—Injection, anesthetic agent; other peripheral nerve or branch

 A video showing headache nerve block injections can be found in the companion eBook.

REFERENCES

1. Blumenfeld A, Ashkenazi A, Napchan U, et al. Expert consensus recommendations for the performance of peripheral nerve blocks for headaches—A narrative review. *Headache*. 2013;53(3):437–446.
2. Lauretti GR, Correa SW, Mattos AL. Efficacy of the greater occipital nerve block for cervicogenic headache: Comparing classical and subcompartmental techniques. *Pain Pract*. 2015;15(7):654–661.
3. Ruiz Pinero M, Mulero Carrillo P, et al. Pericranial nerve blockade as a preventive treatment for migraine: Experience in 60 patients. *Neurologia*. 2016;31(7):445–451.
4. Allen SM, Mookadam F, Cha SS, et al. Greater occipital nerve block for acute treatment of migraine headache. *J Am Board Fam Med*. 2018;31(2):211–218.
5. Ebied AM, Nguyen DT, Dang T. Evaluation of occipital nerve blocks for acute pain relief of migraines. *J Clin Pharmacol*. 2020;60(3):378–383.
6. Gonen M, Balgetir F, Aytac E, et al. Suboccipital steroid injection alone as a preventive treatment for cluster headache. *J Clin Neurosci*. 2019;68:140–145.
7. Robbins MS, Starling AJ, Pringsheim TM, et al. Treatment of cluster headache: The American Headache Society Evidence-Based Guidelines. *Headache*. 2016;56(7):1093–1106.
8. Lambru G, Abu Bakar N, Stahlhut L, et al. Greater occipital nerve blocks in chronic cluster headache: A prospective open-label study. *Eur J Neurol*. 2014;21(2):338–343.
9. Cortijo E, Guerrero-Peral AL, Herrero-Velazquez S, et al. Hemicrania continua: Characteristics and therapeutic experience in a series of 36 patients. *Rev Neurol*. 2012;55(5):270–278.
10. Tobin J, Flitman S. Occipital nerve blocks: When and what to inject? *Headache*. 2009;49(10):1521–1533.
11. Szperka CL, Gelfand AA, Hershey AD. Patterns of use of peripheral nerve blocks and trigger point injections for pediatric headache: Results of a survey of the American Headache Society Pediatric and Adolescent Section. *Headache*. 2016;56(10):1597–1607.
12. Puledda F, Goadsby PJ, Prabhakar P. Treatment of disabling headache with greater occipital nerve injections in a large population of childhood and adolescent patients: A service evaluation. *J Headache Pain*. 2018;19(1):5.
13. Govindappagari S, Grossman TB, Dayal AK, et al. Peripheral nerve blocks in the treatment of migraine in pregnancy. *Obstet Gynecol*. 2014;124(6):1169–1174.
14. Miller S, Lagrata S, Matharu M. Multiple cranial nerve blocks for the transitional treatment of chronic headaches. *Cephalalgia*. 2019;39(12):1488–1499.
15. Davies RJ. Buffering the pain of local anaesthetics: A systematic review. *Emerg Med (Fremantle)*. 2003;15(1):81–88.
16. Bancroft JW, et al. Neutralized lidocaine: Use in pain reduction in local anesthesia. *J Vasc Interv Radiol*. 1992;3(1):107–109.

8

Chalazion

James W. McNabb

A chalazion is an acute or chronic granuloma that forms due to inflammation and obstruction in the meibomian glands (or tarsal glands) on the conjunctival surface of either the upper or the lower eyelids. The obstruction in these small sebaceous glands may occur due to allergy, acne in adolescence, or rosacea. A chalazion contains many steroid-responsive immune cells including macrophages, plasma cells, polymorphonuclear cells, and eosinophils. Patients with this condition present occasionally to the primary care office, and although considered self-limited, it may last for weeks to months before spontaneously disappearing. Traditional conservative treatment includes the application of local heat, lubricant eye drops, careful cleansing of the eyelid, and topical antibiotics (although this condition, unlike a hordeolum, is not an infectious process). Lesions that persist after more than 2 months of conservative therapy should be treated with surgery or a corticosteroid injection.[1]

An often unrecognized procedure is the simple injection of a small amount of corticosteroid (4 mg of triamcinolone) into or around the chalazion lesion. Studies show that the procedure is quick, well tolerated, and safe. It results in greater than 80% resolution of the chalazion lesion within days of administration.[2-5] Response rates mirror that of surgical treatment with incision and curettage.[6] Additional advantages of this technique over traditional incision and curettage include its simplicity, less pain, considerably decreased cost, no requirement of special instruments, no need for postoperative eye patching, and convenience for both the provider and the patient.

Indications	ICD-10 Code
Chalazion	H00.19

Relevant Anatomy: (Fig. 8.1)

PATIENT POSITION

- Supine on the examination table with the head of the bed elevated 30 degrees.
- The patient's hands are folded in his or her lap.
- The clinician stands lateral to the patient, on the same side as the chalazion.

ANESTHESIA

- Injection of local anesthetic into the skin of the eyelid prior to injection of the corticosteroid is not used because it causes local swelling that obliterates the location of the chalazion.

FIGURE 8.1 • Superior eyelid. The tarsus forms the skeleton of the eyelid and contains the tarsal glands.

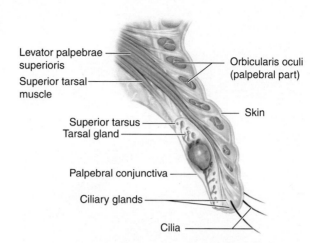

Levator palpebrae superioris

Superior tarsal muscle

Orbicularis oculi (palpebral part)

Skin

Superior tarsus

Tarsal gland

Palpebral conjunctiva

Ciliary glands

Cilia

- Topical corneal anesthesia is never provided so that inadvertent introduction of the needle through the eyelid, through the conjunctiva, and into the globe cannot occur.
- Topical vapocoolant spray cannot be sprayed directly around the eyes.
- Topical vapocoolant spray can be sprayed on a cotton swab until saturated, and the swab is then applied directly to the injection site.
- Alternatively, a supraorbital nerve block provides anesthesia of the upper eyelid, and an infraorbital nerve block provides anesthesia for the lower eyelid.

EQUIPMENT

- (Optional) Corneal eye shield protectors (Kolberg Optical Supplies, Inc. http://www. corneaprotectors.com/)
- (Optional) Chalazion clamp
- Topical vapocoolant spray
- 3-mL syringe
- 30-gauge, 1/2-in. needle
- 0.1 mL (4 mg) of the steroid solution (40 mg/mL of triamcinolone acetonide)
- One alcohol prep pad
- Two povidone–iodine prep pads
- Sterile gauze pads

TECHNIQUE

1. Provide adequate anesthesia to the upper eyelid by performing supraorbital and supratrochlear nerve blocks or the lower eyelid by performing an infraorbital nerve block. See chapter 7.
2. (Optional) Corneal eye shield protectors may be used to protect the cornea and globe.
3. Identify the injection site a few millimeters lateral to the chalazion. Prep the insertion site with alcohol followed by the povidone–iodine pads.
4. (Optional) A chalazion clamp may also be used, if desired, to stabilize the lesion. However, use of this instrument requires both nerve block(s) and topical corneal anesthesia.
5. With your fingertips, apply lateral traction to the eyelid to stretch and fix the skin.
6. Approach the eyelid from a lateral to a medial direction.

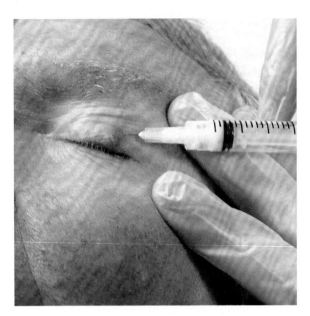

FIGURE 8.2 ● Chalazion injection.

7. To ensure safety, make sure that the needle is oriented parallel to the surface of the globe of the eye. The operator should also rest his or her injection hand on the patient's face to stabilize the needle.
8. In order to provide topical anesthesia, spray PainEase mist onto a sterile cotton swab until saturated. Then, apply the swab just lateral to the chalazion.
9. Using the no-touch technique, insert the needle through the skin external to the eyelid about 2 to 3 mm lateral to the chalazion (Fig. 8.2).
10. Advance the needle slowly and carefully into the center of the chalazion.
11. After insertion into the chalazion, confirm accurate placement by moving the needle slightly from side to side to ensure that the lesion moves with the needle.
12. Inject 0.1 mL (4 mg) of the steroid solution (40 mg/mL of triamcinolone acetonide) into the chalazion. Swelling of the chalazion will occur.
13. Remove the needle and apply gentle direct pressure with the gauze pad.

AFTERCARE

- None needed.
- Consider follow-up examination in 1 week.

CPT code:
- 68200—Subconjunctival injection

PEARLS

- After the needle has been inserted into the chalazion, confirm accurate placement by moving the needle slightly from side to side to ensure that the nodule moves with the needle.
- One-third of the cases may require a second injection at a later date.
- If the chalazion continues to recur after two injections, it should be evaluated for malignancy. In this case, referral to a subspecialist colleague is recommended for more aggressive measures such as primary excision or curettage through a cruciform incision.

• Potential complications may include inadvertent corneal injury, penetration of the globe, cataract from administration of steroid in the globe, persistent triamcinolone deposits,[7] and skin depigmentation.

 A video showing a chalazion injection can be found in the companion eBook.

REFERENCES

1. Wu AY, Gervasio KA, Gergoudis KN, et al. Conservative therapy for chalazia: Is it really effective? *Acta Ophthalmol*. 2018;96(4):e503–e509.
2. Wong MY, Yau GS, Lee JW, et al. Intralesional triamcinolone acetonide injection for the treatment of primary chalazions. *Int Ophthalmol*. 2014;34(5):1049–1053.
3. Ben Simon GJ, Rosen N, Rosner M, et al. Intralesional triamcinolone acetonide injection versus incision and curettage for primary chalazia: A prospective, randomized study. *Am J Ophthalmol*. 2011;151(4):714–718.
4. Goawalla A, Lee V. A prospective randomized treatment study comparing three treatment options for chalazia: Triamcinolone acetonide injections, incision and curettage and treatment with hot compresses. *Clin Experiment Ophthalmol*. 2007;35(8):706–712.
5. Chung CF, Lai JS, Li PS. Subcutaneous extralesional triamcinolone acetonide injection versus conservative management in the treatment of chalazion. *Hong Kong Med J*. 2006;12(4):278–281.
6. Singhania R, Sharma N, Vashisht S, et al. Intralesional triamcinolone acetonide (TA) versus incision and curettage (I & C) for medium and large size chalazia. *Nepal J Ophthalmol*. 2018;10(19):3–10.
7. Wolkow N, Jakobiec FA, Hatton MP. A common procedure with an uncommon pathology: Triamcinolone acetonide eyelid injection. *Ophthalmic Plast Reconstr Surg*. 2018;34(3):e72–e73.

Keloid Scar

Keloid scars occur as the result of an abnormal overgrowth of dense fibrous tissue that develops in areas of prior skin trauma. The tissue elevates above the surface of the surrounding skin, extends beyond the borders of the original wound, does not regress spontaneously, and often recurs after excision. Keloids usually occur during the second and third decades of life, with a higher prevalence in persons with darker pigmented skin. They are most commonly asymptomatic but can present with itching and pain if they become inflamed or enlarge.

Since primary surgical excision may result in worsening of the keloid scar, many other therapeutic modalities for keloids and hypertrophic scars are used in clinical practice. These include ablative laser, fractional laser, photodynamic therapy, silicone gel application, and cryosurgery.

Intralesional injection of therapeutic agents is the most commonly used treatment. The primary injectable agent for many years has been corticosteroids. Corticosteroids reduce excessive scarring by decreasing collagen synthesis, suppressing vascular endothelial growth factor, and decreasing production of inflammatory mediators and fibroblast proliferation during wound healing. In a recent study by Huu and colleagues, the optimal dose for treatment of a keloid was determined to be 7.5 mg/1 cm^2 scar.[1] Complications of repeated corticosteroid injections may include skin atrophy, telangiectasia formation, hypopigmentation, and a depressed scar.

Combinations of various therapies may produce an even greater benefit. Triamcinolone used in combination with 5-flurouracil results in improved scar regression and reduced recurrence of keloids.[2,3] Combined injection of intralesional steroids with botulinum toxin-A appears to be superior to either therapy alone.[4] A recent network meta-analysis showed that injection of intralesional botulinum toxin type A combined with corticosteroids was more effective and had fewer side effects. The optimal treatment course was monthly intralesional injections of triamcinolone acetonide 40 mg/mL (0.1 mL/cm^3) mixed with botulinum toxin type A (2.5 IU/cm^3) for a total of three treatments.[5] Combining intralesional platelet-rich plasma with triamcinolone could yield cosmetically better outcomes in keloid treatment with lower incidence of corticosteroid-induced side effects, especially atrophy and hypopigmentation.[6] Finally, combination therapy with intralesional cryosurgery followed by injected steroids,[7] and surgical excision followed by corticosteroid injections,[8,9] have also been shown to be effective.

Indications	ICD-10 Code
Keloid scar	L91.0

PATIENT POSITION

- Supine on the examination table.

- Rotate the patient's head away from the side that is being injected. This minimizes anxiety and pain perception.
- The clinician stands on the side of the patient that allows best access to the keloid scar.

ANESTHESIA

- Local anesthesia of the injection site with topical vapocoolant spray

EQUIPMENT

- Topical vapocoolant spray
- 3-mL syringe
- 25-gauge, 1- or 1½-in. needle depending on the size of the keloid
- 0.25 to 1 mL of the steroid solution (40 mg/mL of triamcinolone acetonide)
- (Optional) 0.25 to 1 mL of 5-fluorouracil solution (50 mg/mL)
- (Optional) 0.1 to 1 mL of onabotulinumtoxinA solution (100 units/mL)
- One alcohol prep pad
- Two povidone–iodine prep pads
- Sterile gauze pads
- Sterile adhesive bandage

TECHNIQUE

1. Prep the insertion site with alcohol followed by the povidone–iodine pads.
2. Achieve good local anesthesia by using topical vapocoolant spray.
3. Position the needle and syringe parallel to the surface of the skin at the edge of the keloid with the tip of the needle directed toward the center of the keloid scar.
4. Using the no-touch technique, introduce the needle at the edge of the keloid (Fig. 8.3).
5. Advance the needle into the lesion.

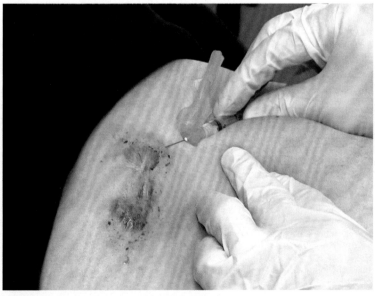

FIGURE 8.3 ● Keloid injection.

6. Withdraw the plunger of the syringe to ensure that there is no blood return.
7. Perform a uniform injection of 0.25 to 1 mL of steroid solution (10 to 40 mg of triamcinolone acetonide—see above for dosing) (and/or optionally, 0.25 to 1 mL [12.5 to 50 mg] of 5-fluorouracil solution) (and/or optionally, 10 to 100 units of ona-botulinumtoxinA solution—see above for dosing) into the substance of the keloid at a depth that is half the thickness of the keloid.
8. Avoid injection into the subcutaneous fat or surrounding normal skin.
9. Following injection, withdraw the needle.
10. Apply a sterile adhesive bandage.

AFTERCARE

- None needed
- Follow-up examination in 4 to 6 weeks

CPT codes:

- 11900—Intralesional injections (1 to 7 lesions)
- 11901—Intralesional injections (>7 lesions)

PEARLS

- If the keloid continues to recur after several injections, more aggressive measures may be used, as noted above.
- Avoid superficial injections as they may increase the likelihood of dermal complications.

 A video showing a keloid scar injection can be found in the companion eBook.

REFERENCES

1. Huu ND, Huu SN, Thi XL, et al. Successful treatment of intralesional triamcinolone acetonide injection in keloid patients. *Open Access Maced J Med Sci.* 2019;7(2):275–278.
2. Davison SP, Dayan JH, Clemens MW, et al. Efficacy of intralesional 5-fluorouracil and triamcinolone in the treatment of keloids. *Aesthet Surg J.* 2009;29(1):40–46.
3. Darougheh A, Asilian A, Shariati F. Intralesional triamcinolone alone or in combination with 5-fluoroura-cil for the treatment of keloid and hypertrophic scars. *Clin Exp Dermatol.* 2009;34(2):219–223.
4. Gamil HD, Khattab FM, El Fawal MM, et al. Comparison of intralesional triamcinolone acetonide, botulinum toxin type A, and their combination for the treatment of keloid lesions. *J Dermatolog Treat.* 2020;31(5):535–544.
5. Sun P, Lu X, Zhang H, Hu Z. The efficacy of drug injection in the treatment of pathological scar: A net-work meta-analysis. *Aesthetic Plast Surg.* 2019 Dec 18. doi: 10.1007/s00266-019-01570-8. Epub ahead of print. PMID: 31853608.
6. Hewedy ES, Sabaa BEI, Mohamed WS, et al. Combined intralesional triamcinolone acetonide and platelet rich plasma versus intralesional triamcinolone acetonide alone in treatment of keloids. *J Dermatolog Treat.* 2020;1–7.
7. Weshahy AH, Abdel Hay R. Intralesional cryosurgery and intralesional steroid injection: A good combina-tion therapy for treatment of keloids and hypertrophic scars. *Dermatol Ther.* 2012;25(3):273–276.
8. Hayashi T, Furukawa H, Oyama A, et al. A new uniform protocol of combined corticosteroid injections and ointment application reduces recurrence rates after surgical keloid/hypertrophic scar excision. *Dermatol Surg.* 2012;38(6):893–897.
9. Park TH, Seo SW, Kim JK, et al. Clinical characteristics of facial keloids treated with surgical exci-sion followed by intra- and postoperative intralesional steroid injections. *Aesthetic Plast Surg.* 2012;36(1):169–173.

Common Warts

Patients very often present to the primary care office for evaluation of common warts. These verrucous structures are the focal dermal expression of human papillomavirus infections. Common warts may be treated with various modalities, including cryosurgery, electrosurgery, laser ablation, cautery, curettage, and injection therapy.

Immunotherapy achieved by injecting *Candida albicans*; measles, mumps, and rubella; Trichophyton; and tuberculin antigens intradermally at the edge of a wart incites a host immune response that is mediated through stimulation of T helper-1 cell cytokines.[1] This commonly results in spontaneous regression of the treated warts. In addition, an HPV-directed cell-mediated immune response plays a role in the resolution of distant untreated warts. There is a growing body of literature that documents effectiveness and safety of intralesional and/or perilesional injection therapy with *Candida*[2] and measles–mumps–rubella[3] antigens. A large study yielded a 70% complete response to intralesional injections of *Candida* antigen for children with multiple recalcitrant cutaneous warts.[4] Compared to liquid nitrogen cryotherapy, intralesional injection of *Candida* antigen has a better therapeutic response, needs fewer sessions, and is capable of treating distant warts.[5]

Candida antigen is available as "Candin" (Nielsen BioSciences, Inc. 11125 Flintkote Ave, San Diego, CA 92121, phone: 858-571-2726, web site: https://nielsenbio.com/candin-hcp/) or the generic (Hollister Stier Allergy. 3525 N. Regal St, Spokane, WA 99207, phone: 509-489-5656, web site: http://www.hsallergy.com/).

Indications	ICD-10 Code
Common warts	B07.8
Genital warts	A63.0
Plantar warts	B07.0

PATIENT POSITION

- Supine on the examination table.
- Rotate the patient's head away from the side that is being injected. This minimizes anxiety and pain perception.

ANESTHESIA

- Local anesthesia of the skin using topical vapocoolant spray

EQUIPMENT

- Topical vapocoolant spray
- 3-mL syringe

- 30-gauge, 1/2-in. needle
- Up to 1 mL of the *Candida* antigen
- Up to 1 mL of 1% lidocaine without epinephrine
- One alcohol prep pad
- Sterile gauze pads
- Sterile adhesive bandage
- Nonsterile, clean chucks pad

TECHNIQUE

1. Prepare the injection solution: Mix equal parts of up to 1 mL of *Candida* antigen and up to 1 mL of 1% lidocaine without epinephrine.
2. Prep the insertion site(s) with alcohol pads.
3. Achieve good local anesthesia by using topical vapocoolant spray.
4. Position the needle and syringe at a 10-degree angle to the surface of the skin at the edge of the wart with the tip of the needle directed toward the wart.
5. Using the no-touch technique, introduce the needle about 5 mm from the edge of the wart (Fig. 8.4).
6. Advance the needle into the dermis to the edge of the wart.
7. Withdraw the plunger of the syringe to ensure that there is no blood return.
8. Perform an intradermal injection immediately adjacent to the wart using 0.1 mL of the solution per wart. Limit the total amount at any one visit to 1 mL of the *Candida* antigen.
9. Avoid injection into the subcutaneous tissues.
10. Following injection of the solution, withdraw the needle.
11. Apply a sterile adhesive bandage.

AFTERCARE

- None needed.
- Instruct the patient to expect these local symptoms following injection as the immune system is reacting to the antigen: localized erythema, itching, drying of the wart, lesion turning a black color, peeling of the treated tissue, or simply (and most commonly) spontaneous regression.

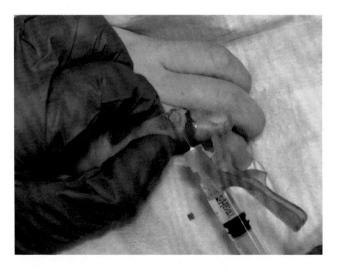

FIGURE 8.4 ● Common wart injection using *Candida* antigen.

- Adverse reactions may also include rash, adenopathy, and persistence of wart(s).
- Consider follow-up examination in 3 weeks.

CPT codes:
- 11900—Intralesional injections (1 to 7 lesions)
- 11901—Intralesional injections (>7 lesions)

PEARLS

- *Candida* antigen should not be used after a previous unacceptable adverse reaction such as extreme hypersensitivity or allergy to this antigen or to a similar product.
- Repeat injection in 3 weeks if there is any residual wart.
- Sixty-five to seventy-five percent of warts treated with *Candida* antigen injection resolve after the first injection.[6]
- Fifty percent of the remaining warts respond after a second injection.[7]
- Antigen injection of warts is an "off-label" use of *Candida* and mumps antigens, and there is no J code listed for these antigens. Thus, insurance companies do not provide reimbursement for the antigen used in this procedure. Unfortunately, the injection code does not include this cost, and the antigen itself is more expensive than the payment for the procedure. Therefore, if providing this treatment, consider asking the patient to fill a prescription at a reputable pharmacy, bring the unopened injectable to the office, and then perform the procedure.

 A video showing common wart injections can be found in the companion eBook.

REFERENCES

1. Nofal A, Salah E, Nofal E, et al. Intralesional antigen immunotherapy for the treatment of warts: Current concepts and future prospects. *Am J Clin Dermatol*. 2013;14(4):253–260.
2. Alikhan A, Griffin JR, Newman CC. Use of *Candida* antigen injections for the treatment of verruca vulgaris: A two-year Mayo Clinic experience. *J Dermatolog Treat*. 2016;27(4):355–358.
3. Vania R, Pranata R, Tan ST. Intralesional measles-mumps-rubella is associated with a higher complete response in cutaneous warts: A systematic review and meta-analysis of randomized controlled trial including GRADE qualification. *J Dermatolog Treat*. 2020:1–8.
4. Muñoz Garza FZ, Roé Crespo E, Torres Pradilla M, et al. Intralesional *Candida* antigen immunotherapy for the treatment of recalcitrant and multiple warts in children. *Pediatr Dermatol*. 2015;32(6):797–801.
5. Khozeimeh F, Jabbari Azad F, Mahboubi Oskouei Y, et al. Intralesional immunotherapy compared to cryotherapy in the treatment of warts. *Int J Dermatol*. 2017;56(4):474–478.
6. Phillips R, Pfenninger JL, et al. *Candida* antigen for the treatment of verruca. *Arch Dermatol*. 2000;136:1274–1275.
7. Singhania R, Sharma N, Vashisht S, et al. Intralesional triamcinolone acetonide (TA) versus incision and curettage (I & C) for medium and large size chalazia. *Nepal J Ophthalmol*. 2018;10(19):3–10.

Granuloma Annulare and Other Thin, Benign, Inflammatory Dermatoses

Granuloma annulare is an example of a *thin* benign inflammatory dermatosis. This is associated with many conditions such as malignancy, trauma, thyroid disease, diabetes mellitus, and HIV infection. In the most common localized form, it presents as skin-colored or erythematous dermal papules and ring-shaped lesions up to 5 cm in diameter (Fig. 8.5). The localized variant has a predilection for the feet, ankles, lower limbs, and wrists and generally self-resolves within 2 years without treatment. However, the generalized form is more chronic and less responsive to therapy.[1] Treatment is not evidence based and is determined by provider preference, expert opinion, and case reports. Potent topical corticosteroids or intralesional corticosteroids are most commonly utilized. There are a myriad of other treatment options, including liquid nitrogen cryosurgery, photodynamic therapy, hydroxychloroquine, dapsone, tacrolimus, pimecrolimus, and imiquimod.[2]

Indications	ICD-10 Code
Alopecia areata	L63.9

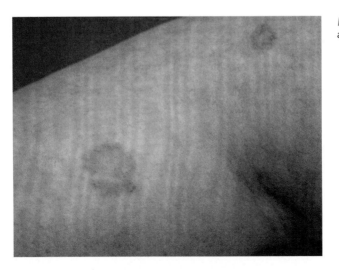

FIGURE 8.5 ● Granuloma annulare lesion.

PATIENT POSITION

- Supine on the examination table with the head of the bed elevated 30 degrees.
- The patient's hands are folded in his or her lap.
- The clinician stands lateral to the patient, on the same side as the affected area.

ANESTHESIA

- Local anesthesia of the injection site with topical vapocoolant spray

EQUIPMENT

- Topical vapocoolant spray
- 0.5-mL insulin syringe with its attached 8-mm, 31-gauge needle
- Steroid solution (10 mg/mL of triamcinolone acetonide)
- One alcohol prep pad
- Sterile gauze pads
- Sterile adhesive bandage

TECHNIQUE

1. Over the lesion, plot out a grid at 1-cm intervals using a ruler and surgical marking pen.
2. Prep the site with an alcohol pad.
3. Achieve good local anesthesia by using Gebauer's Pain Ease Mist topical vapocoolant spray (Fig. 8.6).
4. Position the needle and syringe at about a 20-degree angle to the surface of the skin at each injection site.
5. Using the no-touch technique, quickly introduce the needle into the skin.
6. Advance the needle to the mid to deep dermis.
7. Withdraw the plunger of the syringe to ensure that there is no blood return.
8. Inject 0.02 to 0.05 mL of the steroid solution (10 mg/mL of triamcinolone acetonide) (Fig. 8.7).

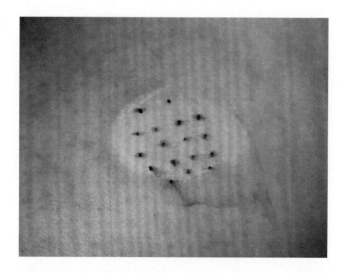

FIGURE 8.6 ● Granuloma annulare lesion with 1-cm grid markings—immediately after Pain Ease Mist topical vapocoolant spray.

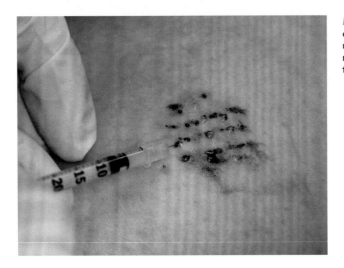

FIGURE 8.7 ● Injections of granuloma annulare lesion using an insulin syringe/ needle with small volumes of triamcinolone.

9. Repeat the injections to cover the entire lesion.
10. Following the injections of the corticosteroid solution, withdraw the needle, and apply direct pressure with the gauze pad.
11. Apply a sterile adhesive bandage.
12. The injections may be repeated every 4 to 6 weeks until the lesion resolves (Fig. 8.8).

AFTERCARE

- None needed.
- Schedule follow-up examination in 4 to 6 weeks.

CPT codes:
- 11900—Intralesional injections (1 to 7 lesions)
- 11901—Intralesional injections (>7 lesions)

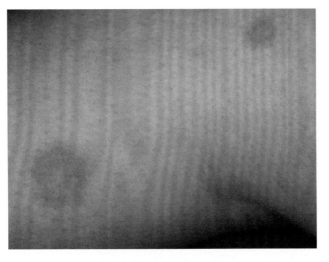

FIGURE 8.8 ● Resolving granuloma annulare lesion 7 days after corticosteroid injection.

PEARLS

• Avoid injection into the epidermis or subcutaneous tissues.

 A video showing injections for thin, benign, inflammatory dermatoses can be found in the companion eBook.

REFERENCES

1. Wang J, Khachemoune A. Granuloma annulare: A focused review of therapeutic options. *Am J Clin Dermatol*. 2018;19(3):333–344.
2. Thornsberry LA, English JC III. Etiology, diagnosis, and therapeutic management of granuloma annulare: An update. *Am J Clin Dermatol*. 2013;14(4):279–290.

Prurigo Nodularis and Other Thick, Benign, Inflammatory Dermatoses

Prurigo nodularis (PN) is an example of a *thick* benign inflammatory dermatosis. It can occur spontaneously, or as an expression of underlying conditions such as atopic dermatitis, chronic kidney disease, and neurological diseases. There is also a strong association with psychiatric disease. PN is a chronic, highly pruritic condition characterized by the presence of generally symmetric, hyperkeratotic, excoriated, hyperpigmented, firm, intensely pruritic nodules. Chronic and repetitive scratching or picking of the nodules causes permanent skin changes, including nodular lichenification, hyperkeratosis, hyperpigmentation, and skin thickening. Unhealed, excoriated lesions are often scaling and crusted. They can involve any part of the body, but generally begin on the arms and legs. PN appears to have a neuropathic origin, with alterations in the dermal and epidermal small diameter nerve fibers.[1] The diagnosis is based on the physical features of the nodules and the presence of itching. A skin biopsy is often performed to exclude other diseases.

PN often has a tremendous impact on the quality of life. Unfortunately, few randomized controlled trials are available to guide therapy.[2] Intralesional steroids are highly effective, and triamcinolone acetonide is commonly used. A total dose of up to 20 mg for adults may need to be repeated monthly for a maximum of 4 months to achieve a good clinical result.[3] More severe or recalcitrant cases may necessitate the use of phototherapy, systemic immunosuppressives, thalidomide, lenalidomide, opioid receptor antagonists, or neurokinin-1 receptor antagonists.[4] Regardless of the intervention, effective management of PN involves consideration of any associated psychological factors.[5]

Indications	ICD-10 Code
Prurigo nodularis	L28.1

PATIENT POSITION

- Usually supine on the examination table.
- Rotate the patient's head away from the side that is being injected. This minimizes anxiety and pain perception.
- The clinician stands on the side of the patient that allows best access to the PN lesion.

ANESTHESIA

- Local anesthesia of the injection site with topical vapocoolant spray

EQUIPMENT

- Topical vapocoolant spray
- 3-mL syringe
- 25-gauge, 1-in. needle
- 0.25 to 1 mL of the steroid solution (10 to 40 mg/mL of triamcinolone acetonide)
- One alcohol prep pad
- Two povidone–iodine prep pads
- Sterile gauze pads
- Sterile adhesive bandage

TECHNIQUE

1. Prep the insertion site with alcohol.
2. Achieve good local anesthesia by using topical vapocoolant spray.
3. Position the needle and syringe at a 10- to 45-degree angle to the surface of the skin at the edge of the lesion with the tip of the needle directed toward the center of the nodule.
4. Using the no-touch technique, introduce the needle at the edge of the lesion (Fig. 8.9).
5. Advance the needle into the lesion.
6. Withdraw the plunger of the syringe to ensure that there is no blood return.
7. Perform injection(s) of 0.1 mL to a maximum of 1 mL (40 mg/mL of triamcinolone acetonide) into the base of the lesion to uniformly infuse the entire lesion.
8. Avoid injection into the epidermis or subcutaneous tissues.
9. Following the injection of the corticosteroid solution, withdraw the needle.
10. Apply a sterile adhesive bandage.

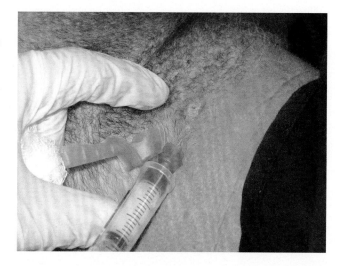

FIGURE 8.9 ● Injection of prurigo nodularis lesion using a 25-gauge needle with triamcinolone.

AFTERCARE

- None needed.
- Schedule a follow-up examination in 4 to 6 weeks.

CPT codes:
- 11900—Intralesional injections (1 to 7 lesions)
- 11901—Intralesional injections (>7 lesions)

PEARLS

- Avoid injection into the epidermis or subcutaneous tissues.

 A video showing an injection for thick, benign, inflammatory dermatoses can be found in the companion eBook.

REFERENCES

1. Fostini AC, Girolomoni G, Tessari G. Prurigo nodularis: An update on etiopathogenesis and therapy. *J Dermatolog Treat.* 2013;24(6):458–462.
2. Wu AY, Gervasio KA, Gergoudis KN, et al. Conservative therapy for chalazia: Is it really effective? *Acta Ophthalmol.* 2018;96(4):e503–e509.
3. Richards RN. Update on intralesional steroid: Focus on dermatoses. *J Cutan Med Surg.* 2010;14(1):19–23.
4. Kowalski EH, Kneiber D, Valdebran M, et al. Treatment-resistant prurigo nodularis: Challenges and solutions. *Clin Cosmet Investig Dermatol.* 2019;12:163–172.
5. Lotti T, Buggiani G, Prignano F. Prurigo nodularis and lichen simplex chronicus. *Dermatol Ther.* 2008;21(1):42–46.

Temporomandibular Joint

James W. McNabb

Patients commonly present to the primary care office for evaluation of jaw pain from temporomandibular joint (TMJ) dysfunction and/or arthritis. Arthrocentesis of the TMJ combined with intra-articular washout and intra-articular injection of pharmacological agents has been used for many years. There is literature support for injecting corticosteroids in pediatric patients with juvenile idiopathic arthritis.[1] However, a recent systematic review of randomized controlled trials in adults shows that intra-articular injections with corticosteroids seem to result in similar findings to those with other therapeutic drugs, with no significant differences.[2] Furthermore, adverse effects limit their usefulness.[3]

Although not approved by the US Food and Drug Administration, there is an increasing body of evidence that both hyaluronic acid[4,5] and especially platelet-rich plasma intra-articular injections[6,7] are effective in treating the pain of TMJ disorders in the medium and long term.[8] These injections appear significantly more effective than conservative treatments for both pain reduction and improvement of TMJ function. Therefore, injections should be implemented as first-line treatments or should be considered early, if patients do not show a clear benefit from initial conservative treatment.[9]

Ultrasound guidance of the procedure significantly improves localization of TMJ intra-articular injections,[10] especially in the pediatric population.[11,12]

Indications	ICD-10 Code
Temporomandibular joint pain	M26.629
Temporomandibular joint arthritis	M26.69
TMJ joint osteoarthritis, primary	M19.91
TMJ joint osteoarthritis, posttraumatic	M26.69

Relevant Anatomy: (Fig. 9.1)

PATIENT POSITION

- Sitting on the examination table.
- The patient's hands are folded in his or her lap.

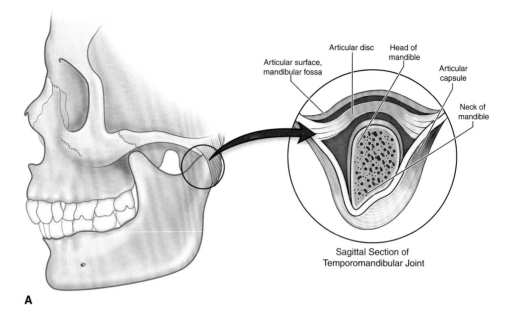

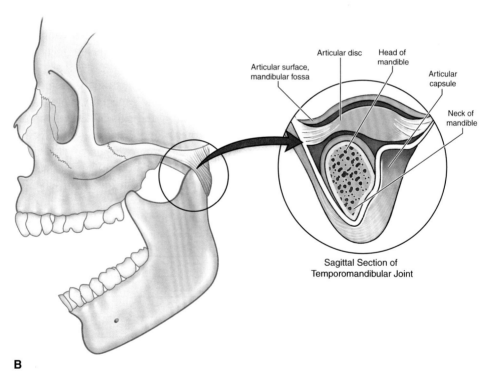

B

FIGURE 9.1 ● Sagittal view of the temporomandibular joint. **A:** Jaw closed. **B:** Jaw open.

LANDMARKS

1. With the patient seated on the examination table, the clinician stands lateral and posterior to the affected jaw.
2. Palpate the TMJ with the mouth in the closed and then the fully open positions.

3. Identify the sulcus that forms with jaw opening and mark that spot with ink.
4. At that site, press firmly on the skin with the retracted tip of a ballpoint pen. This indention represents the entry point for the needle.
5. After the landmarks are identified, the patient should not move the jaw.
6. The patient must keep his or her mouth open until the completion of the procedure.

ANESTHESIA

- Local anesthesia of the skin using topical vapocoolant spray may be used but is not necessary in most patients. If using a spray, make sure that "overspray" of the vapocoolant chemical does not enter the patient's eyes or external ear canal.

EQUIPMENT

- Topical vapocoolant spray
- 3-mL syringe
- 25-gauge, 1-in. needle
- 0.5 mL of 1% mepivacaine without epinephrine
- 0.5 mL of the steroid solution (20 mg of triamcinolone acetonide)
- One alcohol prep pad
- Two povidone–iodine prep pads
- Sterile gauze pads
- Sterile adhesive bandage

TECHNIQUE

1. Prep the insertion site with alcohol followed by the povidone–iodine pads.
2. Achieve good local anesthesia by using topical vapocoolant spray.
3. Position the needle and syringe from a posterior approach at a 30-degree angle to the sagittal plane into the sulcus with the tip of the needle directed anteromedial toward the posterior aspect of the TMJ.
4. Using the no-touch technique, introduce the needle at the insertion site (Fig. 9.2).
5. Advance the needle toward the joint until the needle tip is located in the joint capsule. There will be a decrease in resistance when entering the joint capsule. After

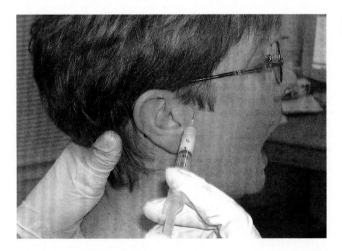

FIGURE 9.2 ● Temporomandibular joint injection.

entering the joint space, the needle will touch the articular surface or the articular disk. Back up the needle 1 to 2 mm.

6. Withdraw the plunger of the syringe to ensure that there is no blood return.
7. Inject the mepivacaine/corticosteroid solution as a bolus into the TMJ articular capsule. The injected solution should flow smoothly into the space. If increased resistance is encountered, advance or withdraw the needle slightly before attempting further injection.
8. Following injection, withdraw the needle.
9. Apply a sterile adhesive bandage.
10. Instruct the patient to move his or her jaw through its full range of motion. This movement distributes the mepivacaine/corticosteroid solution throughout the joint capsule.
11. Reexamine the TMJ in 5 min to assess pain relief.

AFTERCARE

- Avoid excessive use of the jaw by avoiding chewing gum, chewing tough foods, and excessive talking over the next 2 weeks.
- Nonsteroidal anti-inflammatory drugs (NSAIDs), ice, and/or physical therapy as indicated.
- Consider follow-up examination in 2 weeks.

CPT codes:
- 20605—Arthrocentesis, aspiration and/or injection, intermediate joint or bursa; without ultrasound guidance
- 20606—With ultrasound guidance, with permanent recording and reporting

PEARLS

- Be aware that there are reports of articular degeneration following corticosteroid joint injections—especially in adult patients.

 A video showing a TMJ injection can be found in the companion eBook.

REFERENCES

1. Stoll ML, Good J, Sharpe T, et al. Intra-articular corticosteroid injections to the temporomandibular joints are safe and appear to be effective therapy in children with juvenile idiopathic arthritis. *J Oral Maxillofac Surg.* 2012;70(8):1802–1807.
2. Davoudi A, Khaki H, Mohammadi I, et al. Is arthrocentesis of temporomandibular joint with corticosteroids beneficial? A systematic review. *Med Oral Patol Oral Cir Bucal.* 2018;23(3):e367–e375.
3. Isacsson G, Schumann M, Nohlert E, et al. Pain relief following a single-dose intra-articular injection of methylprednisolone in the temporomandibular joint arthralgia—A multicentre randomised controlled trial. *J Oral Rehabil.* 2019;46(1):5–13.
4. Manfredini D, Piccotti F, Guarda-Nardini L. Hyaluronic acid in the treatment of TMJ disorders: A systematic review of the literature. *Cranio.* 2010;28(3):166–176.
5. Guarda-Nardini L, Cadorin C, Frizziero A, et al. Comparison of 2 hyaluronic acid drugs for the treatment of temporomandibular joint osteoarthritis. *J Oral Maxillofac Surg.* 2012;70(11):2522–2530.
6. Haigler MC, Abdulrehman E, Siddappa S, et al. Use of platelet-rich plasma, platelet-rich growth factor with arthrocentesis or arthroscopy to treat temporomandibular joint osteoarthritis: Systematic review with meta-analyses. *J Am Dent Assoc.* 2018;149(11):940–952.e2.
7. Chung PY, Lin MT, Chang HP. Effectiveness of platelet-rich plasma injection in patients with temporomandibular joint osteoarthritis: A systematic review and meta-analysis of randomized controlled trials. *Oral Surg Oral Med Oral Pathol Oral Radiol.* 2019;127(2):106–116.

8. Li F, Wu C, Sun H, et al. Effect of platelet-rich plasma injections on pain reduction in patients with temporomandibular joint osteoarthrosis: A meta-analysis of randomized controlled trials. *J Oral Facial Pain Headache*. 2020;34(2):149–156.

9. Al-Moraissi EA, Wolford LM, Ellis E III, et al. The hierarchy of different treatments for arthrogenous temporomandibular disorders: A network meta-analysis of randomized clinical trials. *J Craniomaxillofac Surg*. 2020;48(1):9–23.

10. Champs B, Corre P, Hamel A, et al. US-guided temporomandibular joint injection: Validation of an in-plane longitudinal approach. *J Stomatol Oral Maxillofac Surg*. 2019;120(1):67–70.

11. Young CM, Shiels WE II, Coley BD. Ultrasound-guided corticosteroid injection therapy for juvenile idiopathic arthritis: 12-year care experience. *Pediatr Radiol*. 2012;42(12):1481–1489.

12. Habibi S, Ellis J, Strike H, et al. Safety and efficacy of US-guided CS injection into temporomandibular joints in children with active JIA. *Rheumatology (Oxford)*. 2012;51(5):874–877.

Suprascapular Nerve

Patients uncommonly present to the primary care office for evaluation of suprascapular neuropathy. It is an underdiagnosed disorder that is the result of nerve entrapment and compression. The suprascapular nerve is vulnerable as it passes through the suprascapular notch and again at the spinoglenoid notch. Entrapment at the former leads to weakness of the supraspinatus and infraspinatus muscles as well as vague posterior unilateral shoulder pain that is described as a deep, dull, aching discomfort that is exacerbated with overhead throwing motions. Entrapment at the latter causes weakness of the infraspinatus muscle and is generally painless. The most common causes of suprascapular neuropathy are acute trauma, inflammatory processes (i.e., brachial neuritis), a spinoglenoid notch cyst, and rotator cuff tears and overuse.[1] Spinoglenoid notch cysts and suprascapular notch entrapment respond best to surgical decompression, while overuse and viral etiologies respond best to conservative measures.[2] A nerve block at the suprascapular notch can be used in the conservative management of this condition as well as to treat shoulder pain following surgery,[3] hemiplegic shoulder pain following strokes,[4,5] and pain associated with adhesive capsulitis.[6] Ultrasound-guided suprascapular nerve blocks are more effective and safer than nonguided techniques to treat suprascapular entrapment shoulder pain.[7]

Indication	ICD-10 Code
Suprascapular neuropathy	G56.80

Relevant Anatomy: (Fig. 9.3)

PATIENT POSITION

- Sitting on an examination stool, with arms resting on the examination table and neck in a neutral position.

LANDMARKS

1. With the patient sitting on an examination stool, the clinician stands posterior to the affected scapula.
2. Find the midpoint between the tip of the acromion and the medial aspect of the spine of the scapula, and mark it with an ink pen.
3. Find the coracoid process, and mark it with an ink pen.
4. Draw a line between these two points, and mark the midposition of this line.
5. At that site, press firmly on the skin with the retracted tip of a ballpoint pen. This indention represents the entry point for the needle.
6. After the landmarks are identified, the patient should not move.

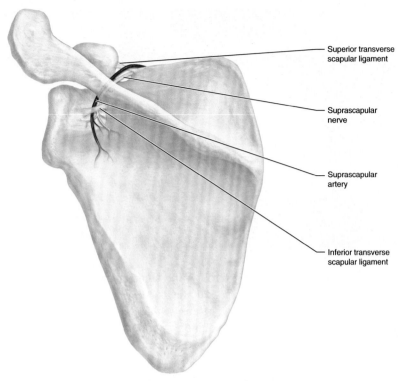

Superior transverse
scapular ligament

Suprascapular
nerve

Suprascapular
artery

Inferior transverse
scapular ligament

FIGURE 9.3 ● Nerves and vessels of left posterior scapular region.

ANESTHESIA

• Local anesthesia of the skin using topical vapocoolant spray

EQUIPMENT

• Topical vapocoolant spray
• 3-mL syringe
• 25-gauge, 1½ in. needle
• 1 mL of 1% lidocaine without epinephrine
• 1 mL of the steroid solution (40 mg of triamcinolone acetonide)
• One alcohol prep pad
• Two povidone–iodine prep pads
• Sterile gauze pads
• Sterile, adhesive bandage

TECHNIQUE

1. Prep the insertion site with alcohol followed by the povidone–iodine pads.
2. Achieve good local anesthesia by using topical vapocoolant spray.
3. Position the needle and syringe perpendicular to the skin with the tip of the needle directed toward the suprascapular notch.
4. Using the no-touch technique, introduce the needle at the insertion site (Fig. 9.4).

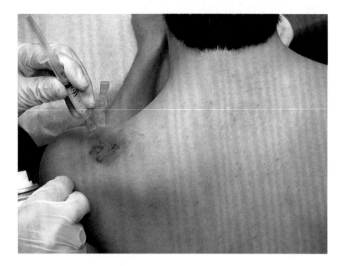

FIGURE 9.4 ● Suprascapular nerve injection.

5. Advance the needle completely through the supraspinatus muscle and touch the bone of the suprascapular fossa. Back up the needle 1 to 2 mm.
6. Withdraw the plunger of the syringe to ensure that there is no blood return.
7. Inject the lidocaine/corticosteroid solution as a bolus into the muscle around the suprascapular nerve. The injected solution should flow smoothly into this area. If increased resistance is encountered, advance or withdraw the needle slightly before attempting further injection.
8. Following injection, withdraw the needle.
9. Apply a sterile adhesive bandage.
10. Instruct the patient to move his or her shoulder through its full range of motion in external rotation and abduction. This movement distributes the lidocaine/corticosteroid solution throughout the suprascapular fossa.
11. Reexamine the shoulder and scapula in 5 min to assess pain relief.

AFTERCARE

- Avoid excessive abduction, external rotation, and overhead throwing motions of the shoulder over the next 2 weeks.
- NSAIDs, ice, and/or physical therapy as indicated.
- Consider follow-up examination in 2 weeks.

CPT codes:
- 64418—Introduction/injection of anesthetic agent (nerve block), diagnostic or therapeutic procedures on the somatic nerves
- 76942 (optional)—Ultrasonic guidance for needle placement with imaging supervision and interpretation with permanent recording

PEARLS

- Consider ultrasound guidance to enhance the safety of this procedure—particularly to avoid pneumothorax and/or vascular injury.
- Always aspirate before injecting to make sure that the needle tip is not in the suprascapular artery.

- If there is no significant improvement in pain or weakness, and the diagnosis has been confirmed by EMG, then refer the patient for surgical decompression of the superior or inferior transverse scapular ligaments.

 A video showing a suprascapular nerve injection can be found in the companion eBook.

REFERENCES

1. Hill LJ, Jelsing EJ, Terry MJ, et al. Evaluation, treatment, and outcomes of suprascapular neuropathy: A 5-year review. *PM R*. 2014;6(9):774–780. pii:S1934-1482(14)00071-9.
2. Antoniou J, Tae SK, Williams GR, et al. Suprascapular neuropathy. Variability in the diagnosis, treatment, and outcome. *Clin Orthop Relat Res*. 2001;(386):131–138.
3. Jerosch J, Saad M, Greig M, et al. Suprascapular nerve block as a method of preemptive pain control in shoulder surgery. *Knee Surg Sports Traumatol Arthrosc*. 2008;16(6):602–607.
4. Picelli A, Bonazza S, Lobba D, et al. Suprascapular nerve block for the treatment of hemiplegic shoulder pain in patients with long-term chronic stroke: A pilot study. *Neurol Sci*. 2017;38(9):1697–1701.
5. Adey-Wakeling Z, Crotty M, Shanahan EM. Suprascapular nerve block for shoulder pain in the first year after stroke: A randomized controlled trial. *Stroke*. 2013;44(11):3136–3141.
6. Jones DS, Chattopadhyay C. Suprascapular nerve block for the treatment of frozen shoulder in primary care: A randomized trial. *Br J Gen Pract*. 1999;49(438):39–41.
7. Aydın T, Şen Eİ, Yardımcı MY, et al. Efficacy of ultrasound-guided suprascapular nerve block treatment in patients with painful hemiplegic shoulder. *Neurol Sci*. 2019;40(5):985–991.

Scapulothoracic Syndrome

Scapulothoracic syndrome is a relatively uncommon problem in general clinical practice. It primarily affects middle-aged persons whose occupations require them to extend their arms for prolonged periods of time. This can also occur as a complication from preexisting shoulder lesions or in disabled patients who are unable to control the scapulothoracic relationship. The abnormal positioning causes bursitis because of altered biomechanics of the scapula and the underlying posterior chest wall. Scapulothoracic syndrome is characterized by pain that may be localized to the medial superior border of the scapula or may radiate to the neck and shoulder. Nonsurgical therapy utilizing scapular stabilization, postural exercises, and/or local corticosteroid injections can be effective for symptoms due to scapular dyskinesis or benign, nonosseous lesions.[1] However, these techniques are less successful than surgical management in patients with anatomic abnormalities.[2] In patients with normal anatomy, this condition can be successfully treated with a local corticosteroid injection at site of maximum tenderness at the medial superior scapular border.[3] Ultrasound guidance improves the accuracy and safety of scapulothoracic bursa injections.[4]

Indications	ICD-10 Code
Scapulothoracic syndrome	G56.80
Scapulothoracic bursitis	M75.50

Relevant Anatomy: (Fig. 9.5)

PATIENT POSITION

- Sitting erect on an examination stool, with ipsilateral hand on the contralateral shoulder.

LANDMARKS

1. With the patient seated on the examination stool, the clinician stands or sits behind the affected scapula.
2. Palpate to determine the area of most intense pain. This is usually along the medial superior border of the scapula. Mark this location with an ink pen.
3. At that site, press firmly on the skin with the retracted tip of a ballpoint pen. This indention represents the entry point for the needle.
4. After the landmarks are identified, the patient should not move.

ANESTHESIA

- Local anesthesia of the skin using topical vapocoolant spray

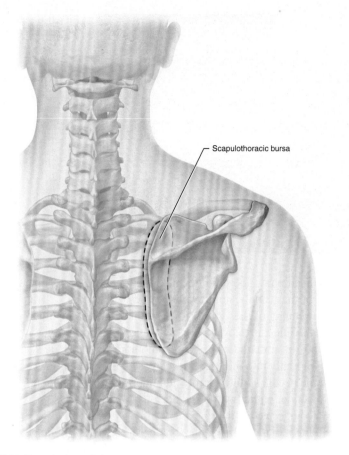

FIGURE 9.5 ● Scapulothoracic bursa.

EQUIPMENT

- Topical vapocoolant spray
- 3-mL syringe
- 25-gauge, 1½ in. needle
- 1 mL of 1% lidocaine without epinephrine
- 1 mL of the steroid solution (40 mg of triamcinolone acetonide)
- One alcohol prep pad
- Two povidone–iodine prep pads
- Sterile gauze pads
- Sterile adhesive bandage

TECHNIQUE

1. Prep the insertion site with alcohol followed by the povidone–iodine pads.
2. Achieve good local anesthesia by using topical vapocoolant spray.
3. Position the needle and syringe at a 20-degree angle to the skin with the tip of the needle directed toward the area of tenderness in the scapulothoracic space.
4. Using the no-touch technique, introduce the needle at the insertion site (Fig. 9.6).

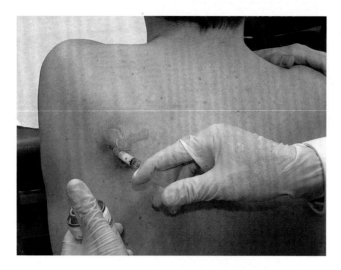

FIGURE 9.6 ● Scapulo-thoracic bursa injection.

5. Advance the needle into the point of maximal tenderness in a plane parallel to the undersurface of the scapula, not toward the chest wall.
6. Withdraw the plunger of the syringe to ensure that there is no blood return.
7. Inject half of the lidocaine/corticosteroid solution as a bolus at the point of maximal tenderness and the remainder in the scapulothoracic space. The injected solution should flow smoothly into the space. If increased resistance is encountered, advance or withdraw the needle slightly before attempting further injection.
8. Following injection, withdraw the needle.
9. Apply a sterile adhesive bandage.
10. Instruct the patient to move his or her shoulder through its full range of motion. This movement distributes the lidocaine/corticosteroid solution throughout the area.
11. Reexamine the scapula in 5 min to assess pain relief.

AFTERCARE

- Avoid excessive shoulder abduction, protraction, retraction, or pushing, pulling, and overhead throwing motions over the next 2 weeks.
- NSAIDs, ice, and/or physical therapy as indicated.
- Consider follow-up examination in 2 weeks.

CPT codes:
- 20610—Arthrocentesis, aspiration, and/or injection, major joint or bursa; without ultrasound guidance
- 20611—With ultrasound guidance, with permanent recording and reporting

PEARLS

- Consider ultrasound guidance to enhance the safety of this procedure to avoid pneumothorax.
- Avoid advancing the needle so deeply as to risk the complication of pneumothorax.

 A video showing a scapulothoracic bursa injection can be found in the companion eBook.

REFERENCES

1. Osias W, Matcuk GR Jr, Skalski MR, et al. Scapulothoracic pathology: Review of anatomy, pathophysiology, imaging findings, and an approach to management. *Skeletal Radiol.* 2018;47(2):161–171.
2. Gaskill T, Millett PJ. Snapping scapula syndrome: Diagnosis and management. *J Am Acad Orthop Surg.* 2013;21(4):214–224.
3. Boneti C, Arentz C, Klimberg VS. Scapulothoracic bursitis as a significant cause of breast and chest wall pain: Underrecognized and undertreated. *Ann Surg Oncol.* 2010;17(Suppl 3):321–324.
4. Walter WR, Burke CJ, Adler RS. Ultrasound-guided therapeutic scapulothoracic interval injections. *J Ultrasound Med.* 2019;38(7):1899–1906.

Sacroiliac Joint

Pain involving the sacroiliac joint(s) is a common condition seen by primary care physicians.[1] Sacroiliac joint pain may be caused by acute or repetitive trauma, spondyloarthropathies, degenerative arthritis, pregnancy, and rarely by an infection of the joint. Injection into the SI joint(s) can be both diagnostic and therapeutic. Corticosteroid injections are an effective conservative treatment option for sacroiliitis.[2] These can be safely and effectively performed using landmark-guided techniques because significant extra-articular sources of sacroiliac region pain exist.[3,4] However, ultrasound-guided SI joint injections are shown to increase the accuracy[5] and improve the treatment effect of pain relief and function. In addition, ultrasound may improve safety by facilitating the identification and avoidance of critical vessels around or within the SI joints.[6] Other agents including platelet-rich plasma,[7] botulinum toxin injections,[8] and prolotherapy[9] utilizing dextrose show promise for the treatment of sacroiliac joint pain.

Indications	ICD-10 Code
SI pain	M53.3
Sacroiliitis	M46.1
Sacroiliac joint arthritis	M47.818
Sacroiliac joint arthropathy	M47.818

Relevant Anatomy: (Fig. 9.7)

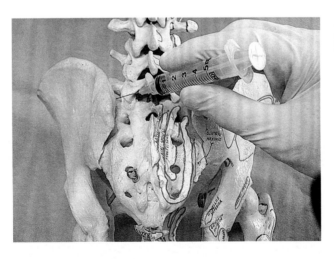

FIGURE 9.7 ● Sacroiliac anatomy—note the angle of insertion.

PATIENT POSITION

- Patient is standing and leaning over an examination table with the forearms supported by the table. The back is held in a position of 45 degrees of forward flexion.

LANDMARKS

1. With the patient standing fully upright, the clinician stands directly behind the patient.
2. Identify tenderness over the sacroiliac joint.
3. While continuously palpating the location of the SI joint, have the patient lean forward, to 45 degrees of forward flexion, over the examination table and support the upper body with the forearms.
4. Mark the location of the SI joint with ink.
5. At that site, press firmly on the skin with the retracted tip of a ballpoint pen. This indention represents the entry point for the needle.

ANESTHESIA

- Local anesthesia of the skin using Pain Ease Mist topical vapocoolant spray

EQUIPMENT

- Topical vapocoolant spray
- 3-mL syringe
- 25-gauge, 2 in. needle
- 1 mL of 1% mepivacaine without epinephrine
- 1 mL of the steroid solution (40 mg of triamcinolone acetonide)
- One alcohol prep pad
- Two povidone–iodine prep pads
- Sterile gauze pads
- Sterile adhesive bandage

TECHNIQUE

1. Prep the insertion site with alcohol followed by the povidone–iodine pads.
2. Achieve good local anesthesia by using Pain Ease Mist topical vapocoolant spray.
3. Position the 25-gauge, 2 in. needle at a 30-degree angle laterally, relative to the sagittal plane, and 15 degrees inferiorly, relative to the transverse plane, with the tip of the needle directed toward the sacroiliac joint.
4. Using the no-touch technique, introduce the needle at the insertion site (Fig. 9.8).
5. Advance the needle slowly and carefully into the SI joint.
6. Withdraw the plunger of the syringe to ensure that there is no blood return.
7. Inject the mepivacaine/corticosteroid solution as a bolus into the sacroiliac joint. The injected solution should flow smoothly into the space. If increased resistance is encountered, advance or withdraw the needle slightly before attempting further injection.
8. Following injection, withdraw the needle.
9. Apply a sterile adhesive bandage.
10. Reexamine the sacroiliac joint in 5 min to assess pain relief.

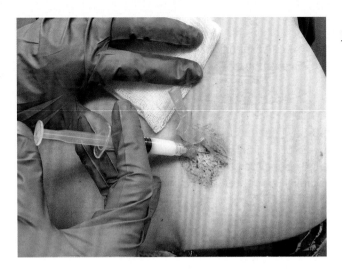

FIGURE 9.8 ● Sacroiliac joint injection.

AFTERCARE

- NSAIDs, ice, and/or physical therapy as indicated.
- Treatment of the underlying condition.
- Consider follow-up examination in 2 weeks.

CPT codes:
- 20552—Injection of single or multiple trigger point(s) without imaging guidance
- 27096—Injection of SI joint using anesthetic agents and/or steroid, with imaging guidance and permanent recording

PEARLS

- The successful placement of this injection may require ultrasound guidance.
- Use Pain Ease Mist spray to provide a topical vapocoolant anesthetic effect. Both Ethyl Chloride and Pain Ease Stream Spray run down the skin. In this location, the product will follow gravity and accumulate in the patients' groin, thus turning this injection into a very uncomfortable experience!

 A video showing a sacroiliac joint injection can be found in the companion eBook.

REFERENCES

1. Wu L, Varacallo M. Sacroiliac joint injection. *StatPearls* [Internet]. Treasure Island, FL: StatPearls Publishing, 2020 Jan. Available at http://www.ncbi.nlm.nih.gov/books/NBK513245/. Accessed on February 13, 2020.
2. Hawkins J, Schofferman J. Serial therapeutic sacroiliac joint injections: A practice audit. *Pain Med.* 2009;10(5):850–853.
3. Borowsky CD, Fagen G. Sources of sacroiliac region pain: Insights gained from a study comparing standard intra-articular injection with a technique combining intra- and peri-articular injection. *Arch Phys Med Rehabil.* 2008;89(11):2048–2056.
4. Hartung W, Ross CJ, Straub R, et al. Ultrasound-guided sacroiliac joint injection in patients with established sacroiliitis: Precise IA injection verified by MRI scanning does not predict clinical outcome. *Rheumatology (Oxford).* 2010;49(8):1479–1482.

5. De Luigi AJ, Saini V, Mathur R, et al. Assessing the accuracy of ultrasound-guided needle placement in sacroiliac joint injections. *Am J Phys Med Rehabil.* 2019;98(8):666–670.

6. Jee H, Lee JH, Park KD, et al. Ultrasound-guided versus fluoroscopy-guided sacroiliac joint intra-articular injections in the noninflammatory sacroiliac joint dysfunction: A prospective, randomized, single-blinded study. *Arch Phys Med Rehabil.* 2014;95(2):330–337.

7. Mohi Eldin M, Sorour OO, Hassan ASA, et al. Percutaneous injection of autologous platelet-rich fibrin versus platelet-rich plasma in sacroiliac joint dysfunction: An applied comparative study. *J Back Musculoskelet Rehabil.* 2019;32(3):511–518.

8. Lee JH, Lee SH, Song SH. Clinical effectiveness of botulinum toxin A compared to a mixture of steroid and local anesthetics as a treatment for sacroiliac joint pain. *Pain Med.* 2010;11(5):692–700.

9. Kim WM, Lee HG, Jeong CW, et al. A randomized controlled trial of intra-articular prolotherapy versus steroid injection for sacroiliac joint pain. *J Altern Complement Med.* 2010;16(12):1285–1290.

10

Subacromial Space Injection—Posterior Approach

James W. McNabb

Patients very commonly present to the primary care medical office for evaluation of shoulder pain. Almost all shoulder disorders that can be treated by injection therapy involve the rotator cuff complex. These disorders may occur due to acute trauma, overuse injury, and/or chronic degenerative changes. Since the subacromial space affords access to the rotator cuff complex, it allows easy access to these structures for injection treatment. In patients with degenerative disease, the subacromial bursa may perforate into and communicate with the GH joint. In this case, a well-placed subacromial space injection provides therapy to the rotator cuff, GH joint, and the proximal aspect of the long head of the biceps tendon.[1]

Lateral, anterior, and posterior approaches to the subacromial space can be used; however, the **posterior approach is preferred**. This is the easiest to perform and is well accepted by patients. Since they cannot see the approaching needle, anxiety is diminished. Of the three standard portals, it holds an additional advantage over the others. When using the posterior approach, the needle is directed cephalad piercing the deltoid muscle, passing over the supraspinatus muscle/tendon, entering the subacromial space, and then touching the underside of the acromion. Therefore, accurate placement is confirmed. When utilizing the anterior and lateral approaches without ultrasound guidance, the operator cannot be assured that the corticosteroid is not being deposited into the supraspinatus muscle/tendon. Inadvertent deposition of steroid into the tendon may lead to further tendinopathy or even rupture. A longer needle must be used in the posterior approach.[2] A small-diameter needle is selected since this technique is used to inject anesthetic and/or steroid solution into the subacromial space. A large-diameter needle is infrequently used since a significant amount of fluid rarely collects in the space.

The medical literature indicates that low-volume corticosteroid injections[3] in the subacromial space are effective in the short- to medium-term treatment of rotator cuff disorders[4,5] and for the treatment of adhesive capsulitis.[6,7] On the other hand, a meta-analysis showed that corticosteroid injections provide only small and transient pain relief in patients with rotator cuff tendinosis.[8] In studies of optimal corticosteroid dosing, there was no difference in pain or function between intra-articular injections of 20 or 40 mg of triamcinolone acetonide.[9,10] Safety has also been established as use of corticosteroid injections in patients with subacromial impingement does not result in an increase in rotator cuff tears.[11] Platelet-rich plasma injections are an emerging therapeutic option.[12] Hyaluronic acid viscosupplementation has been studied and shown to be effective at 12 weeks.[13–16] However, this has not been approved by the FDA for use outside of osteoarthritis of the knee. The use of ultrasound improves the accuracy[17] and efficacy of therapeutic injections.[18]

A subacromial injection performed using local anesthetic without steroid can help the clinician differentiate the cause of nonlocalized shoulder pain. The injected mepivacaine removes pain from subacromial impingement as a confounding factor and allows the clinician to physically test the integrity of the rotator cuff complex by asking the patient to abduct the shoulder. This is known as the "impingement injection test." Injection of local anesthetic does not cause muscle weakness and therefore does not affect the validity of this test.[19]

Indications	ICD-10 Code
Shoulder pain	M25.519
Shoulder impingement syndrome	M75.40
Rotator cuff tendonitis	M75.80

Relevant Anatomy: (Figs. 10.1 and 10.2)

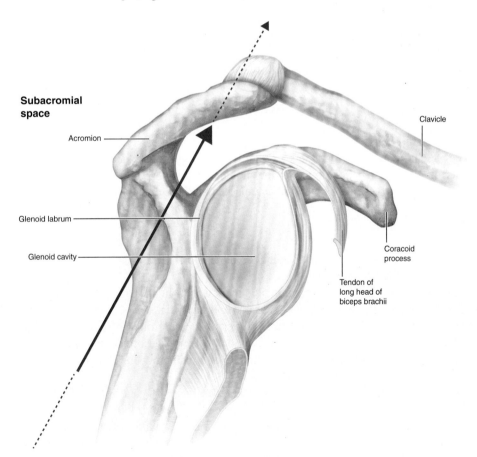

FIGURE 10.1 ● Lateral aspect of right shoulder (*red arrow* indicates path of the needle). (From Agur AM, Dalley AF. *Grant's Atlas of Anatomy*, 14th Ed. Philadelphia, PA: Wolters Kluwer, 2016.)

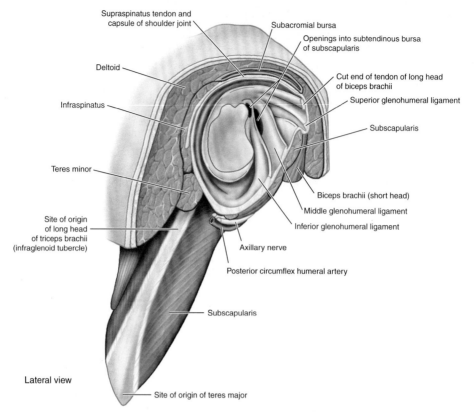

Supraspinatus tendon and
capsule of shoulder joint

Subacromial bursa

Openings into subtendinous bursa
of subscapularis

Deltoid

Cut end of tendon of long head
of biceps brachii

Superior glenohumeral ligament

Infraspinatus

Subscapularis

Teres minor

Biceps brachii (short head)

Middle glenohumeral ligament

Site of origin
of long head
of triceps brachii
(infraglenoid tubercle)

Inferior glenohumeral ligament

Axillary nerve

Posterior circumflex humeral artery

Subscapularis

Lateral view

Site of origin of teres major

FIGURE 10.2 ● Interior of right shoulder. (From Agur AM, Dalley AF. *Grant's Atlas of Anatomy*, 14th Ed. Philadelphia, PA: Wolters Kluwer, 2016.)

PATIENT POSITION

- Sitting on the examination table.
- The patient's hands are folded in his or her lap with fingers interlaced.
- This allows consistent positioning of the shoulder so that the landmarks do not change from the time that they are identified and marked until the time of injection.

LANDMARKS

1. With the patient seated on the examination table, the clinician stands lateral and posterior to the affected shoulder.
2. Find the lateral edge of the acromion, and mark it with an ink pen.
3. Palpate the posterior border of the acromion and mark that.
4. Having identified the posterior lateral corner of the acromion, drop a vertical line down from that point and mark a spot 2 cm below the posterior lateral corner.
5. At that site, press firmly with the retracted tip of a ballpoint pen. This indention represents the entry point for the needle.
6. Next, identify the target site by placing the index finger of your nondominant hand over the superior aspect of the acromion posterior to the AC joint. As you palpate, please realize that the acromion has length and width. The target site is in the center of the acromion. This will be the target for the tip of the needle (Fig. 10.3). If your index finger is at the target site—on top of the acromion—it will be protected from accidental needlestick.
7. After the landmarks are identified, the patient should not move the shoulder or arm.

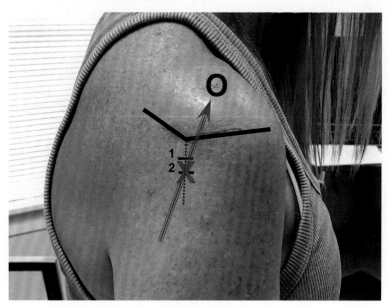

FIGURE 10.3 ● Right shoulder injection landmarks.

ANESTHESIA

- Tactile skin distraction is administered by firmly stroking the skin outside of the injection point as the small diameter needle is quickly introduced into the skin. Topical vapocoolant spray or injection of a local anesthetic is unnecessary in almost all patients.

EQUIPMENT

- 5-mL syringe
- 25-gauge, 2-in. needle (Consider a 3½-in., 22-gauge spinal needle in large individuals.)
- 1 mL of 1% mepivacaine without epinephrine
- 0.5 mL of the steroid solution (20 mg of triamcinolone acetonide)
- One alcohol prep pad
- Two povidone–iodine prep pads
- Sterile gauze pads
- Sterile adhesive bandage

TECHNIQUE

1. Prep the insertion site with alcohol followed by the povidone–iodine pads.
2. Position the needle and syringe at about a 30-degree angle to the skin with the needle tip directed cephalad toward the acromion.
3. Using the no-touch technique, introduce the needle at the insertion site (Fig. 10.4).
4. Direct the needle underneath the acromion, and advance it toward the target until the needle tip touches the undersurface of the acromion. Back up the needle 1 to 2 mm.
5. Withdraw the plunger of the syringe to ensure that there is no blood return.
6. Inject the mepivacaine/corticosteroid solution as a bolus into the subacromial space. The injected solution should flow smoothly into the space. Increased resistance may indicate that the injected fluid is entering the supraspinatus muscle or tendon. In that case, advance or withdraw the needle slightly before attempting further injection.

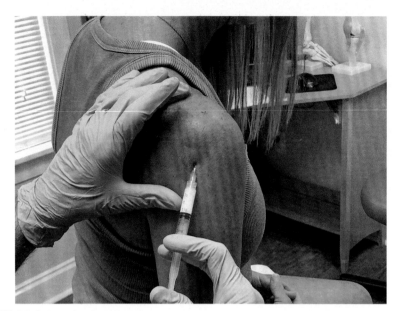

FIGURE 10.4 ● Right shoulder subacromial space injection.

7. Following injection, withdraw the needle.
8. Apply a sterile adhesive bandage.
9. Instruct the patient to move his or her shoulder through its full range of motion. This movement distributes the mepivacaine/corticosteroid solution throughout the subacromial space.
10. Reexamine the shoulder in 5 min to assess pain relief.

AFTERCARE

- Avoid excessive use of the shoulder over the next 2 weeks.
- Consider the use of an arm sling.
- Nonsteroidal anti-inflammatory drugs (NSAIDs), ice, and/or physical therapy as indicated.
- Consider follow-up examination in 2 weeks.

CPT codes:
- 20610—Arthrocentesis, aspiration and/or injection, major joint or bursa; without ultrasound guidance
- 20611—With ultrasound guidance, with permanent recording and reporting

PEARLS

- The correct identification of the acromion landmarks is more difficult than many primary care providers realize. Make sure to take your time and recheck the landmarks before proceeding with the injection.
- When palpating to determine the anatomy of the acromion, use the tips of your index, middle, and ring fingers positioned in a straight line. Firmly, carefully, and methodically move in a distal-to-proximal direction. Mark the site where your fingers contact the lateral and posterior margins of the acromion.

- Use a long 2-in., 25-gauge needle for this injection.
- Ensure that the needle is underneath the acromion before advancing it toward the target finger.
- Always keep your target finger over the acromion to protect it from accidental needlestick.

 A video showing a subacromial space injection can be found in the companion eBook.

REFERENCES

1. Gofeld M, Hurdle MF, Agur A. Biceps tendon sheath injection: An anatomical conundrum. *Pain Med.* 2019;20(1):138–142.
2. Sardelli M, Burks RT. Distances to the subacromial bursa from 3 different injection sites as measured arthroscopically. *Arthroscopy.* 2008;24(9):992–996.
3. Boonard M, Sumanont S, Arirachakaran A, et al. Short-term outcomes of subacromial injection of combined corticosteroid with low-volume compared to high-volume local anesthetic for rotator cuff impingement syndrome: A randomized controlled non-inferiority trial. *Eur J Orthop Surg Traumatol.* 2018;28(6):1079–1087.
4. Gialanella B, Prometti P. Effects of corticosteroids injection in rotator cuff tears. *Pain Med.* 2011;12(10):1559–1565.
5. Karthikeyan S, Kwong HT, Upadhyay PK, et al. A double-blind randomised controlled study comparing subacromial injection of tenoxicam or methylprednisolone in patients with subacromial impingement. *J Bone Joint Surg Br.* 2010;92(1):77–82.
6. Shin SJ, Lee SY. Efficacies of corticosteroid injection at different sites of the shoulder for the treatment of adhesive capsulitis. *J Shoulder Elbow Surg.* 2013;22(4):521–527.
7. Oh JH, Oh CH, Choi JA, et al. Comparison of glenohumeral and subacromial steroid injection in primary frozen shoulder: A prospective, randomized short-term comparison study. *J Shoulder Elbow Surg.* 2011;20(7):1034–1040.
8. Mohamadi A, Chan JJ, Claessen FM, et al. Corticosteroid injections give small and transient pain relief in rotator cuff tendinosis: A meta-analysis. *Clin Orthop Relat Res.* 2017;475(1):232–243.
9. Hong JY, Yoon SH, Moon DJ, et al. Comparison of high- and low-dose corticosteroid in subacromial injection for periarticular shoulder disorder: A randomized, triple-blind, placebo-controlled trial. *Arch Phys Med Rehabil.* 2011;92(12):1951–1960.
10. Carroll MB, Motley SA, Smith B, et al. Comparing corticosteroid preparation and dose in the improvement of shoulder function and pain: A randomized, single-blind pilot study. *Am J Phys Med Rehabil.* 2018;97(6):450–455.
11. Bhatia M, Singh B, Nicolaou N, et al. Correlation between rotator cuff tears and repeated subacromial steroid injections: A case-controlled study. *Ann R Coll Surg Engl.* 2009;91(5):414–416.
12. Šmíd P, Hart R, Komzák M, et al. Treatment of the shoulder impingement syndrome with PRP injection. *Acta Chir Orthop Traumatol Cech.* 2018;85(4):261–265.
13. Jiménez I, Marcos-García A, Muratore-Moreno G, et al. Subacromial sodium hyaluronate injection for the treatment of chronic shoulder pain: A prospective series of eighty patients. *Acta Ortop Mex.* 2018;32(2):70–75.
14. Kim YS, Park JY, Lee CS, et al. Does hyaluronate injection work in shoulder disease in early stage? A multicenter, randomized, single blind and open comparative clinical study. *J Shoulder Elbow Surg.* 2012;21(6):722–727.
15. Merolla G, Bianchi P, Porcellini G. Ultrasound-guided subacromial injections of sodium hyaluronate for the management of rotator cuff tendinopathy: A prospective comparative study with rehabilitation therapy. *Musculoskelet Surg.* 2013;97(Suppl 1):49–56.
16. Noël E, Hardy P, Hagena FW, et al. Efficacy and safety of Hylan G-F 20 in shoulder osteoarthritis with an intact rotator cuff. Open-label prospective multicenter study. *Joint Bone Spine.* 2009;76(6):670–673.
17. Daley EL, Bajaj S, Bisson LJ, et al. Improving injection accuracy of the elbow, knee, and shoulder: Does injection site and imaging make a difference? A systematic review. *Am J Sports Med.* 2011;39(3):656–662.
18. Messina C, Banfi G, Orlandi D, et al. Ultrasound-guided interventional procedures around the shoulder. *Br J Radiol.* 2016;89(1057):20150372.
19. Farshad M, Jundt-Ecker M, Sutter R, et al. Does subacromial injection of a local anesthetic influence strength in healthy shoulders? A double-blinded, placebo-controlled study. *J Bone Joint Surg Am.* 2012;94(19):1751–1755.

Glenohumeral Joint— Posterior Approach

The glenohumeral (GH) joint is a relatively common injection site for most primary care providers. It is typically used for the treatment of adhesive capsulitis as well as GH osteoarthritis. Both anterior and posterior approaches can be used. However, the **posterior approach to the GH joint is preferred** for reasons listed in the previous chapter, safety considerations, and to avoid confusion with other pain generators that are located over the anterior aspect of the GH joint (subscapularis tendon and proximal aspect of the long head of the biceps). One uses the same injection site identified in the "Subacromial Space Injection" chapter. Since the long head of the biceps tendon has its origin within the GH joint capsule, this injection may offer an alternative approach to injecting this structure.[1]

Intra-articular corticosteroid injections are more effective in pain relief in the short term (8 to 12 weeks), but not long term. But, they provide greater passive range of motion[2] and overall function.[3] In a study of optimal corticosteroid dosing, there was no difference in pain or function between intra-articular injections of 20 or 40 mg of triamcinolone acetonide.[4] Thus, the smaller dose is recommended. Providers may consider corticosteroid injection to treat adhesive capsulitis, especially in the early stages when pain is the predominant presentation.[5]

A small-diameter needle is selected since this technique is used to inject steroid solution into the joint space. A large-diameter needle is infrequently used since a significant amount of fluid rarely collects in the joint capsule. There is a growing body of literature supporting injection therapy using platelet-rich plasma[6] and other biologics.[7] The use of ultrasound improves the accuracy[8] and efficacy of therapeutic injections.[9]

Indications	ICD-10 Code
Shoulder pain	M25.519
Shoulder adhesive capsulitis	M75.00
GH joint arthritis, unspecified	M19.019
GH joint osteoarthritis, primary	M19.019
GH joint osteoarthritis, posttraumatic	M19.119
GH joint arthrosis, secondary	M19.219

Relevant Anatomy: (Figs. 10.5 and 10.6)

PATIENT POSITION

- Sitting on the examination table.
- The patient's hands are folded in his or her lap with fingers interlaced.

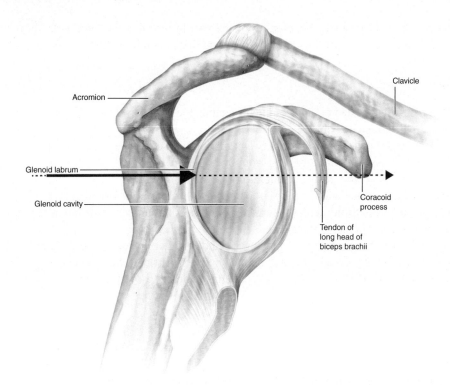

FIGURE 10.5 ● Lateral aspect of right shoulder (*red arrow* indicates path of the needle). (From Agur AM, Dalley AF. *Grant's Atlas of Anatomy*, 14th Ed. Philadelphia, PA: Wolters Kluwer, 2016.)

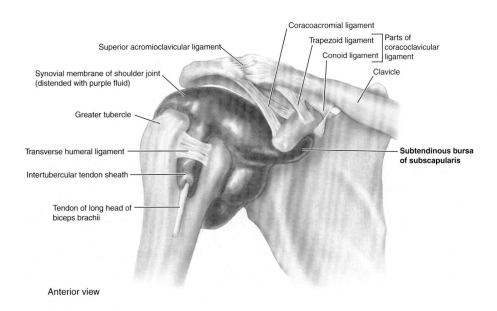

FIGURE 10.6 ● Right glenohumeral joint capsule. (From Agur AM, Dalley AF. *Grant's Atlas of Anatomy*, 14th Ed. Philadelphia, PA: Wolters Kluwer, 2016.)

- This allows consistency of positioning of the shoulder so that the landmarks do not change from the time that they are identified and marked until the time of injection.

LANDMARKS

1. With the patient seated on the examination table, the clinician stands lateral and posterior to the affected shoulder.
2. Find the lateral edge of the acromion, and mark it with an ink pen.
3. Palpate the posterior border of the acromion and mark that.
4. Having identified the posterior lateral corner of the acromion, drop a vertical line down from that point and mark a spot 2 cm below the posterior lateral corner.
5. At that site, press firmly with the retracted tip of a ballpoint pen. This indention represents the entry point for the needle.
6. Next, identify the target site by placing the index finger of your nondominant hand over the coracoid process. This will be the target for the tip of the needle.
7. After the landmarks are identified, the patient should not move the shoulder or arm.

ANESTHESIA

- Tactile skin distraction is administered by firmly stroking the skin outside of the injection point as the needle is quickly introduced into the skin. Topical vapocoolant spray or injection of a local anesthetic is unnecessary in almost all patients.

EQUIPMENT

- 3-mL syringe
- 25-gauge, 1½-in. needle
- 1 mL of 1% mepivacaine without epinephrine
- 0.5 mL of the steroid solution (20 mg of triamcinolone acetonide)
- One alcohol prep pad
- Two povidone–iodine prep pads
- Sterile gauze pads
- Sterile adhesive bandage

TECHNIQUE

1. Prep the insertion site with alcohol followed by the povidone–iodine pads.
2. Position the needle and syringe perpendicular to the skin with the needle tip directed anterior toward the coracoid process.
3. Using the no-touch technique, introduce the needle at the insertion site (Fig. 10.7).
4. Advance the needle toward the target until the needle tip touches the humeral head. Back up the needle 1 to 2 mm.
5. Withdraw the plunger of the syringe to ensure that there is no blood return.
6. Inject the mepivacaine/corticosteroid solution as a bolus into the GH joint. The injected solution should flow smoothly into the joint space. If increased resistance is encountered, advance or withdraw the needle slightly before attempting further injection.
7. Following injection, withdraw the needle.
8. Apply a sterile adhesive bandage.

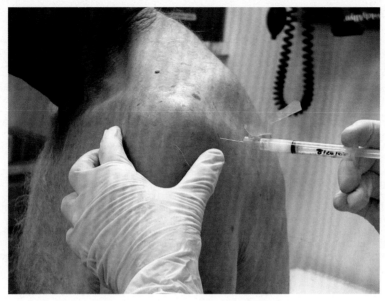

FIGURE 10.7 • Glenohumeral joint injection—posterior approach.

9. Instruct the patient to move his or her shoulder through its full range of motion. This movement distributes the mepivacaine/corticosteroid solution throughout the subacromial space.
10. Reexamine the shoulder in 5 min to assess pain relief.

AFTERCARE

- Avoid excessive use of the shoulder over the next 2 weeks.
- Consider the use of an arm sling.
- NSAIDs, ice, and/or physical therapy as indicated.
- Consider follow-up examination in 2 weeks.

CPT codes:
- 20610—Arthrocentesis, aspiration and/or injection, major joint or bursa; without ultrasound guidance
- 20611—With ultrasound guidance, with permanent recording and reporting

PEARLS

- The correct identification of the acromion landmarks is more difficult than many primary care providers realize. Make sure to take your time and recheck the landmarks before proceeding with the injection.
- When palpating to determine the anatomy of the acromion, use the tips of your index, middle, and ring fingers positioned in a straight line. Firmly, carefully, and methodically move in a distal-to-proximal direction. Mark the site where your fingers contact the lateral and posterior margins of the acromion.

A video showing a posterior glenohumeral joint injection can be found in the companion eBook.

REFERENCES

1. Gofeld M, Hurdle MF, Agur A. Biceps tendon sheath injection: An anatomical conundrum. *Pain Med.* 2019;20(1):138–142.
2. Wang W, Shi M, Zhou C, et al. Effectiveness of corticosteroid injections in adhesive capsulitis of shoulder: A meta-analysis. *Medicine (Baltimore).* 2017;96(28):e7529.
3. Ranalletta M, Rossi LA, Bongiovanni SL, et al. Corticosteroid injections accelerate pain relief and recovery of function compared with oral NSAIDs in patients with adhesive capsulitis: A randomized controlled trial. *Am J Sports Med.* 2016;44(2):474–481.
4. Yoon SH, Lee HY, Lee HJ, et al. Optimal dose of intra-articular corticosteroids for adhesive capsulitis: A randomized, triple-blind, placebo-controlled trial. *Am J Sports Med.* 2013;41(5):1133–1139.
5. Koh KH. Corticosteroid injection for adhesive capsulitis in primary care: A systematic review of randomised clinical trials. *Singapore Med J.* 2016;57(12):646–657.
6. Barman A, Mukherjee S, Sahoo J, et al. Single intra-articular platelet-rich plasma versus corticosteroid injections in the treatment of adhesive capsulitis of the shoulder: A cohort study. *Am J Phys Med Rehabil.* 2019;98(7):549–557.
7. Carr JB II, Rodeo SA. The role of biologic agents in the management of common shoulder pathologies: Current state and future directions. *J Shoulder Elbow Surg.* 2019;28(11):2041–2052.
8. Daley EL, Bajaj S, Bisson LJ, et al. Improving injection accuracy of the elbow, knee, and shoulder: Does injection site and imaging make a difference? A systematic review. *Am J Sports Med.* 2011;39(3):656–662.
9. Messina C, Banfi G, Orlandi D, et al. Ultrasound-guided interventional procedures around the shoulder. *Br J Radiol.* 2016;89(1057):20150372.

Acromioclavicular Joint

The acromioclavicular (AC) joint is a common injection site for most primary care providers. Despite its superficial location, accurate identification and successful injection can be challenging.[1] In addition, clinical trials demonstrate effectiveness of a corticosteroid injection into the AC joint in only a minority of patients.[2] This is most likely a result of inaccurate needle placement due to the small size of the joint.[3] Multiple studies show that this is a difficult injection to perform successfully, with only about 40% of injections actually reaching the intended intra-articular target.[4] Ultrasound guidance greatly improves accuracy to nearly 100%.[5] US-guided AC joint intra-articular injections have also been demonstrated to result in better pain and functional status improvement than palpation-guided injections.[6] An emerging therapeutic option is ultrasound-guided prolotherapy with a 15% dextrose solution for treatment of AC joint arthropathy.[7]

Indications	ICD-10 Code
AC joint pain	M25.519
AC joint arthritis, unspecified	M12.9
AC joint osteoarthritis, primary	M19.019
AC joint osteoarthritis, posttraumatic	M19.119
AC joint osteoarthritis, secondary	M19.219

Relevant Anatomy: (Fig. 10.8)

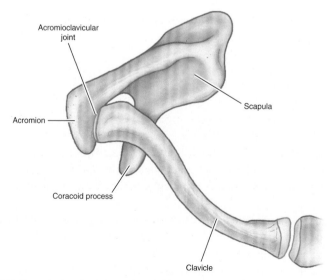

FIGURE 10.8 ● Right AC joint. (Modified from Agur AM, Dalley AF. *Grant's Atlas of Anatomy,* 14th Ed. Philadelphia, PA: Wolters Kluwer, 2016.)

PATIENT POSITION

- Sitting or lying supine on the examination table.
- The patient's hands are folded in his or her lap with fingers interlaced.
- This allows consistency of positioning of the shoulder so that the landmarks do not change from the time that they are identified and marked until the time of injection.
- Rotate the patient's head away from the side that is being injected. This minimizes anxiety and pain perception.

LANDMARKS

1. With the patient seated or lying supine on the examination table, the clinician stands lateral and anterior to the affected shoulder.
2. Identify the AC joint. Palpate the clavicle in a medial-to-lateral direction. At the lateral aspect of the clavicle, there is a small depression that will be tender in the above conditions.
3. The injection point is located directly over the AC joint. At that site, press firmly with the retracted tip of a ballpoint pen. As an alternative, pressure can be placed with the fingernail or a paperclip positioned across the AC joint. These indentions represent the entry point for the needle.
4. Once the landmarks are identified, the patient should not move the chest or shoulder.

ANESTHESIA

- Local anesthesia of the skin using topical vapocoolant spray.

EQUIPMENT

- Topical vapocoolant spray
- 3-mL syringe
- 25-gauge, 5/8-in. needle
- 0.5 mL of 1% mepivacaine without epinephrine
- 0.5 mL of the steroid solution (20 mg of triamcinolone acetonide)
- One alcohol prep pad
- Two povidone–iodine prep pads
- Sterile gauze pads
- Sterile adhesive bandage

TECHNIQUE

1. Prep the insertion site with alcohol followed by the povidone–iodine pads.
2. Achieve good local anesthesia by using topical vapocoolant spray.
3. Position the needle and syringe perpendicular to the skin with the needle tip directed caudad.
4. Using the no-touch technique, introduce the needle at the insertion site (Fig. 10.9).
5. Advance the needle into the AC joint. If the needle does not "drop" into the AC joint, then "walk" the needle in the area until it does so.
6. Withdraw the plunger of the syringe to ensure that there is no blood return.
7. Inject the mepivacaine/corticosteroid solution as a bolus into the AC joint. The injected solution should flow smoothly into the joint space. If increased resistance

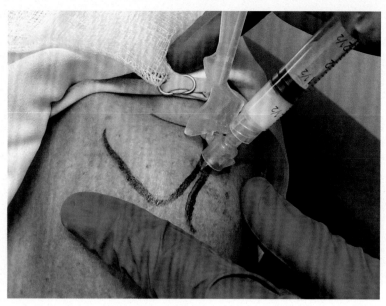

FIGURE 10.9 ● AC joint injection with landmarks.

is encountered, advance or withdraw the needle slightly before attempting further injection. If the needle will not drop into the joint, then employ the aid of ultrasound imaging, or as a last resort, perform a periarticular injection.

8. Following injection, withdraw the needle.
9. Apply a sterile adhesive bandage.
10. Instruct the patient to move his or her shoulder through its full range of motion. This movement distributes the mepivacaine/corticosteroid solution throughout the AC joint.
11. Reexamine the shoulder in 5 min to assess pain relief.

AFTERCARE

- Avoid excessive use of the shoulder over the next 2 weeks.
- Consider the use of an arm sling.
- NSAIDs, ice, and/or physical therapy as indicated.
- Consider follow-up examination in 2 weeks.

CPT codes:
- 20605—Arthrocentesis, aspiration and/or injection, intermediate joint or bursa; without ultrasound guidance
- 20606—With ultrasound guidance, with permanent recording and reporting

PEARLS

- The AC joint is superficial. Depositing corticosteroid in the subcutaneous tissues can result in the complication of skin atrophy and hypopigmentation. Avoid the development of a subdermal wheal while performing all injections of corticosteroid solutions.
- Perform the "pinch technique" as described in the "Lateral Epicondylitis" chapter.

A video showing an acromioclavicular joint injection can be found in the companion eBook.

REFERENCES

1. Scillia A, Issa K, McInerney VK, et al. Accuracy of in vivo palpation-guided acromioclavicular joint injection assessed with contrast material and fluoroscopic evaluations. *Skeletal Radiol*. 2015;44(8):1135–1139.
2. van Riet RP, Goehre T, Bell SN. The long term effect of an intra-articular injection of corticosteroids in the acromioclavicular joint. *J Shoulder Elbow Surg*. 2012;21(3):376–379.
3. Javed S, Sadozai Z, Javed A, et al. Should all acromioclavicular joint injections be performed under image guidance? *J Orthop Surg (Hong Kong)*. 2017;25(3):2309499017731633.
4. Wasserman BR, Pettrone S, Jazrawi LM, et al. Accuracy of acromioclavicular joint injections. *Am J Sports Med*. 2013;41(1):149–152.
5. Sabeti-Aschraf M, Lemmerhofer B, Lang S, et al. Ultrasound guidance improves the accuracy of the acromioclavicular joint infiltration: A prospective randomized study. *Knee Surg Sports Traumatol Arthrosc*. 2011;19(2):292–295.
6. Park KD, Kim TK, Lee J, et al. Palpation versus ultrasound-guided acromioclavicular joint intra-articular corticosteroid injections: A retrospective comparative clinical study. *Pain Physician*. 2015;18(4):333–341.
7. Hsieh PC, Chiou HJ, Wang HK, et al. Ultrasound-guided prolotherapy for acromial enthesopathy and acromioclavicular joint arthropathy: A single-arm prospective study. *J Ultrasound Med*. 2019;38(3):605–612.

Sternoclavicular Joint

The sternoclavicular (SC) joint is a rare injection site for most primary care providers. Successful injection can be difficult because of the small joint space. There is only a single study that describes accurate injection technique utilizing ultrasound guidance in cadavers.[1] There is one other study that details CT-guided injections.[2] In this trial, two-thirds of patients had short-term symptom relief of pain only with no statistically significant relief in long-term pain.

Indications	ICD-10 Code
SC joint pain	M25.519
SC joint subluxation	S43.203
SC joint arthritis, unspecified	M19.019
SC joint osteoarthritis, primary	M19.019
SC joint osteoarthritis, posttraumatic	M19.119
SC joint osteoarthritis, secondary	M19.219

Relevant Anatomy: (Fig. 10.10)

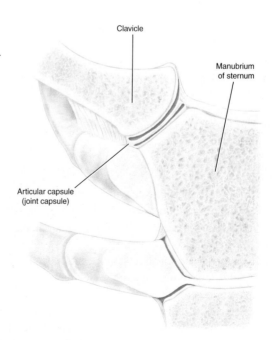

FIGURE 10.10 ● Sternoclavicular joint. (From Gest TR. *Lippincott Atlas of Anatomy*, 2nd Ed. Philadelphia, PA: Wolters Kluwer, 2019.)

Clavicle

Manubrium of sternum

Articular capsule (joint capsule)

PATIENT POSITION

- Supine on the examination table.
- The patient's hands are folded in his or her lap with fingers interlaced.
- Rotate the patient's head away from the side that is being injected. This minimizes anxiety and pain perception.

LANDMARKS

1. With the patient supine on the examination table, the clinician stands to the patient's affected side.
2. Identify the SC joint. Palpate the clavicle in a lateral-to-medial direction. At the medial aspect of the clavicle, there is a small depression that represents the SC joint. This structure will be tender.
3. It may be helpful to move the ipsilateral shoulder in order to more easily identify the SC joint.
4. The injection point is located directly over the SC joint. At that site, press firmly with the retracted tip of a ballpoint pen. As an alternative, pressure can be placed with the fingernail or a paperclip positioned across the SC joint. These indentions represent the entry point for the needle.
5. After the landmarks are identified, the patient should not move the chest or shoulder.

ANESTHESIA

- Local anesthesia of the skin using topical vapocoolant spray.

EQUIPMENT

- Topical vapocoolant spray
- 3-mL syringe
- 25-gauge, 5/8-in. or 1-in. needle
- 0.5 mL of 1% mepivacaine without epinephrine
- 0.5 mL of the steroid solution (20 mg of triamcinolone acetonide)
- One alcohol prep pad
- Two povidone–iodine prep pads
- Sterile gauze pads
- Sterile adhesive bandage

TECHNIQUE

1. Prep the insertion site with alcohol followed by the povidone–iodine pads.
2. Achieve good local anesthesia by using topical vapocoolant spray.
3. Position the needle and syringe perpendicular to the skin with the needle tip directed posteriorly.
4. Using the no-touch technique, introduce the needle at the insertion site (Fig. 10.11).
5. Advance the needle into the SC joint space.
6. Withdraw the plunger of the syringe to ensure that there is no blood return.
7. Inject the mepivacaine/corticosteroid solution as a bolus into the SC joint. The injected solution should flow smoothly into the joint space. If increased resistance is encountered, advance or withdraw the needle slightly before attempting further

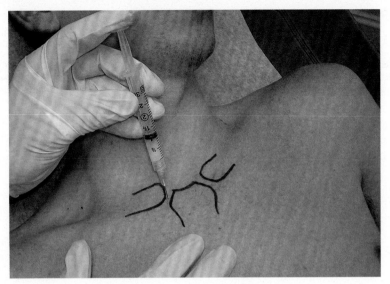

FIGURE 10.11 ● Sternoclavicular joint injection with landmarks.

injection. If the needle will not drop into the joint, then employ the aid of ultrasound imaging, or as a last resort, perform a periarticular injection.

8. Following injection of the mepivacaine/corticosteroid solution, withdraw the needle.
9. Apply a sterile adhesive bandage.
10. Instruct the patient to move his or her shoulder through its full range of motion. This movement distributes the mepivacaine/corticosteroid solution throughout the SC joint.
11. Reexamine the SC joint in 5 min to assess pain relief.

AFTERCARE

- Avoid excessive use of the shoulder over the next 2 weeks.
- Consider use of an arm sling.
- NSAIDs, ice, and/or physical therapy as indicated.
- Consider follow-up examination in 2 weeks.

CPT codes:
- 20605—Arthrocentesis, aspiration and/or injection, intermediate joint or bursa; without ultrasound guidance
- 20606—With ultrasound guidance, with permanent recording and reporting

PEARLS

- The SC joint is superficial. Depositing corticosteroid in the subcutaneous tissues can result in the complication of skin atrophy and hypopigmentation. Avoid the development of a subdermal wheal while performing all injections of corticosteroid solutions.
- Perform the "pinch technique" as described in the "Lateral Epicondylitis" chapter.

 A video showing a sternoclavicular joint injection can be found in the companion eBook.

REFERENCES

1. Pourcho AM, Sellon JL, Smith J. Sonographically guided sternoclavicular joint injection: Description of technique and validation. *J Ultrasound Med.* 2015;34(2):325–331.
2. Peterson CK, Saupe N, Buck F, et al. CT-guided sternoclavicular joint injections: Description of the procedure, reliability of imaging diagnosis, and short-term patient responses. *AJR Am J Roentgenol.* 2010;195(6):W435–W439.

Biceps Tendon—Long Head

Patients occasionally present to the primary care office for evaluation and treatment of the pain of tendinopathy of the long head of biceps. This is an inflammatory and degenerative condition more frequently seen in the long head rather than the short head of the biceps brachii muscle. It develops either from direct acute trauma or chronic overuse in throwing athletes and nonathletes who use their arms to do repetitive biceps contraction, resisted forearm supination, or overhead work. Biceps tendinopathy is frequently diagnosed in association with rotator cuff disease as a component of the impingement syndrome or secondary to intra-articular pathology, such as labral tears. Local tenderness is usually located over the bicipital groove of the humerus. Conservative management of biceps tendon pain usually consists of rest, ice, oral analgesics, physical therapy, or corticosteroid injections.

As demonstrated in the literature, physicians have difficulty correctly identifying the intertubercular groove that contains the tendon of the long head of the biceps. Localization attempts are usually far medial of its actual location.[1] Consequently, clinicians should exercise caution when relying on clinical palpation to perform a biceps long head tendon sheath injection. Ultrasound guidance significantly improves injection accuracy[2] and clinical response.[3,4]

Indication	ICD-10 Code
Biceps tenosynovitis	M75.20

Relevant Anatomy: (Fig. 10.12)

PATIENT POSITION

- Supine on the examination table with the head of the bed elevated 30 degrees.
- The patient's hands are placed in a position of supination at his or her side with slight external rotation of the arm.
- Rotate the patient's head away from the side that is being injected. This minimizes anxiety and pain perception.

LANDMARKS

1. With the patient lying supine on the examination table, the clinician stands lateral to the affected arm.
2. Instruct the patient to flex the elbow and contract the biceps muscle.
3. Palpate the course of the long head of the bicipital tendon over the anterior aspect of the upper arm.
4. Determine the location of maximal tenderness, which will most likely be under the edge of the pectoralis major muscle. Mark that spot with an ink pen.

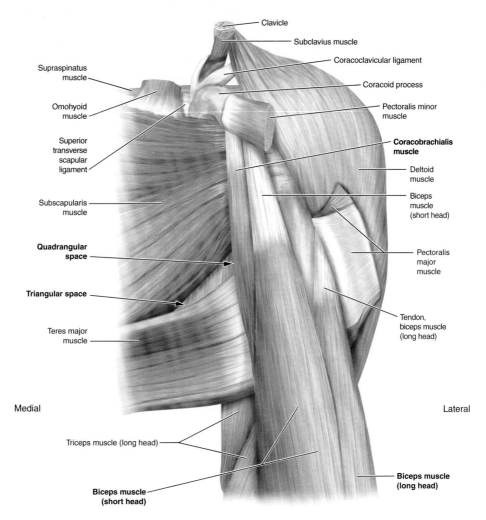

FIGURE 10.12 ● Muscles of anterior left arm. (Modified from Paulsen F, Waschke J. *Sobotta Atlas of Human Anatomy*, 16th Ed. 2018 © Elsevier GmbH, Urban & Fischer, Munich.)

5. At that site, press firmly on the skin with the retracted tip of a ballpoint pen. This indention represents the entry point for the needle.
6. After the landmarks are identified, the patient should not move the shoulder or arm.

ANESTHESIA

• Local anesthesia of the skin using topical vapocoolant spray.

EQUIPMENT

• Topical vapocoolant spray
• 3-mL syringe
• 25-gauge, 1½-in. needle
• 1 mL of 1% lidocaine without epinephrine
• 0.5 to 1 mL of the steroid solution (20 to 40 mg of triamcinolone acetonide)
• One alcohol prep pad

- Two povidone–iodine prep pads
- Sterile gauze pads
- Sterile adhesive bandage

TECHNIQUE

1. Prep the insertion site with alcohol followed by the povidone–iodine pads.
2. Achieve good local anesthesia by using topical vapocoolant spray.
3. Position the needle and syringe at a 45-degree angle to the skin with the needle tip directed proximally.
4. Using the no-touch technique, introduce the needle at the insertion site (Fig. 10.13).
5. Advance the needle until the needle tip touches the tendon. (An increase in resistance will be detected.) Back up the needle 1 to 2 mm.
6. Withdraw the plunger of the syringe to ensure that there is no blood return.
7. Inject the lidocaine/corticosteroid solution as a bolus around the bicipital tendon. The injected solution should flow smoothly into the tenosynovial sheath. If increased resistance is encountered, advance or withdraw the needle slightly before attempting further injection.
8. Following injection of the lidocaine/corticosteroid solution, withdraw the needle.
9. Apply a sterile adhesive bandage.
10. Instruct the patient to move his or her biceps muscle and shoulder through their full range of motion. This movement distributes the lidocaine/corticosteroid solution throughout the tenosynovial sheath.
11. Reexamine the arm in 5 min to assess pain relief.

AFTERCARE

- Avoid all throwing and excessive use of the arm and shoulder over the next 2 weeks.
- NSAIDs, ice, and/or physical therapy as indicated.
- Consider follow-up examination in 2 weeks.

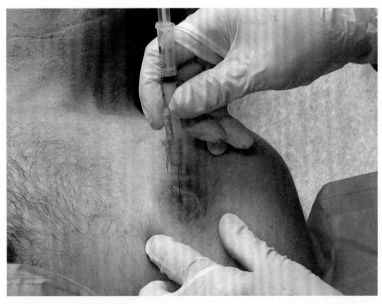

FIGURE 10.13 ● Injection of the tendon of the long head of the biceps brachii muscle.

CPT codes:
- 20550—Injection(s); single tendon sheath, or ligament, aponeurosis
- 76942 (optional)—Ultrasonic guidance for needle placement with imaging supervision and interpretation with permanent recording

PEARLS

- Failure to recognize or treat this condition may lead to rupture of the tendon of the long head of the biceps brachii.
- Make sure to place the injection around the tendon and not into the substance of the tendon in order to avoid iatrogenic degeneration of the tendon and subsequent rupture.
- Subacromial or GH joint corticosteroid injections may be considered for persistent cases of biceps tendinitis.

 A video showing an injection of the tendon of the long head of the biceps muscle can be found in the companion eBook.

REFERENCES

1. Gazzillo GP, Finnoff JT, Hall MM, et al. Accuracy of palpating the long head of the biceps tendon: An ultrasonographic study. *PM R*. 2011;3(11):1035–1040.
2. Hashiuchi T, Sakurai G, Morimoto M, et al. Accuracy of the biceps tendon sheath injection: Ultrasound guided or unguided injection? A randomized controlled trial. *J Shoulder Elbow Surg*. 2011;20(7):1069–1073.
3. Zhang J, Ebraheim N, Lause GE. Ultrasound-guided injection for the biceps brachii tendinitis: Results and experience. *Ultrasound Med Biol*. 2011;37(5):729–733.
4. Petscavage-Thomas J, Gustas C. Comparison of ultrasound-guided to fluoroscopy-guided biceps tendon sheath therapeutic injection. *J Ultrasound Med*. 2016;35(10):2217–2221.

Cubital Tunnel Syndrome

Cubital tunnel syndrome is an uncommon condition encountered by primary care providers. It develops when the ulnar nerve becomes entrapped in the cubital tunnel posterior to the medial epicondyle. Nonsurgical treatment, aiming to decrease both compression and traction on the ulnar nerve about the elbow, is successful in most patients with mild nerve dysfunction.[1] Conservative measures usually involve activity modification by the avoidance of predisposing repetitive movements and nighttime application of an elbow splint/brace. The clinician may wish to attempt to provide relief of pain by administration of a corticosteroid injection in carefully selected patients. Unfortunately, a single randomized controlled trial did not demonstrate a positive effect of ultrasound-guided corticosteroid injections compared with placebo.[2] Successful treatment may require surgical referral for transposition of the ulnar nerve in order to relocate it over the medial epicondyle.

Indication	ICD-10 Code
Cubital tunnel syndrome	G56.20

Relevant Anatomy: (Fig. 10.14)

PATIENT POSITION

- Supine on the examination table with the head of the bed elevated 30 degrees.
- Shoulder at 30 degrees of abduction and full external rotation.
- The affected elbow is flexed at 90 degrees.
- The wrist is in a neutral position.
- The elbow is supported with the placement of chucks pads or towels.
- Rotate the patient's head away from the side that is being injected. This minimizes anxiety and pain perception.

LANDMARKS

1. With the patient supine on the examination table, the clinician stands lateral to the affected elbow.
2. Identify and mark the medial epicondyle of the humerus.
3. Identify and mark the course of the ulnar nerve in the ulnar groove posterior to the medial epicondyle.
4. Mark the point of maximal tenderness over the ulnar nerve. This is usually just posterior to the medical epicondyle.
5. At that site, press firmly on the skin with the retracted tip of a ballpoint pen. This indention represents the entry point for the needle.
6. After the landmarks are identified, the patient should not move the elbow.

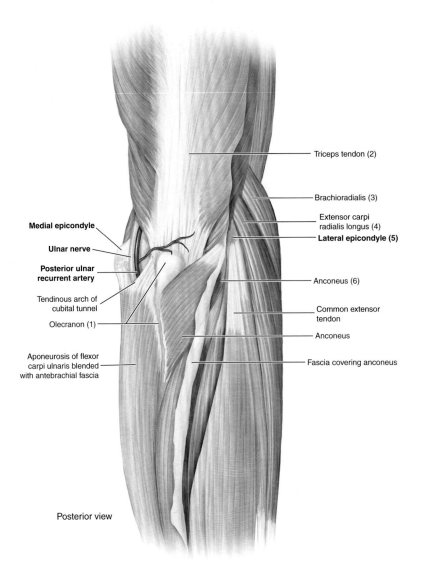

Posterior view

FIGURE 10.14 ● Posterior aspect of right elbow.

ANESTHESIA

- Local anesthesia of the skin using topical vapocoolant spray.

EQUIPMENT

- Topical vapocoolant spray
- 3-mL syringe
- 25-gauge, 1-in. needle
- 1 mL of 1% lidocaine without epinephrine
- 1 mL of the steroid solution (40 mg of triamcinolone acetonide)
- One alcohol prep pad

- Two povidone–iodine prep pads
- Sterile gauze pads
- Sterile adhesive bandage
- Nonsterile, clean chucks pad

TECHNIQUE

1. Prep the insertion site with alcohol followed by the povidone–iodine pads.
2. Achieve good local anesthesia by using topical vapocoolant spray.
3. Position the needle and syringe at a 30-degree angle to the skin with the tip of the needle directed distally along the ulnar nerve.
4. Using the no-touch technique, introduce the needle at the insertion site (Fig. 10.15).
5. Advance the needle slowly at a shallow angle to a position just along the side of the ulnar nerve.
6. If any pain, paresthesias, or numbness is encountered, withdraw the needle slightly and redirect the needle tip using a slightly different angle.
7. When the needle is placed along the ulnar nerve, withdraw the plunger of the syringe to ensure that there is no blood return.
8. Slowly inject the lidocaine/corticosteroid solution as a bolus around that structure. If increased resistance is encountered, advance or withdraw the needle slightly before attempting further injection.
9. Following injection, withdraw the needle.
10. Apply a sterile adhesive bandage.
11. Instruct the patient to move his or her elbow through its full range of motion. This movement distributes the lidocaine/corticosteroid solution along the course of the ulnar nerve in the cubital tunnel.
12. Reexamine the elbow in 5 min to assess pain relief and the development of numbness in the distribution of the ulnar nerve from the local anesthetic.

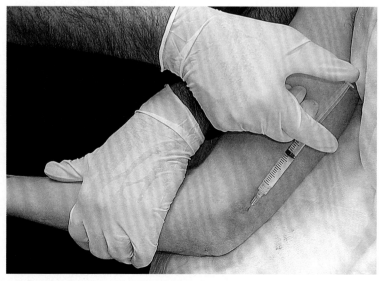

FIGURE 10.15 ● Right cubital tunnel injection.

AFTERCARE

- Avoid further overuse mechanisms of injury.
- Use an elbow extension brace while sleeping to avoid excessive elbow flexion.
- NSAIDs, ice, and/or physical therapy as indicated.
- Consider follow-up examination in 2 weeks.

CPT codes:

- 64450—Injection, nerve block, therapeutic, other peripheral nerve or branch
- 76942 (optional)—Ultrasonic guidance for needle placement with imaging supervision and interpretation with permanent recording

 A video showing a cubital tunnel syndrome injection can be found in the companion eBook.

REFERENCES

1. Staples JR, Calfee R. Cubital tunnel syndrome: Current concepts. *J Am Acad Orthop Surg.* 2017;25(10):e215–e224.
2. vanVeen KE, Alblas KC, Alons IM, et al. Corticosteroid injection in patients with ulnar neuropathy at the elbow: A randomized, double-blind, placebo-controlled trial. *Muscle Nerve.* 2015;52(3):380–385.

Elbow Joint

Aspiration and injection of the elbow joint is an uncommon procedure in most primary care practices. A tense collection of blood distending the elbow joint develops with intra-articular fractures. Significant pain relief may follow aspiration. Arthritis in the elbow with fluid accumulation may occur with gout, rheumatoid arthritis, and osteoarthritis. This may respond to corticosteroid injection, but this aspiration and injection procedure is not described in any clinical trials.

There are two common approaches to the elbow joint. Either the humero-ulnar or the radio-humeral articulations can be used. The joint between the humerus and the ulna offers the largest area of joint space and is therefore easy to perform with a higher degree of success than attempting needle entry via the joint space between the radial head and the humerus. High-resolution ultrasonography can help clinicians visualize key anatomic structures of the elbow and guide periarticular and intra-articular injections.[1]

Indications	ICD-10 Code
Elbow pain	M25.529
Elbow joint arthritis, unspecified	M19.029
Elbow joint osteoarthritis, primary	M19.029
Elbow joint osteoarthritis, posttraumatic	M19.129
Elbow joint osteoarthritis, secondary	M19.229

Relevant Anatomy: (Fig. 10.16)

PATIENT POSITION

- Supine on the examination table with the head of the bed elevated 30 degrees.
- The elbow is positioned at 45 degrees of flexion.
- The wrist is in a neutral position.
- The elbow is supported with the placement of chucks pads or towels.
- Rotate the patient's head away from the side that is being injected. This minimizes anxiety and pain perception.

LANDMARKS

1. With the patient supine on the examination table, the clinician stands lateral to the affected elbow.
2. (Humero-ulnar articulation) This approach generally gives the easiest access to the largest accessible entry point to the elbow joint. Locate the lateral epicondyle. Slide your fingertip over and down the epicondyle until it sits in the sulcus between the epicondyle and the ulna. Mark the deepest point of the sulcus with ink.

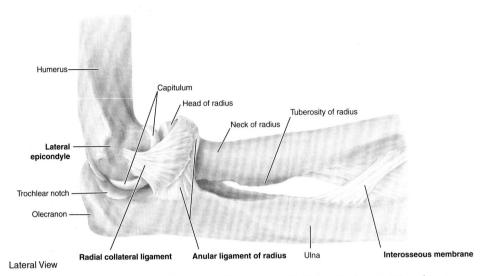

Humerus

Capitulum

Head of radius

Tuberosity of radius

Neck of radius

Lateral epicondyle

Trochlear notch

Olecranon

Radial collateral ligament   **Anular ligament of radius**   Ulna   **Interosseous membrane**

Lateral View

FIGURE 10.16 ● Right lateral elbow joint. (From Agur AM, Dalley AF. *Grant's Atlas of Anatomy*, 14th Ed. Philadelphia, PA: Wolters Kluwer, 2016.)

3. (Radio-humeral articulation) Alternatively, find the radial head by palpating over the lateral aspect of the elbow joint while supinating and pronating the wrist. Find the depression immediately proximal to the radial head and mark it with ink.
4. At the selected site, press firmly on the skin with the retracted tip of a ballpoint pen. This indention represents the entry point for the needle.
5. After the landmarks are identified, the patient should not move the elbow.

ANESTHESIA

- Local anesthesia of the skin using topical vapocoolant spray.

EQUIPMENT

- Topical vapocoolant spray
- 3-mL syringe
- 10-mL syringe—for optional aspiration
- 25-gauge, 1-in. needle
- 20-gauge, 1-in. needle—for optional aspiration
- 0.5 mL of 1% mepivacaine without epinephrine
- 0.5 mL of the steroid solution (20 mg of triamcinolone acetonide)
- One alcohol prep pad
- Two povidone–iodine prep pads
- Sterile gauze pads
- Sterile adhesive bandage
- Nonsterile, clean chucks pad

TECHNIQUE

1. Prep the insertion site with alcohol followed by the povidone–iodine pads.
2. Achieve good local anesthesia by using topical vapocoolant spray.

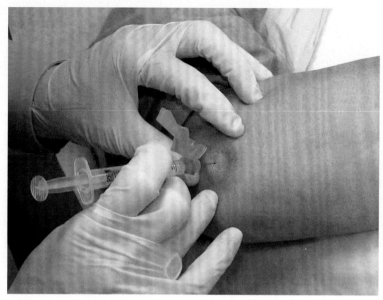

FIGURE 10.17 ● Left elbow joint injection.

3. Position the needle and syringe perpendicular to the skin with the needle tip directed medially toward the elbow joint.
4. Using the no-touch technique, introduce the needle at the insertion site (Fig. 10.17).
5. Advance the needle into the elbow joint. This places the needle tip between the humeral lateral condyle and either the ulna or the radial head.
6. If aspirating, withdraw fluid using a 20-gauge, 1-in. needle with the 10-mL syringe.
7. If injection of corticosteroid is to follow the aspiration, grasp the needle firmly, remove the 10-mL syringe from the 20-gauge needle, and then attach the 3-mL syringe filled with the mepivacaine/corticosteroid mixture.
8. If only injecting the mepivacaine/corticosteroid mixture, use a 25-gauge, 1-in. needle with the 3-mL syringe.
9. Inject the mepivacaine/corticosteroid solution as a bolus into the elbow joint. The injected solution should flow smoothly into the space. If increased resistance is encountered, advance or withdraw the needle slightly before attempting further injection.
10. Following injection, withdraw the needle.
11. Apply a sterile adhesive bandage.
12. Instruct the patient to move his or her elbow through its full range of motion. This movement distributes the mepivacaine/corticosteroid solution throughout the elbow joint.
13. Reexamine the elbow in 5 min to assess pain relief.

AFTERCARE

- Do not brace or rest the elbow. A study showed a significantly higher rate of synovitis relapse in patients following corticosteroid injection who were rested for 48 hours in an elbow sling versus normal activity without restrictions.[2]
- Consider use of a neoprene elbow sleeve.
- Avoid vigorous use of the elbow over the next 2 weeks.
- NSAIDs, ice, and/or physical therapy as indicated.
- Consider follow-up examination in 2 weeks.

CPT codes:
- 20605—Arthrocentesis, aspiration and/or injection, intermediate joint or bursa; without ultrasound guidance
- 20606—With ultrasound guidance, with permanent recording and reporting

PEARLS

- The joint space at the radial head can be "opened up" by extending the elbow.
- Since the elbow has a narrow joint space, a 20-gauge needle is used for aspiration instead of the larger diameter, 18-gauge needle.
- If a fracture is suspected, do not inject corticosteroid.

 A video showing an elbow joint injection can be found in the companion eBook.

REFERENCES

1. Sussman WI, Williams CJ, Mautner K. Ultrasound-guided elbow procedures. *Phys Med Rehabil Clin N Am.* 2016;27(3):573–587.
2. Weitoft T, Forsberg C. Importance of immobilization after intraarticular glucocorticoid treatment for elbow synovitis: A randomized controlled study. *Arthritis Care Res (Hoboken).* 2010;62(5):735–737.

Olecranon Bursa

Olecranon bursitis is a relatively common aspiration and injection site for primary care providers. The subcutaneous olecranon bursa may become inflamed and accumulate fluid when subjected to repeated excessive pressure or friction. The fluid may consist of blood in acute trauma, thick proteinaceous mucoid fluid after repetitive injury, or purulent fluid if infected.

In most cases, a conservative treatment regimen should be pursued, following bursal aspirate-based differentiation between septic and nonseptic bursitis.[1] Successful aspiration is usually easily accomplished because the location of the bursa is superficial and easily identified. In a recent study, evaluating treatment options of olecranon bursitis, there were no differences in efficacy between compression bandaging with NSAIDs, aspiration, and aspiration with steroid injection.[2] Injected corticosteroids may be considered in select cases of inflammatory olecranon bursitis such as that seen with gout or rheumatoid arthritis. However, steroids should not be administered if septic bursitis is suspected.

Indication	ICD-10 Code
Olecranon bursitis	M70.20

Relevant Anatomy: (Fig. 10.18)

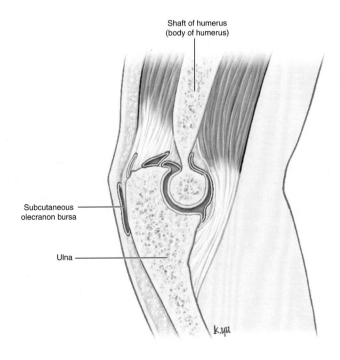

FIGURE 10.18 ● Lateral aspect of right elbow. (From Agur AM, Dalley AF. *Grant's Atlas of Anatomy*, 14th Ed. Philadelphia, PA: Wolters Kluwer, 2016.)

Shaft of humerus
(body of humerus)

Subcutaneous
olecranon bursa

Ulna

PATIENT POSITION

- Supine on the examination table with the head of the bed elevated 30 degrees.
- The affected elbow is maximally flexed.
- The elbow is supported with the placement of chucks pads or towels.
- Rotate the patient's head away from the side that is being injected. This minimizes anxiety and pain perception.

LANDMARKS

1. With the patient supine on the examination table, the clinician stands lateral to the affected elbow.
2. The point of maximal fluctuance is identified.
3. At that site, press firmly on the skin with the retracted tip of a ballpoint pen. This indention represents the entry point for the needle.
4. After the landmarks are identified, the patient should not move the elbow.

ANESTHESIA

- Local anesthesia of the skin using topical vapocoolant spray.

EQUIPMENT

- Topical vapocoolant spray
- 20-mL syringe—for aspiration
- 3-mL syringe—for optional injection
- 18-gauge, 1½-in. needle
- 1 mL of 1% lidocaine without epinephrine—for optional injection
- 0.5 mL of the steroid solution (20 mg of triamcinolone acetonide)—for optional injection
- One alcohol prep pad
- Two povidone–iodine prep pads
- Sterile gauze pads
- Sterile adhesive bandage
- Nonsterile, clean chucks pad

TECHNIQUE

1. Prep the insertion site with alcohol followed by the povidone–iodine pads.
2. Achieve good local anesthesia by using topical vapocoolant spray.
3. Grasp the bursa with the thumb and index finger of your nondominant hand to stabilize the structure and facilitate stable needle entry.
4. Position the 18-gauge needle and syringe with the needle tip directed toward the area of maximal fluid collection.
5. Using the no-touch technique, introduce the needle at the insertion site (Fig. 10.19).
6. Advance the needle into the center of the bursa.
7. Aspiration should be easy accomplished. Use multiple syringes if the effusion is large.

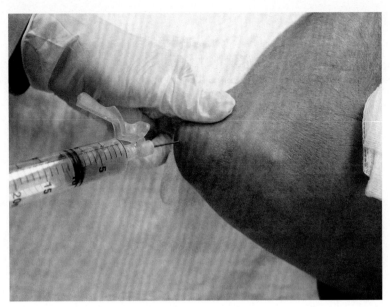

FIGURE 10.19 ⦿ Olecranon bursa aspiration.

8. If injection following aspiration is elected, grasp the hub of the needle, remove the large syringe, and then attach the 3-mL syringe filled with the lidocaine/corticosteroid solution.
9. The injected solution should flow smoothly into the space. If increased resistance is encountered, advance or withdraw the needle slightly before attempting further injection.
10. Following complete aspiration, and possible injection, withdraw the needle.
11. Apply a sterile adhesive bandage followed by a compressive elastic bandage.

AFTERCARE

- Avoid excessive use of the elbow over the next 2 weeks.
- Consider the use of a neoprene elbow sleeve or elastic compression bandage.
- NSAIDs, ice, and/or physical therapy as indicated.
- Consider follow-up examination in 2 weeks.

CPT codes:
- 20605—Arthrocentesis, aspiration and/or injection, intermediate joint or bursa; without ultrasound guidance
- 20606—With ultrasound guidance, with permanent recording and reporting

PEARLS

- If the olecranon bursitis is due to an infection or acute hemorrhagic event, do not follow aspiration with corticosteroid injection.
- Injection of corticosteroid is usually reserved for inflammatory bursitis.

 A video showing an olecranon bursitis aspiration can be found in the companion eBook.

REFERENCES

1. Baumbach SF, Lobo CM, Badyine I. Prepatellar and olecranon bursitis: Literature review and development of a treatment algorithm. *Arch Orthop Trauma Surg*. 2014;134(3):359–370.
2. Kim JY, Chung SW, Kim JH. A randomized trial among compression plus nonsteroidal antiinflammatory drugs, aspiration, and aspiration with steroid injection for nonseptic olecranon bursitis. *Clin Orthop Relat Res*. 2016;474(3):776–783.

Lateral Epicondyle

Lateral epicondylitis is one of the most common soft tissue conditions treated by primary care providers. This is a misnomer and actually involves a noninflammatory tendinosis with collagen disarray—principally involving the extensor carpi radialis brevis (ECRB) tendon. It usually is the result of an overuse injury, frequently associated with degenerative microtears to the hypovascular origins of the wrist extensor and supinator muscle groups that originate at the lateral condyle of the distal humerus.

Injection of various therapeutics to treat this condition has been extensively reported in the literature. Although corticosteroid injections have been used for years, it appears that they are beneficial only in the short term.[1,2] Long-term results are no better than placebo and may in fact be worse.[3,4] In addition, corticosteroid injections used in treating tennis elbow may have both systemic and local adverse effects, to include well-described atrophy[5] and hypopigmentation.[6]

In actuality, there is no injection or physiotherapy intervention that has consistently shown treatment efficacy in the medium to long term in patients diagnosed with lateral epicondylitis.[7–9] In the long-term, platelet-rich plasma injections may show greater improvement in pain and function than corticosteroid injections,[10,11] but not all studies are favorable.[12] Botulinum toxin has also been used with promising results.[13–15] More research is needed to determine how to best use orthobiologics and other interventions in the treatment of lateral epicondylitis.[16]

A reduction in the corticosteroid injection rate would be expected following the publication of high-level evidence demonstrating a lack of efficacy; however, this has not been the case.[17,18] The authors suspect that this is due to the positive short-term benefit of corticosteroids on pain. Perhaps investigation should shift to the effect of combination therapies rather than individual treatments for this condition.

Indication	ICD-10 Code
Lateral epicondylitis	M77.10

Relevant Anatomy: (Fig. 10.20)

PATIENT POSITION

- Supine on the examination table with the head of the bed elevated 30 degrees.
- The affected elbow is slightly flexed.
- The wrist is in a neutral to slightly pronated position.
- The elbow is supported with the placement of chucks pads or towels.
- Rotate the patient's head away from the side that is being injected. This minimizes anxiety and pain perception.

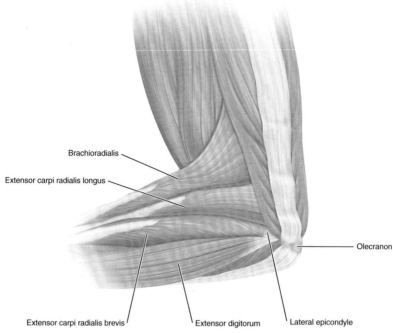

Brachioradialis

Extensor carpi radialis longus

Olecranon

Extensor carpi radialis brevis

Extensor digitorum

Lateral epicondyle

FIGURE 10.20 ● Lateral view of muscular structures at left elbow.

LANDMARKS

1. With the patient supine on the examination table, the clinician stands lateral to the affected elbow.
2. Identify and mark the point of maximal tenderness adjacent to the lateral epicondyle.
3. At that site, press firmly on the skin with the retracted tip of a ballpoint pen. This indention represents the entry point for the needle.
4. After the landmark is identified, the patient should not move the elbow.

ANESTHESIA

• Local anesthesia of the skin using topical vapocoolant spray.

EQUIPMENT

• Topical vapocoolant spray
• 3-mL syringe
• 25-gauge, 1-in. needle
• 1 mL of 1% lidocaine without epinephrine
• 0.5 to 1 mL of the steroid solution (20–40 mg of triamcinolone acetonide)—if desired
• One alcohol prep pad
• Two povidone–iodine prep pads
• Sterile gauze pads
• Sterile adhesive bandage
• Nonsterile, clean chucks pad

TECHNIQUE

1. Prep the insertion site with alcohol followed by the povidone–iodine pads.
2. Achieve good local anesthesia by using topical vapocoolant spray.
3. Position the needle and syringe perpendicular to the skin with the needle tip directed medially toward the lateral epicondyle.
4. Using the no-touch technique, introduce the needle at the insertion site (Fig. 10.21).
5. Advance the needle to the bone of the lateral epicondyle.
6. Withdraw the needle 1 to 2 mm.
7. Perform the "pinch technique" (see description in "Pearls" section).
8. Withdraw the plunger of the syringe to ensure that there is no blood return.
9. Inject the lidocaine/corticosteroid or other therapeutic solution steadily into this area. If increased resistance is encountered, advance or withdraw the needle slightly before attempting further injection.
10. Following injection, withdraw the needle.
11. Apply a sterile adhesive bandage.
12. Instruct the patient to move his or her wrist and elbow through their full range of motion.
13. Reexamine the elbow in 5 min to assess pain relief.

AFTERCARE

- Avoid excessive wrist extension and supination over the next 2 weeks.
- Consider the use of a neoprene elbow sleeve or elastic compression bandage.
- Consider the use of a wrist brace to limit wrist extension.
- NSAIDs, ice, heat, and/or physical therapy as indicated.
- Consider follow-up examination in 2 weeks.
- Consider treatment using alternative modalities if initial therapy is not effective.

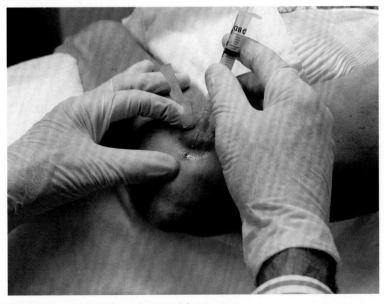

FIGURE 10.21 ● Left elbow lateral epicondyle injection.

CPT codes:
- 20551—Injection; single tendon origin/insertion
- 76942 (optional)—Ultrasonic guidance for needle placement with imaging supervision and interpretation with permanent recording

PEARLS

- Entrapment of branches of the radial nerve in the elbow and forearm can mimic the pain of lateral epicondylitis. Radial tunnel syndrome is most commonly caused by entrapment of the deep radial nerve as it enters the supinator muscle at the arcade of Frohse. Pain in this condition occurs about 4 cm distal to the lateral epicondyle.
- The lateral epicondylitis injection can be superficial—especially in thin persons. Depositing corticosteroid in the subcutaneous tissues commonly results in skin atrophy and hypopigmentation. This particular injection is notorious for the development of this complication. Avoid the development of a subdermal wheal while performing all injections of corticosteroid solutions.
- In order to prevent this dermal complication, one can use the pinch technique (Fig. 10.22). After insertion, gently grasp the skin on either side of the needle, pinch the soft tissue and push it up the needle toward the syringe. This provides a greater distance between the skin and the actual injection site at the epicondyle, thus minimizing the chance of developing atrophy and hypopigmentation.

 A video showing a lateral epicondyle injection can be found in the companion eBook.

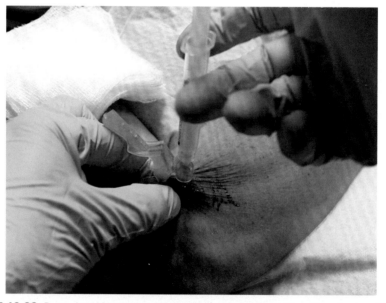

FIGURE 10.22 ● Pinch up the tissue to avoid subcutaneous deposition of corticosteroid.

REFERENCES

1. Krogh TP, Fredberg U, Stengaard-Pedersen K, et al. Treatment of lateral epicondylitis with platelet-rich plasma, glucocorticoid, or saline: A randomized, double-blind, placebo-controlled trial. *Am J Sports Med.* 2013;41(3):625–635.
2. Coombes BK, Bisset L, Vicenzino B. Efficacy and safety of corticosteroid injections and other injections for management of tendinopathy: A systematic review of randomised controlled trials. *Lancet.* 2010;376(9754):1751–1767.
3. Sardelli M, Burks RT. Distances to the subacromial bursa from 3 different injection sites as measured arthroscopically. *Arthroscopy.* 2008;24(9):992–996.
4. Coombes BK, Bisset L, Brooks P, et al. Effect of corticosteroid injection, physiotherapy, or both on clinical outcomes in patients with unilateral lateral epicondylalgia: A randomized controlled trial. *JAMA.* 2013;309(5):461–469.
5. Pace CS, Blanchet NP, Isaacs JE. Soft tissue atrophy related to corticosteroid injection: Review of the literature and implications for hand surgeons. *J Hand Surg Am.* 2018;43(6):558–563.
6. Freire V, Bureau NJ. Injectable corticosteroids: Take precautions and use caution. *Semin Musculoskelet Radiol.* 2016;20(5):401–408.
7. Gao B, Dwivedi S, DeFroda S, et al. The therapeutic benefits of saline solution injection for lateral epicondylitis: A meta-analysis of randomized controlled trials comparing saline injections with nonsurgical injection therapies. *Arthroscopy.* 2019;35(6):1847–1859.e12.
8. Krogh TP, Bartels EM, Ellingsen T, et al. Comparative effectiveness of injection therapies in lateral epicondylitis: A systematic review and network meta-analysis of randomized controlled trials. *Am J Sports Med.* 2013;41(6):1435–1446.
9. Wolf JM, Ozer K, Scott F, et al. Comparison of autologous blood, corticosteroid, and saline injection in the treatment of lateral epicondylitis: A prospective, randomized, controlled multicenter study. *J Hand Surg Am.* 2011;36(8):1269–1272.
10. Li A, Wang H, Yu Z, et al. Platelet-rich plasma vs corticosteroids for elbow epicondylitis: A systematic review and meta-analysis. *Medicine (Baltimore).* 2019;98(51):e18358.
11. Xu Q, Chen J, Cheng L. Comparison of platelet rich plasma and corticosteroids in the management of lateral epicondylitis: A meta-analysis of randomized controlled trials. *Int J Surg.* 2019;67:37–46.
12. Franchini M, Cruciani M, Mengoli C, et al. Efficacy of platelet-rich plasma as conservative treatment in orthopaedics: A systematic review and meta-analysis. *Blood Transfus.* 2018;16(6):502–513.
13. Galván Ruiz A, Vergara Díaz G, Rendón Fernández B, et al. Effects of ultrasound-guided administration of botulinum toxin (IncobotulinumtoxinA) in patients with lateral epicondylitis. *Toxins (Basel).* 2019;11(1):46.
14. Kalichman L, Bannuru RR, Severin M, et al. Injection of botulinum toxin for treatment of chronic lateral epicondylitis: Systematic review and meta-analysis. *Semin Arthritis Rheum.* 2011;40(6):532–538.
15. Lin C, Tu YK, Chen SS, et al. Comparison between botulinum toxin and corticosteroid injection in the treatment of acute and subacute tennis elbow: A prospective, randomized, double-blind, active drug-controlled pilot study. *Am J Phys Med Rehabil.* 2010;89(8):653–659.
16. Calandruccio JH, Steiner MM. Autologous blood and platelet-rich plasma injections for treatment of lateral epicondylitis. *Orthop Clin North Am.* 2017;48(3):351–357.
17. Fujihara Y, Huetteman HE, Chung TT, et al. The effect of impactful articles on clinical practice in the united states: Corticosteroid injection for patients with lateral epicondylitis. *Plast Reconstr Surg.* 2018;141(5):1183–1191.
18. Vicenzino B, Britt H, Pollack AJ, et al. No abatement of steroid injections for tennis elbow in Australian General Practice: A 15-year observational study with random general practitioner sampling. *PLoS One.* 2017;12(7):e0181631.

Medial Epicondyle

Medial epicondylitis is a fairly common soft tissue condition encountered by primary care physicians. Pathologically similar to lateral epicondylitis, this condition also involves a noninflammatory tendinosis with collagen disarray. It usually is the result of an overuse injury with microtears to the hypovascular origins of the wrist flexor and pronator muscle groups. As with lateral epicondylitis, there is no consistent medical literature that is available to guide treatment with any injectable medication or intervention. A single study suggests short-term improvement only with use of corticosteroids.[1] Once the acute symptomology is alleviated, focus is turned to flexor–pronator mass rehabilitation and injury prevention.[2]

Indication	ICD-10 Code
Medial epicondylitis	M77.00

Relevant Anatomy: (Fig. 10.23)

PATIENT POSITION

- Supine on the examination table with the head of the bed elevated 30 degrees.
- Shoulder at 30 degrees of abduction and full external rotation.
- The affected elbow is flexed at 90 degrees.
- The wrist is in a neutral position.
- The elbow is supported with the placement of chucks pads or towels.
- Rotate the patient's head away from the side that is being injected. This minimizes anxiety and pain perception.

LANDMARKS

1. With the patient supine on the examination table, the clinician stands lateral to the affected elbow.
2. Identify and mark the point of maximal tenderness adjacent to the medial epicondyle.
3. At that site, press firmly on the skin with the retracted tip of a ballpoint pen. This indention represents the entry point for the needle.
4. After the landmarks are identified, the patient should not move the elbow.

ANESTHESIA

- Local anesthesia of the skin using topical vapocoolant spray.

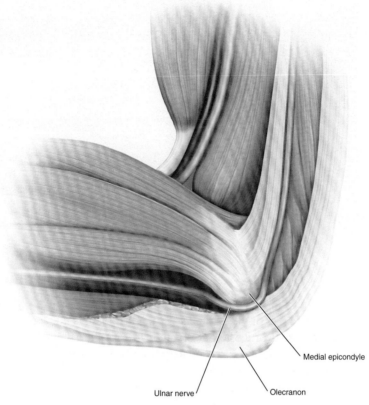

Medial epicondyle

Ulnar nerve

Olecranon

FIGURE 10.23 ● Medial view of muscular structures at right elbow.

EQUIPMENT

- Topical vapocoolant spray
- 3-mL syringe
- 25-gauge, 1-in. needle
- 1 mL of 1% lidocaine without epinephrine
- 0.5 to 1 mL of the steroid solution (20 to 40 mg of triamcinolone acetonide)
- One alcohol prep pad
- Two povidone–iodine prep pads
- Sterile gauze pads
- Sterile adhesive bandage
- Nonsterile, clean chucks pad

TECHNIQUE

1. Prep the insertion site with alcohol followed by the povidone–iodine pads.
2. Achieve good local anesthesia by using topical vapocoolant spray.
3. Position the needle and syringe perpendicular to the skin with the needle tip directed laterally toward the medial epicondyle.
4. Using the no-touch technique, introduce the needle at the insertion site (Fig. 10.24).
5. Advance the needle to the bone of the medial epicondyle.

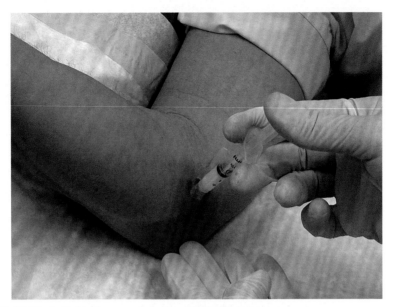

FIGURE 10.24 ● Right elbow medial epicondylitis injection.

6. Withdraw the needle 1 to 2 mm.
7. Withdraw the plunger of the syringe to ensure that there is no blood return.
8. Inject the lidocaine/corticosteroid or other therapeutic solution steadily into this area. If increased resistance is encountered, advance or withdraw the needle slightly before attempting further injection.
9. Following injection, withdraw the needle.
10. Apply a sterile adhesive bandage.
11. Instruct the patient to move his or her wrist and elbow through their full range of motion.
12. Reexamine the elbow in 5 min to assess pain relief.

AFTERCARE

- Avoid excessive wrist flexion or pronation over the next 2 weeks.
- Consider the use of a neoprene elbow sleeve or elastic compression bandage.
- Consider the use of a wrist brace to limit wrist flexion.
- NSAIDs, ice, heat, and/or physical therapy as indicated.
- Consider follow-up examination in 2 weeks.
- Consider treatment using alternative modalities if initial therapy is not effective.

CPT codes:
- 20551—Injection; single tendon origin/insertion
- 76942 (optional)—Ultrasonic guidance for needle placement with imaging supervision and interpretation with permanent recording

PEARLS

- The ulnar nerve travels in close proximity to this injection. It courses just posterior and inferior to the medial epicondyle. On occasion, the local anesthetic spreading out from a properly placed injection may involve the ulnar nerve. The patient should be warned that transient numbness might occur in the lateral aspect of the hand as well as the ring and little fingers.

 A video showing a medial epicondyle injection can be found in the companion eBook.

REFERENCES

1. Stahl S, Kaufman T. The efficacy of an injection of steroids for medial epicondylitis: A prospective study of sixty elbows. *J Bone Joint Surg Am.* 1997;79(11):1648–1652.
2. Amin NH, Kumar NS, Schickendantz MS. Medial epicondylitis: Evaluation and management. *J Am Acad Orthop Surg.* 2015;23(6):348–355.

Radial Nerve Entrapment

Patients uncommonly present to the primary care office for treatment of radial nerve entrapment in the forearm. This syndrome is caused by entrapment of the deep branch of the radial nerve (posterior interosseous nerve) as it enters the supinator muscle at the arcade of Frohse. Compression or scarring of the posterior interosseous nerve may cause denervation of extensor/supinator muscles and numbness or paresthesias in the distribution of the radial sensory nerve. The result can be pain, weakness, and dysfunction. Pain in this condition occurs about 4 cm distal to the lateral epicondyle. A nerve block injection utilizing local anesthetic can be given to help confirm diagnosis, and corticosteroid may be added for conservative management.[1] Alternative therapies include dry needling[2] and radial nerve hydrodissection. Successful treatment often requires surgical release.

Indication	ICD-10 Code
Radial nerve entrapment syndrome	G56.30

Relevant Anatomy: (Fig. 10.25)

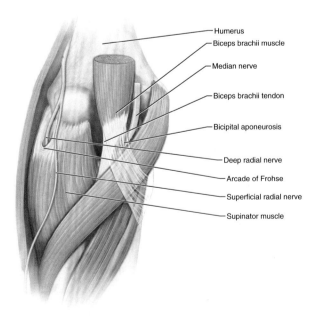

Humerus
Biceps brachii muscle
Median nerve
Biceps brachii tendon
Bicipital aponeurosis
Deep radial nerve
Arcade of Frohse
Superficial radial nerve
Supinator muscle

FIGURE 10.25 ● Anterior aspect of right elbow. (Modified from Paulsen F, Waschke J. *Sobotta Atlas of Human Anatomy*, 16th Ed. 2018 © Elsevier GmbH, Urban & Fischer, Munich)

PATIENT POSITION

- Supine on the examination table with the head of the bed elevated 30 degrees.
- The affected elbow is slightly flexed.
- The wrist is in a neutral to slightly pronated position.
- The elbow is supported with the placement of chucks pads or towels.
- Rotate the patient's head away from the side that is being injected. This minimizes anxiety and pain perception.

LANDMARKS

1. With the patient supine on the examination table, the clinician stands lateral to the affected forearm.
2. Identify the lateral epicondyle.
3. The point of maximal tenderness is usually located about 4 cm distal and anterior to the lateral epicondyle.
4. Identify and mark the point of maximal tenderness.
5. At that site, press firmly on the skin with the retracted tip of a ballpoint pen. This indention represents the entry point for the needle.
6. After the landmarks are identified, the patient should not move the elbow.

ANESTHESIA

- Local anesthesia of the skin using topical vapocoolant spray.

EQUIPMENT

- Topical vapocoolant spray
- 3-mL syringe
- 25-gauge, 1-in. needle
- 1 mL of 1% lidocaine without epinephrine
- 1 mL of the steroid solution (40 mg of triamcinolone acetonide)
- One alcohol prep pad
- Two povidone–iodine prep pads
- Sterile gauze pads
- Sterile adhesive bandage
- Nonsterile, clean chucks pad

TECHNIQUE

1. Prep the insertion site with alcohol followed by the povidone–iodine pads.
2. Achieve good local anesthesia by using topical vapocoolant spray.
3. Position the needle and syringe perpendicular to the skin with the needle tip directed posteriorly.
4. Using the no-touch technique, introduce the needle at the insertion site (Fig. 10.26).
5. Slowly advance the needle until the needle tip is at the anticipated injection site at the radial nerve.
6. If any pain, paresthesias, or numbness is encountered, withdraw the needle slightly.
7. When the needle is placed along the radial nerve, withdraw the plunger of the syringe to ensure that there is no blood return.

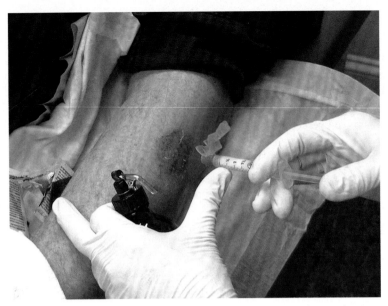

FIGURE 10.26 ● Left arm radial nerve entrapment injection.

8. Slowly inject the lidocaine/corticosteroid solution as a bolus around the radial nerve.
9. If increased resistance is encountered, advance or withdraw the needle slightly before attempting further injection.
10. Following injection, withdraw the needle.
11. Apply a sterile adhesive bandage.
12. Instruct the patient to move his or her wrist and elbow through their full range of motion to distribute the lidocaine/corticosteroid solution along the course of the radial nerve.
13. Reexamine the proximal forearm in 5 min to assess pain relief and the development of numbness in the distribution of the radial nerve from the local anesthetic.

AFTERCARE

- Avoid excessive wrist extension and supination over the next 2 weeks.
- NSAIDs, ice, and/or physical therapy as indicated.
- Consider follow-up examination in 2 weeks.
- Consider treatment using alternative modalities if initial therapy is not effective.

CPT codes:
- 64450—Injection, nerve block, therapeutic, other peripheral nerve or branch
- 76942 (optional)—Ultrasonic guidance for needle placement with imaging supervision and interpretation with permanent recording

PEARLS

- Entrapment of branches of the radial nerve in the elbow and forearm can mimic the pain of lateral epicondylitis.

 A video showing a radial nerve entrapment injection can be found in the companion eBook.

REFERENCES

1. Carter GT, Weiss MD. Diagnosis and treatment of work-related proximal median and radial nerve entrapment. *Phys Med Rehabil Clin N Am.* 2015;26(3):539–549.
2. Anandkumar S. Effect of dry needling on radial tunnel syndrome: A case report. *Physiother Theory Pract.* 2019;35(4):373–382.

Intersection Syndrome

Injection of corticosteroids for the treatment of intersection syndrome is a rare procedure for primary care providers. This is a painful condition that affects the dorsum of the forearm 4 cm proximal to the wrist joint from Lister's tubercle[1] at the intersection of the abductor pollicis longus (APL) and extensor pollicis brevis (EPB) muscles at the point where they cross over (intersect) the extensor carpi radialis longus (ECRL) and the extensor carpi radialis brevis (ECRB) tendons. The mechanism of injury usually involves repetitive resisted wrist extension that occurs in rowers and certain industrial workers. Patients typically describe pain, local swelling, and a rubbing/squeaking sensation when they extend their wrist repeatedly.

Conservative treatment includes rest, activity modification, bracing, and NSAIDs. Alternatively, patients may be treated with a corticosteroid injection or ultrasound-guided saline hydrodissection.[2]

Indication	ICD-10 Code
Intersection syndrome	M65.839

Relevant Anatomy: (Fig. 10.27)

PATIENT POSITION

- Supine on the examination table with the head of the bed elevated 30 degrees.
- The affected wrist is held in a neutral position. The thumb is directed superiorly midway between supination and pronation.

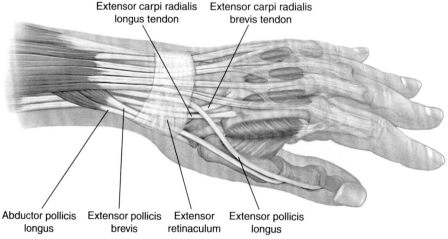

Extensor carpi radialis longus tendon

Extensor carpi radialis brevis tendon

Abductor pollicis longus

Extensor pollicis brevis

Extensor retinaculum

Extensor pollicis longus

FIGURE 10.27 ● Anatomy of muscles and tendons involved with intersection syndrome.

- The wrist is supported with the placement of chucks pads or towels.
- Rotate the patient's head away from the side that is being injected. This minimizes anxiety and pain perception.

LANDMARKS

1. With the patient supine on the examination table, the clinician stands lateral to the affected wrist.
2. Identify the maximal point of tenderness located over the dorsal–radial aspect of the forearm 4 cm proximal to the wrist joint from Lister's tubercle[3] at the intersection of the APL and EPB muscles at the point where they cross over (intersect) the ECRL and the ECRB tendons.
3. Often, the anatomy is more easily identified by asking the patient to repetitively make very small circular motions with the thumb or perform wrist extensions. The area where these structures intersect can be located by finding the maximal area of pain, or palpating for crepitus.
4. At that site, press firmly on the skin with the retracted tip of a ballpoint pen. This indention represents the target point for the needle.
5. Mark a point 1 cm distal to that spot.
6. At that site, press firmly on the skin with the retracted tip of a ballpoint pen. This indention represents the entry point for the needle.
7. After the landmarks are identified, the patient should not move the wrist or thumb.

ANESTHESIA

- Local anesthesia of the skin using topical vapocoolant spray.

EQUIPMENT

- Topical vapocoolant spray
- 3-mL syringe
- 25-gauge, 1-in. needle
- 0.5 mL of 1% lidocaine without epinephrine
- 0.25 to 0.5 mL of the steroid solution (10 to 20 mg of triamcinolone acetonide)
- One alcohol prep pad
- Two povidone–iodine prep pads
- Sterile gauze pads
- Sterile adhesive bandage
- Nonsterile, clean chucks pad

TECHNIQUE

1. Prep the insertion site with alcohol followed by the povidone–iodine pads.
2. Achieve good local anesthesia by using topical vapocoolant spray.
3. Position the needle and syringe 1 cm distal to the marked target site—at a 45-degree angle to the skin with the needle tip directed proximally.
4. Using the no-touch technique, introduce the needle at the insertion site (Fig. 10.28).
5. Advance the needle toward the target that is located about 1 cm deep to the skin.
6. Withdraw the plunger of the syringe to ensure that there is no blood return.

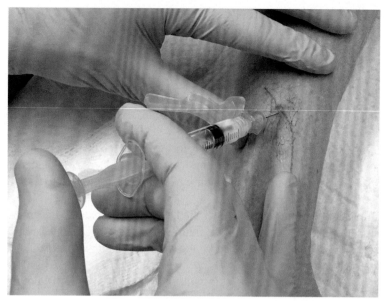

FIGURE 10.28 ● Intersection syndrome injection.

7. Slowly inject the lidocaine/corticosteroid solution as a bolus into the tendon sheath.
8. Following injection, withdraw the needle.
9. Apply a sterile adhesive bandage.
10. Instruct the patient to move his or her thumb and wrist through its full range of motion. This movement distributes the lidocaine/corticosteroid solution throughout the tenosynovial sheath.
11. Reexamine the hand and wrist in 5 min to assess pain relief.

AFTERCARE

- Ensure no excessive wrist or thumb extension/abduction over the next 2 weeks by the application of a wrist thumb spica splint.
- NSAIDs, ice, heat, and/or physical therapy as indicated.
- Consider follow-up examination in 2 weeks.

CPT codes:
- 20550—Injection(s); single tendon sheath, or ligament, aponeurosis
- 76942 (optional)—Ultrasonic guidance for needle placement with imaging supervision and interpretation with permanent recording

PEARLS

- Care should be taken to differentiate this condition from the more common de Quervain's tenosynovitis.
- Ultrasound guidance may offer a significant advantage over landmark-based technique.

 A video showing an intersection syndrome injection can be found in the companion eBook.

REFERENCES

1. Lee RP, Hatem SF, Recht MP. Extended MRI findings of intersection syndrome. *Skeletal Radiol.* 2009;38(2):157–163.
2. Skinner TM. Intersection syndrome: The subtle squeak of an overused wrist. *J Am Board Fam Med.* 2017;30(4):547–551.
3. Lee RP, Hatem SF, Recht MP. Extended MRI findings of intersection syndrome. *Skeletal Radiol.* 2009;38(2):157–163.

de Quervain's Tenosynovitis

Injection of corticosteroids for the treatment of de Quervain's tenosynovitis is a fairly common procedure for primary care providers. This condition represents a stenosing tenosynovitis of the first dorsal compartment over the radial aspect of the wrist. The extensor pollicis brevis (EPB) and abductor pollicis longus (APL) tendons run alongside each other and share a common tendon sheath that occupies the first dorsal compartment of the wrist. Overuse movements that require repetitive extension and abduction of the thumb generally cause this condition. It is commonly seen during pregnancy and especially in the postpartum period.

Studies show that a local injection of corticosteroid leads to a high rate of improvement both in the short and long term with few side effects.[1-3] Ultrasound studies show a 28% to 52% incidence of a tendon sheath septum isolating the EPB from the APL.[4,5] The presence of these subcompartments plays a role in recurrence rates.[6,7] The use of ultrasound has been shown to detect the septum, improve injection accuracy by enabling injection into each subcompartment, and improve clinical outcomes.[8,9]

Indication	ICD-10 Code
de Quervain's tenosynovitis	M65.4

Relevant Anatomy: (Fig. 10.29)

PATIENT POSITION

- Supine on the examination table with the head of the bed elevated 30 degrees.
- The affected wrist is held in a neutral position. The thumb is directed superiorly midway between supination and pronation.
- The wrist is supported with the placement of chucks pads or towels.
- Rotate the patient's head away from the side that is being injected. This minimizes anxiety and pain perception.

LANDMARKS

1. With the patient supine on the examination table, the clinician stands lateral to the affected wrist.
2. Identify tenderness located in the sheath that contains the APL and the EPB tendons.
3. The injection point is located directly between these two tendons. Often, the anatomy is more easily identified by asking the patient to make very small circular motions with the thumb. The two tendons should be easier to identify and the injection point

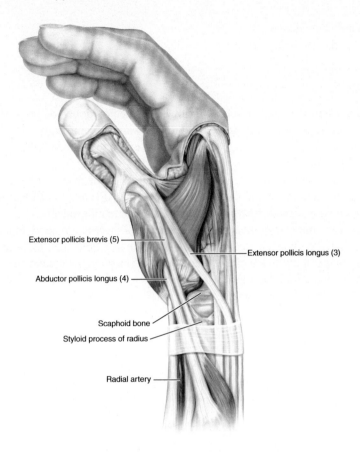

Lateral view

FIGURE 10.29 ● Right hand anatomy. (Modified from Agur AM, Dalley AF. *Grant's Atlas of Anatomy*, 14th Ed. Philadelphia, PA: Wolters Kluwer, 2016.)

marked with an indention made by the fingernail of the examiner placed longitudinally between the APL and EPB tendons. This indention represents the entry point for the needle.
4. After the landmarks are identified, the patient should not move the wrist or thumb.

ANESTHESIA

• Local anesthesia of the skin using topical vapocoolant spray.

EQUIPMENT

• Topical vapocoolant spray
• 3-mL syringe
• 25-gauge, 5/8-in. needle
• 0.5 mL of 1% lidocaine without epinephrine
• 0.25 to 0.5 mL of the steroid solution (10 to 20 mg of triamcinolone acetonide)
• One alcohol prep pad
• Two povidone–iodine prep pads
• Sterile gauze pads

- Sterile adhesive bandage
- Nonsterile, clean chucks pad

TECHNIQUE

1. Prep the insertion site with alcohol followed by the povidone–iodine pads.
2. Achieve good local anesthesia by using topical vapocoolant spray.
3. Position the needle and syringe at a 30-degree angle to the skin with the needle tip directed proximally.
4. Using the no-touch technique, introduce the needle at the insertion site (Fig. 10.30).
5. Advance the needle toward the convergence of the APL and the EPB tendons until the needle tip is located between the tendons in the tendon sheath.
6. Withdraw the plunger of the syringe to ensure that there is no blood return.
7. Slowly inject the lidocaine/corticosteroid solution as a bolus into the tendon sheath. A small bulge in the shape of a sausage often develops in the tendon sheath.
8. Following injection, withdraw the needle.
9. Apply a sterile adhesive bandage.
10. Instruct the patient to move his or her thumb through its full range of motion. This movement distributes the lidocaine/corticosteroid solution throughout the tenosynovial sheath.
11. Reexamine the hand and wrist in 5 min to assess pain relief.

AFTERCARE

- Ensure no excessive wrist flexion or pronation over the next 2 weeks by the application of a wrist thumb spica splint.
- NSAIDs, ice, heat, and/or physical therapy as indicated.
- Consider follow-up examination in 2 weeks.

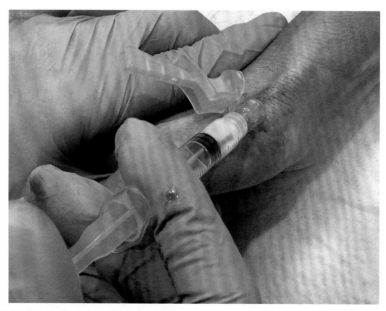

FIGURE 10.30 ● de Quervain's tenosynovitis injection.

CPT codes:

- 20550—Injection(s); single tendon sheath, or ligament, aponeurosis
- 76942 (optional)—Ultrasonic guidance for needle placement with imaging supervision and interpretation with permanent recording

PEARLS

- Care should be taken to differentiate this condition from a painful thumb carpometacarpal joint and the rare intersection syndrome.
- The de Quervain's tenosynovitis injection is superficial—especially in thin persons. Depositing corticosteroid in the subcutaneous tissues can result in the complication of skin atrophy and hypopigmentation. de Quervain's injection is notorious for the development of this complication. Avoid the development of an intradermal wheal while performing all injections of corticosteroid solutions.

 A video showing a de Quervain's injection can be found in the companion eBook.

REFERENCES

1. Peters-Veluthamaningal C, van der Windt DAWM, Winters JC, et al. Corticosteroid injection for de Quervain's tenosynovitis. *Cochrane Database Syst Rev.* 2009;(3):CD005616.
2. Cavaleri R, Schabrun SM, Te M, et al. Hand therapy versus corticosteroid injections in the treatment of de Quervain's disease: A systematic review and meta-analysis. *J Hand Ther.* 2016;29(1):3–11.
3. Abi-Rafeh J, Kazan R, Safran T, et al. Conservative management of de Quervain's stenosing tenosynovitis: Review & presentation of treatment algorithm. *Plast Reconstr Surg.* 2020;146(1):105–126.
4. Mirzanli C, Ozturk K, Esenyel CZ, et al. Accuracy of intrasheath injection techniques for de Quervain's disease: a cadaveric study. *J Hand Surg Eur Vol.* 2012;37(2):155–160.
5. McDermott JD, Ilyas AM, Nazarian LN, et al. Ultrasound-guided injections for de Quervain's tenosynovitis. *Clin Orthop Relat Res.* 2012;470(7):1925–1931.
6. Karthikeyan S, Kwong HT, Upadhyay PK, et al. A double-blind randomised controlled study comparing subacromial injection of tenoxicam or methylprednisolone in patients with subacromial impingement. *J Bone Joint Surg Br.* 2010;92(1):77–82.
7. De Keating-Hart E, Touchais S, Kerjean Y, et al. Presence of an intracompartmental septum detected by ultrasound is associated with the failure of ultrasound-guided steroid injection in de Quervain's syndrome. *J Hand Surg Eur Vol.* 2016;41(2):212–219.
8. Kume K, Amano K, Yamada S, et al. In de Quervain's with a separate EPB compartment, ultrasound-guided steroid injection is more effective than a clinical injection technique: A prospective open-label study. *J Hand Surg Eur Vol.* 2012;37(6):523–527.
9. Kang JW, Park JW, Lee SH, et al. Ultrasound-guided injection for De Quervain's disease: Accuracy and its influenceable anatomical variances in first extensor compartment of fresh cadaver wrists. *J Orthop Sci.* 2017;22(2):270–274.

Carpal Tunnel Syndrome—Preferred Flexor Carpi Radialis Approach

Carpal tunnel syndrome is a very common condition encountered in primary care. It represents a compressive injury to the median nerve as it traverses the carpal tunnel in the wrist. This usually occurs as a result of an overuse injury following repetitive handgrip movements or compression of the contents of the carpal tunnel from various disease processes. Predisposing factors may include previous injury, pregnancy, diabetes, hypothyroidism, rheumatoid arthritis, or amyloidosis. Injection therapy of the carpal tunnel is an effective, but underutilized, treatment option by primary care providers.

In the traditional approach, the needle is inserted 1 cm proximal to the wrist crease and 1 cm ulnar to the palmaris longus tendon, then directed radially and distally at a 30-degree angle to the horizontal. With the preferred flexor carpi radialis (FCR) approach, the needle is inserted 1 cm proximal to the wrist crease, at the ulnar border of the FCR tendon, then in an ulnar direction and distally at a 20-degree angle to the horizontal. Anatomic studies of cadavers have demonstrated a higher risk of ulnar artery and median nerve injury due to the close proximity of those structures as well as median nerve swelling and/or flattening around the distal wrist crease when using the traditional approach.[1-3] The preferred FCR approach gives the highest accuracy rate and is also the safest injection site.[4] Ultrasound guidance further increases the safety[5] and efficacy of this procedure.[6,7]

A single local injection of corticosteroid at or proximal to the carpal tunnel is a remarkably safe procedure.[8] It is more effective than standard conservative therapy[9] and results in long-lasting improvement in at least half of treated patients.[10-13] A second corticosteroid injection appears at least as effective as the first.[14] Favorable prognostic factors include patients with shorter duration of symptoms, no prior injection,[15] electrodiagnostically mild disease,[16] lower symptom severity scores, and lower median nerve ultrasonographic cross-sectional areas at the pisiform bone.[17]

Objective measurable changes following corticosteroid injections include decreased swelling of the median nerve,[18] improvement in distal motor latency of the median nerve,[19] improvement in sonoelasticity of the intracarpal tunnel contents,[20] and decreased vascularity of the median nerve at the distal wrist crease.[21]

Promising alternative therapies of mild to moderate idiopathic carpal tunnel syndrome include nerve hydrodissection[22] as well as injections of platelet-rich plasma[23,24] and dextrose.[25]

Indication	ICD-10 Code
Carpal tunnel syndrome	G56.00

Relevant Anatomy: (Figs. 10.31 and 10.32)

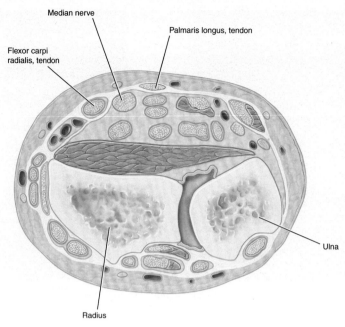

FIGURE 10.31 ● Right wrist cross-section at the level of the distal radioulnar joint. (Modified from Gest TR. *Lippincott Atlas of Anatomy*, 2nd Ed. Philadelphia, PA: Wolters Kluwer, 2019.)

PATIENT POSITION

- Supine on the examination table with the head of the bed elevated at an angle of 30 degrees.
- The elbow is slightly flexed with the wrist in supination.

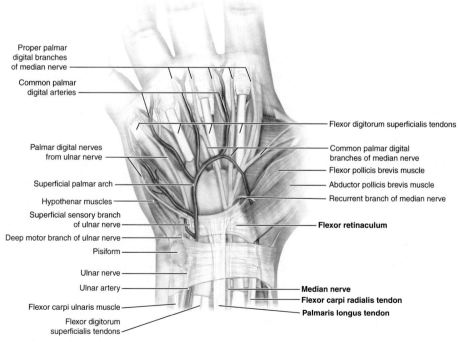

FIGURE 10.32 ● Right wrist—volar aspect.

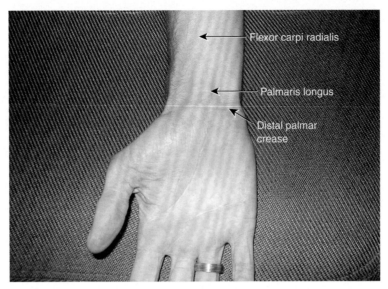

FIGURE 10.33 ● Right hand carpal tunnel injection surface anatomy.

- The wrist is then positioned in slight hyperextension with the placement of chucks pads or towels underneath the supinated wrist.
- Rotate the patient's head away from the side that is being injected. This minimizes anxiety and pain perception.

LANDMARKS

1. With the patient supine on the examination table, the clinician stands lateral to the affected wrist.
2. Identify and mark the distal palmar crease as shown (Fig. 10.33).
3. Identify and mark the course of the palmaris longus and FCR tendons (Fig. 10.34).
4. Mark a point 1 cm proximal to the distal palmar crease on the ulnar border of the FCR tendon. This is the entry point for the needle.
5. At both the entry point and target site, press firmly on the skin with the retracted tip of a ballpoint pen.
6. After the landmarks are identified, the patient should not move the wrist.

ANESTHESIA

- Local anesthesia of the skin using topical vapocoolant spray.

EQUIPMENT

- Topical vapocoolant spray
- 3-mL syringe
- 25-gauge, 1-in. needle
- 1 mL of 1% lidocaine without epinephrine
- 1 mL of the steroid solution (40 mg of triamcinolone acetonide)
- One alcohol prep pad

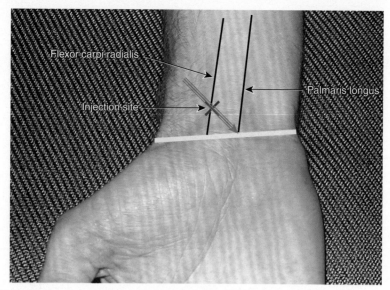

FIGURE 10.34 ● Right hand carpal tunnel injection surface landmarks identified.

- Two povidone–iodine prep pads
- Sterile gauze pads
- Sterile adhesive bandage
- Nonsterile, clean chucks pad

TECHNIQUE

1. Prep the insertion site with alcohol followed by the povidone–iodine pads.
2. Achieve good local anesthesia by using topical vapocoolant spray.
3. Position the needle and syringe at a 20-degree angle to the skin with the needle tip directed in an ulnar and distal direction.
4. Using the no-touch technique, introduce the needle at the insertion site (Fig. 10.35).
5. Very slowly advance the needle approximately 1.5 cm.
6. If any pain, paresthesias, or numbness is encountered, stop the needle advancement and withdraw the needle 1 to 2 mm.
7. Withdraw the plunger of the syringe to ensure that there is no blood return.
8. Slowly inject the lidocaine/corticosteroid solution as a bolus around the median nerve.
9. If increased resistance is encountered, withdraw the needle slightly before attempting further injection.
10. Following injection, withdraw the needle.
11. Apply a sterile adhesive bandage.
12. Reexamine the hand in 5 min to assess pain relief and/or the development of numbness in the distribution of the median nerve from the local anesthetic.

AFTERCARE

- Avoid further overuse mechanisms of injury.
- Use a carpal tunnel wrist brace while sleeping to avoid wrist flexion and extension.
- NSAIDs, ice, and/or physical therapy as indicated.
- Consider follow-up examination in 2 weeks.

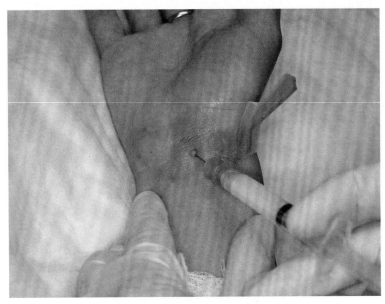

FIGURE 10.35 ● Right hand carpal tunnel injection—preferred FCR approach.

CPT codes:
- 20526—Injection, therapeutic, of carpal tunnel
- 76942 (optional)—Ultrasonic guidance for needle placement with imaging supervision and interpretation with permanent recording

PEARLS

- The preferred FCR approach illustrated here is easy to perform and has few side effects.
- This injection places the steroid solution just proximal to the carpal tunnel. Injections into the carpal tunnel itself may damage the median nerve.
- Warn the patients that the median nerve may be contacted when using this approach.
- Ask them to calmly report any pain or electrical shock sensation without jerking their arm away. If this occurs, simply stop advancing the needle and withdraw the needle 1 to 2 mm before injecting.
- Alternatively, ultrasound guidance of the procedure may be done to increase safety and accuracy of this injection.

 A video showing a carpal tunnel injection using the preferred FCR approach can be found in the companion eBook.

REFERENCES

1. Kim DH, Jang JE, Park BK. Anatomical basis of ulnar approach in carpal tunnel injection. *Pain Physician*. 2013;16(3):E191–E198.
2. Dubert T, Racasan O. A reliable technique for avoiding the median nerve during carpal tunnel injections. *Joint Bone Spine*. 2006;73(1):77–79.
3. MacLennan A, Schimizzi A, Meier KM. Comparison of needle position proximity to the median nerve in 2 carpal tunnel injection methods: A cadaveric study. *J Hand Surg Am*. 2009;34(5):875–879.
4. Ozturk K, Esenyel CZ, Sonmez M, et al. Comparison of carpal tunnel injection techniques: A cadaver study. *Scand J Plast Reconstr Surg Hand Surg*. 2008;42(6):300–304.

5. Gofeld M, Hurdle MF, Agur A. Biceps tendon sheath injection: An anatomical conundrum. *Pain Med.* 2019;20(1):138–142.
6. Babaei-Ghazani A, Roomizadeh P, Forogh B, et al. Ultrasound-guided versus landmark-guided local corticosteroid injection for carpal tunnel syndrome: A systematic review and meta-analysis of randomized controlled trials. *Arch Phys Med Rehabil.* 2018;99(4):766–775.
7. Chen PC, Wang LY, Pong YP, et al. Effectiveness of ultrasound-guided vs direct approach corticosteroid injections for carpal tunnel syndrome: A double-blind randomized controlled trial. *J Rehabil Med.* 2018;50(2):200–208.
8. Kaile E, Bland JDP. Safety of corticosteroid injection for carpal tunnel syndrome. *J Hand Surg Eur Vol.* 2018;43(3):296–302.
9. Chesterton LS, Blagojevic-Bucknall M, Burton C, et al. The clinical and cost-effectiveness of corticosteroid injection versus night splints for carpal tunnel syndrome (INSTINCTS trial): An open-label, parallel group, randomised controlled trial. *Lancet.* 2018;392(10156):1423–1433.
10. Marshall S, Tardif G, Ashworth N. Local corticosteroid injection for carpal tunnel syndrome. *Cochrane Database Syst Rev.* 2007;(2):CD001554.
11. Ly-Pen D, Andréu JL, Millán I, et al. Comparison of surgical decompression and local steroid injection in the treatment of carpal tunnel syndrome: 2-year clinical results from a randomized trial. *Rheumatology (Oxford).* 2012;51(8):1447–1454.
12. Peters-Veluthamaningal C, Winters JC, Groenier KH, et al. Randomised controlled trial of local corticosteroid injections for carpal tunnel syndrome in general practice. *BMC Fam Pract.* 2010;11:54.
13. Dammers JW, Roos Y, Veering MM, et al. Injection with methylprednisolone in patients with the carpal tunnel syndrome: A randomised double blind trial testing three different doses. *J Neurol.* 2006;253(5):574–577.
14. Ashworth NL, Bland JD. Effectiveness of second corticosteroid injections for carpal tunnel syndrome. *Muscle Nerve.* 2013;48(1):122–126.
15. Jerosch-Herold C, Shepstone L, Houghton J, et al. Prognostic factors for response to treatment by corticosteroid injection or surgery in carpal tunnel syndrome (palms study): A prospective multicenter cohort study. *Muscle Nerve.* 2019;60(1):32–40.
16. Visser LH, Ngo Q, Groeneweg SJ, et al. Long term effect of local corticosteroid injection for carpal tunnel syndrome: A relation with electrodiagnostic severity. *Clin Neurophysiol.* 2012;123(4):838–841.
17. Meys V, Thissen S, Rozeman S, et al. Prognostic factors in carpal tunnel syndrome treated with a corticosteroid injection. *Muscle Nerve.* 2011;44(5):763–768.
18. Lee YS, Choi E. Ultrasonographic changes after steroid injection in carpal tunnel syndrome. *Skeletal Radiol.* 2017;46(11):1521–1530.
19. Milo R, Kalichman L, Volchek L, et al. Local corticosteroid treatment for carpal tunnel syndrome: a 6-month clinical and electrophysiological follow-up study. *J Back Musculoskelet Rehabil.* 2009;22(2):59–64.
20. Miyamoto H, Siedentopf C, Kastlunger M, et al. Intracarpal tunnel contents: Evaluation of the effects of corticosteroid injection with sonoelastography. *Radiology.* 2014;270(3):809–815.
21. Cartwright MS, White DL, Demar S, et al. Median nerve changes following steroid injection for carpal tunnel syndrome. *Muscle Nerve.* 2011;44(1):25–29.
22. Wu YT, Chen SR, Li TY, et al. Nerve hydrodissection for carpal tunnel syndrome: A prospective, randomized, double-blind, controlled trial. *Muscle Nerve.* 2019;59(2):174–180.
23. Senna MK, Shaat RM, Ali AAA. Platelet-rich plasma in treatment of patients with idiopathic carpal tunnel syndrome. *Clin Rheumatol.* 2019;38(12):3643–3654.
24. Malahias MA, Chytas D, Mavrogenis AF, et al. Platelet-rich plasma injections for carpal tunnel syndrome: A systematic and comprehensive review. *Eur J Orthop Surg Traumatol.* 2019;29(1):1–8.
25. Wu YT, Ho TY, Chou YC, et al. Six-month efficacy of perineural dextrose for carpal tunnel syndrome: A prospective, randomized, double-blind, controlled trial. *Mayo Clin Proc.* 2017;92(8):1179–1189.

Carpal Tunnel Syndrome— Traditional Approach

Carpal tunnel syndrome is a very common condition encountered in primary care. It represents a compressive injury to the median nerve as it traverses the carpal tunnel in the wrist. This usually occurs as a result of an overuse injury following repetitive handgrip movements or compression of the contents of the carpal tunnel from various disease processes. Predisposing factors may include previous injury, pregnancy, diabetes, hypothyroidism, rheumatoid arthritis, or amyloidosis. Corticosteroid injection of the carpal tunnel is an effective but underutilized treatment option by primary care providers.

This standard technique is the most commonly performed approach to injection of the carpal tunnel. Compared to the preferred FCR approach, it is a bit more awkward to perform. There is also a higher risk for direct needle injury to the ulnar artery and median nerve.

Please read the details concerning carpal tunnel injection that are presented in the preceding chapter.

Indication	ICD-10 Code
Carpal tunnel syndrome	G56.00

Relevant Anatomy: (Fig. 10.27; see previous section)

PATIENT POSITION

- Supine on the examination table with the head of the bed elevated 30 degrees.
- The elbow is slightly flexed with the wrist in supination.
- The wrist is then positioned in slight hyperextension with the placement of chucks pads or towels underneath the supinated wrist.
- Rotate the patient's head away from the side that is being injected. This minimizes anxiety and pain perception.

LANDMARKS

1. With the patient supine on the examination table, the clinician stands lateral to the affected wrist.
2. Identify and mark the distal palmar crease as shown (Fig. 10.33).
3. Identify and mark the intersection of the palmaris longus tendon with the distal palmar crease (Fig. 10.36).
4. Mark a spot 1 cm proximal and 1 cm ulnar to this intersection.

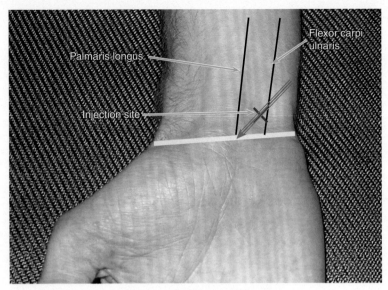

FIGURE 10.36 ● Right hand carpal tunnel injection landmarks.

5. At that site, press firmly with the retracted tip of a ballpoint pen. This indention represents the entry point for the needle.
6. After the landmarks are identified, the patient should not move the wrist.

ANESTHESIA

• Local anesthesia of the skin using topical vapocoolant spray.

EQUIPMENT

• Topical vapocoolant spray
• 3-mL syringe
• 25-gauge, 1-in. needle
• 1 mL of 1% lidocaine without epinephrine
• 1 mL of the steroid solution (40 mg of triamcinolone acetonide)
• One alcohol prep pad
• Two povidone–iodine prep pads
• Sterile gauze pads
• Sterile adhesive bandage
• Nonsterile, clean chucks pad

TECHNIQUE

1. Prep the insertion site with alcohol followed by the povidone–iodine pads.
2. Achieve good local anesthesia by using topical vapocoolant spray.
3. Position the needle and syringe at a 30-degree angle to the skin of the wrist with the needle tip directed toward the base of the thumb.
4. Using the no-touch technique, introduce the needle at the insertion site (Fig. 10.37).
5. Very slowly advance the needle approximately 1 cm toward the base of the thumb.
6. If any pain, paresthesias, or numbness is encountered, stop advancing the needle and withdraw the needle 1 to 2 mm.

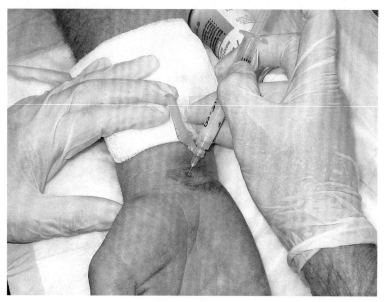

FIGURE 10.37 ● Right hand carpal tunnel injection—traditional approach.

7. Withdraw the plunger of the syringe to ensure that there is no blood return.
8. Slowly inject the lidocaine/corticosteroid solution as a bolus around the median nerve.
9. If increased resistance is encountered, withdraw the needle slightly before attempting further injection.
10. Following injection, withdraw the needle.
11. Apply a sterile adhesive bandage.
12. Reexamine the hand in 5 min to assess pain relief and/or the development of numbness in the distribution of the median nerve from the local anesthetic.

AFTERCARE

- Avoid further overuse mechanisms of injury.
- Use a carpal tunnel wrist brace while sleeping to avoid wrist flexion and extension.
- NSAIDs, ice, and/or physical therapy as indicated.
- Consider follow-up examination in 2 weeks.

CPT codes:
- 20526—Injection, therapeutic, of carpal tunnel
- 76942 (optional)—Ultrasonic guidance for needle placement with imaging supervision and interpretation with permanent recording

PEARLS

- The approach illustrated here is easy to perform and has few side effects.
- However, the possibility of direct needle injury to the median nerve is greater with the traditional technique because the nerve is "fixed" in position by the carpal tunnel.
- Warn the patients that the median nerve may be contacted when using this approach.

- Ask them to calmly report any pain or electrical shock sensation without jerking their arm away. If this occurs, simply stop advancing the needle and withdraw the needle 1 to 2 mm before injecting.
- Alternatively, ultrasound guidance of the procedure may be done to increase safety and accuracy of this injection.

 A video showing a carpal tunnel injection can be found in the companion eBook.

Wrist Joint

Injection of the wrist joint is a relatively uncommon procedure in primary care. Pain and swelling in the wrist may be the result of trauma, osteoarthritis, an infectious etiology, or an inflammatory disorder such as rheumatoid arthritis. A significant number of patients with rheumatoid arthritis on long-term treatment including biologics complain of wrist pain due to synovial proliferation and arthropathic changes. Multiple repeated corticosteroid injections may be safely used to control pain, improve function, and prevent or delay surgery including synovectomy or joint arthroplasty.[1] Occasionally, there will be a small collection of synovial fluid to remove. The success rates of corticosteroid injections can be significantly improved with use of ultrasound guidance.[2–5]

Indications	ICD-10 Code
Wrist pain	M25.539
Wrist joint arthritis, unspecified	M19.039
Wrist joint osteoarthritis, primary	M19.039
Wrist joint osteoarthritis, posttraumatic	M19.139
Wrist joint osteoarthritis, secondary	M19.239

Relevant Anatomy: (Fig. 10.38)

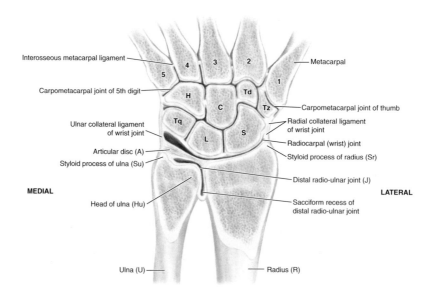

FIGURE 10.38 ● Coronal section of the wrist. (From Gest TR. *Lippincott Atlas of Anatomy*, 2nd Ed. Philadelphia, PA: Wolters Kluwer, 2019.)

PATIENT POSITION

- Supine on the examination table with the head of the bed elevated 30 degrees.
- The elbow is slightly flexed with neutral positioning of the wrist in pronation.
- The wrist is supported with the placement of chucks pads or towels.
- Rotate the patient's head away from the side that is being injected. This minimizes anxiety and pain perception.

LANDMARKS

1. With the patient supine on the examination table, the clinician stands lateral to the affected wrist.
2. Identify and mark the area of maximal tenderness and/or swelling over the dorsal aspect of the wrist joint.
3. At that site, press firmly on the skin with the retracted tip of a ballpoint pen. This indention represents the entry point for the needle.
4. After the landmarks are identified, the patient should not move the wrist.

ANESTHESIA

- Local anesthesia of the skin using topical vapocoolant spray.

EQUIPMENT

- Topical vapocoolant spray
- 3-mL syringe
- 5-mL syringe—for optional aspiration
- 25-gauge, 5/8-in. or 1-in. needle—for injection
- 20-gauge, 1-in. needle—for optional aspiration
- 0.5 mL of 1% mepivacaine without epinephrine
- 0.5 mL of the steroid solution (20 mg of triamcinolone acetonide)
- One alcohol prep pad
- Two povidone–iodine prep pads
- Sterile gauze pads
- Sterile adhesive bandage
- Nonsterile, clean chucks pad

TECHNIQUE

1. Prep the insertion site with alcohol followed by the povidone–iodine pads.
2. Achieve good local anesthesia by using topical vapocoolant spray.
3. Position the needle and syringe perpendicular to the skin with the needle tip directed posteriorly.
4. Using the no-touch technique, introduce the needle at the insertion site (Fig. 10.39).
5. Advance the needle down into the wrist joint.
6. If aspirating, withdraw the fluid using a 20-gauge, 1-in. needle with the 5-mL syringe and then inject through the same needle.
7. If only injecting, use a 25-gauge, 5/8-in. or 1-in. needle with the 3-mL syringe.
8. If injection following aspiration is elected, remove the large syringe from the 20-gauge needle and then attach the 3-mL syringe filled with the mepivacaine/corticosteroid solution.

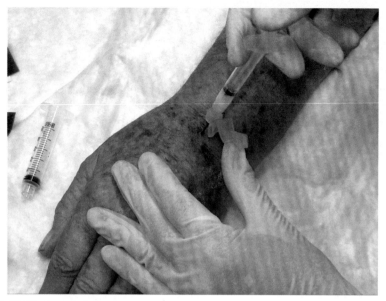

FIGURE 10.39 ● Right dorsal wrist joint injection.

9. Inject the mepivacaine/corticosteroid solution as a bolus into the wrist joint. The injected solution should flow smoothly into the space. If increased resistance is encountered, advance or withdraw the needle slightly before attempting further injection.
10. Following injection, withdraw the needle.
11. Apply a sterile adhesive bandage.
12. Instruct the patient to move his or her wrist through its full range of motion. This movement distributes the mepivacaine/corticosteroid solution throughout the joint.
13. Reexamine the wrist in 5 min to assess pain relief.

AFTERCARE

- Consider the use of a wrist brace.
- Avoid excessive use of the wrist over the next 2 weeks.
- NSAIDs, ice, and/or physical therapy as indicated.
- Consider follow-up examination in 2 weeks.

CPT codes:
- 20605—Arthrocentesis, aspiration and/or injection, intermediate joint or bursa; without ultrasound guidance
- 20606—With ultrasound guidance, with permanent recording and reporting

PEARLS

- There are septa that create multiple partitions within the wrist joint complex. Increasing degrees of synovitis also inhibit flow to all wrist compartments. Therefore, a single injection into a standard injection site in the proximal part of the wrist cannot be assumed to distribute and treat the whole joint.[6] Successful administration of corticosteroid involves pinpoint precision and may require multiple injections during the same office visit.

- Ultrasound guidance will improve accuracy.
- Work on the dorsal aspect of the wrist. The volar aspect contains the radial artery, median nerve, and ulnar artery. These must all be avoided.
- If multiple injections are performed, do not give more than 1 mL of the steroid solution (40 mg of triamcinolone) to the patient at any single office visit.

 A video showing a wrist joint injection can be found in the companion eBook.

REFERENCES

1. Fukui A, Yamada H, Yoshii T. Effect of intraarticular triamcinolone acetonide injection for wrist pain in rheumatoid arthritis patients: A statistical investigation. *J Hand Surg Asian Pac Vol.* 2016;21(2):239–245.
2. Dubreuil M, Greger S, LaValley M, et al. Improvement in wrist pain with ultrasound-guided glucocorticoid injections: A meta-analysis of individual patient data. *Semin Arthritis Rheum.* 2013;42(5):492–497.
3. Smith J, Brault JS, Rizzo M, et al. Accuracy of sonographically guided and palpation guided scaphotrapeziotrapezoid joint injections. *J Ultrasound Med.* 2011;30(11):1509–1515.
4. Cunnington J, Marshall N, Hide G, et al. A randomized, double-blind, controlled study of ultrasound-guided corticosteroid injection into the joint of patients with inflammatory arthritis. *Arthritis Rheum.* 2010;62(7):1862–1869.
5. Lohman M, Vasenius J, Nieminen O. Ultrasound guidance for puncture and injection in the radiocarpal joint. *Acta Radiol.* 2007;48(7):744–747.
6. Boesen M, Jensen KE, Torp-Pedersen S, et al. Intra-articular distribution pattern after ultrasound-guided injections in wrist joints of patients with rheumatoid arthritis. *Eur J Radiol.* 2009;69(2):331–338.

Dorsal Wrist Ganglion Cyst

Aspiration of wrist ganglion cysts is a common procedure for primary care providers. Ganglions are cysts containing clear mucinous, gelatinous fluid. They may originate from the wrist joint or tendon sheaths. A common site of occurrence is along the extensor carpi radialis brevis (ECRB) as it passes over the dorsum of the wrist joint. Although most prevalent in the wrists, ganglion cysts may also occur in other joints. Those located over the dorsal surface of the wrist joint are generally treated with needle aspiration and rarely with corticosteroid.

The very few studies reported in the medical literature suggest a poor response rate to single aspiration attempts with success in only 27% reported by Richman[1] and 42% by Dias.[2] Aspiration combined with corticosteroid injection gave only a 38.5% success rate.[3] In a study by Zubowicz,[4] up to three separate aspirations yielded 85% resolution. The author suspects that the reason for the poor overall response rate is due to incomplete evacuation of the contents of the ganglion cyst with aspiration attempt. Therefore, he developed a technique that combines aspiration with a large-bore needle followed by firm compression of the cyst with the wrist in a flexed position "mash technique." Corticosteroid is not injected. Since employing this technique for more than 15 years, he is aware of only two patients who have failed this conservative treatment. Both were young women with chronic, large dorsal wrist ganglion cysts greater than 1 cm in diameter (anecdotal and unpublished).

Ganglion cysts involving the volar surface of the wrist are intimately associated with the radial artery. Aspiration should never be attempted without ultrasound guidance with color flow Doppler monitoring and are best managed by surgical referral.

Indication	ICD-10 Code
Ganglion cyst of wrist	M67.439

Relevant Anatomy: (Fig. 10.40)

PATIENT POSITION

- Supine on the examination table with the head of the bed elevated 30 degrees.
- For ganglion cysts over the dorsal aspect, the wrist is held in pronation and slight flexion.
- The wrist is supported with the placement of chucks pads or towels.
- Rotate the patient's head away from the side that is being injected. This minimizes anxiety and pain perception.

LANDMARKS

1. With the patient supine on the examination table, the clinician stands lateral to the affected wrist.

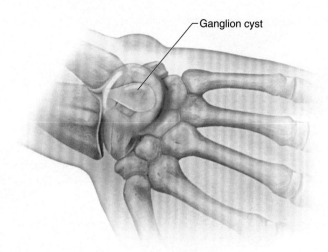

Ganglion cyst

FIGURE 10.40 ● Dorsal wrist ganglion cyst.

2. Position the wrist in flexion.
3. Identify the cystic structure over the dorsal aspect of the wrist joint.
4. The injection point is located directly over the cyst.
5. At that site, press firmly on the skin with the retracted tip of a ballpoint pen. This indention represents the entry point for the needle.
6. After the landmarks are identified, the patient should not move the wrist.

ANESTHESIA

• Local anesthesia of the skin using topical vapocoolant spray.

EQUIPMENT

• Topical vapocoolant spray
• 3-mL syringe
• 18-gauge, 1½-in. needle
• One alcohol prep pad
• Two povidone–iodine prep pads
• Sterile gauze pads
• Sterile adhesive bandage
• Nonsterile, clean chucks pad

TECHNIQUE

1. Prep the insertion site with alcohol followed by the povidone–iodine pads.
2. Achieve good local anesthesia by using topical vapocoolant spray.
3. Position the needle and syringe perpendicular to the skin with the needle tip directed toward the palm.
4. Using the no-touch technique, introduce the needle at the insertion site (Fig. 10.41).
5. Advance the needle quickly but carefully into the cyst.
6. Apply suction with the syringe and withdraw the expected small amount of a clear gel.
7. Following aspiration, withdraw the needle.

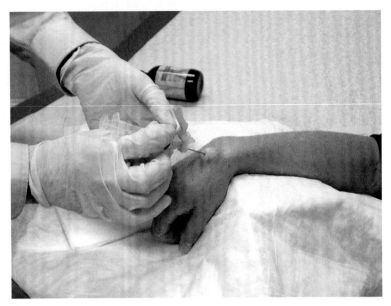

FIGURE 10.41 ● Right wrist dorsal ganglion cyst aspiration.

8. With gloved fingers, apply very firm pressure to the tissues surrounding the punctured cyst "mash technique." Do not contact the injection site with nonsterile gloves. Remove all extruded clear gel with sterile gauze pads (Fig. 10.42).
9. Apply a sterile adhesive bandage.

AFTERCARE

- Consider immobilizing the wrist with a splint for 2 weeks.
- Consider follow-up examination in 2 weeks.

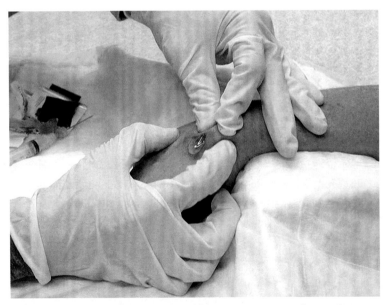

FIGURE 10.42 ● Expression of fluid remaining following aspiration of a ganglion cyst with direct pressure to the surrounding tissues "Mash technique".

CPT codes:

- 20612—Aspiration and/or injection of ganglion cyst(s) any location
- 76942 (optional)—Ultrasonic guidance for needle placement with imaging supervision and interpretation with permanent recording

PEARLS

- Use extreme caution when treating ganglion cysts over the volar aspect of the wrist. These commonly involve the area immediately next to the radial artery. An accidental injury of this artery with an 18-gauge needle can have disastrous results.
- Initial treatment of a symptomatic ganglion cyst usually requires only cyst aspiration with manual extrusion of remaining contents.
- Treatment success may improve with wrist immobilization for 3 weeks.[5]
- Even with proficient technique, ganglion cysts frequently recur and may require surgical referral for definitive management.

 A video showing a dorsal wrist ganglion cyst aspiration can be found in the companion eBook.

REFERENCES

1. Richman JA, Gelberman RH, Engber WD, et al. Ganglions of the wrist and digits: Results of treatment by aspiration and cyst wall puncture. *J Hand Surg Am*. 1987;12:1041–1043.
2. Dias JJ, Dhukaram V, Kumar P. The natural history of untreated dorsal wrist ganglia and patient reported outcome 6 years after intervention. *J Hand Surg Eur Vol*. 2007;32(5):502–508.
3. Limpaphayom N, Wilairatana V. Randomized controlled trial between surgery and aspiration combined with methylprednisolone acetate injection plus wrist immobilization in the treatment of dorsal carpal ganglion. *J Med Assoc Thai*. 2004;87(12):1513–1517.
4. Zubowicz VN. Management of ganglion cysts of the hand by simple aspiration. *J Hand Surg Am*. 1987;12A(4):618.
5. Gofeld M, Hurdle MF, Agur A. Biceps tendon sheath injection: An anatomical conundrum. *Pain Med*. 2019;20(1):138–142.

Thumb Carpometacarpal Joint

The carpometacarpal (CMC) joint of the thumb is a relatively common injection site for most primary care providers. This joint articulates the trapezium and the first metacarpal bone of the thumb. It is the most common site of osteoarthritis in the hand. The diagnosis of thumb CMC osteoarthritis is based on symptoms of localized pain, tenderness, and instability on physical examination as well as radiographic findings.

Review of the medical literature supports the use of corticosteroid injections for short-term[1,2] and perhaps medium- and long-term treatment.[3,4] Improvement is noted in pain, grip strength, and overall hand function. The therapeutic effect may be more beneficial in mild rather than moderate or severe osteoarthritis.[5,6] Hyaluronic acid viscosupplements may play a future role in this condition.[7,8] Autologous fat transplantation may be an interesting alternative, especially in early-stage osteoarthritis of this joint.[9] Thumb CMC injection accuracy can be significantly improved with ultrasound.[10] Those with persistent and recalcitrant symptoms may benefit from surgical intervention.

Indications	ICD-10 Code
Pain of hand joint	M25.549
CMC joint arthritis, unspecified	M18.10
CMC joint osteoarthritis, primary	M18.10
CMC joint osteoarthritis, posttraumatic	M18.30
CMC joint osteoarthritis, secondary	M18.50

Relevant Anatomy: (Fig. 10.43)

PATIENT POSITION

- Supine on the examination table with the head of the bed elevated 30 degrees.
- The affected wrist is held in pronation.
- The wrist is supported with the placement of chucks pads or towels.
- Rotate the patient's head away from the side that is being injected. This minimizes anxiety and pain perception.

LANDMARKS

1. With the patient supine on the examination table, the clinician stands lateral to the affected hand.
2. Locate the CMC joint by palpating the thumb metacarpal bone in a distal-to-proximal direction. At the proximal aspect of the first metacarpal, there will be tenderness as the examiner's finger passes over, then drops into the CMC joint. This is located between the first metacarpal and the trapezium bone. The patient will report tenderness in this joint.

FIGURE 10.43 ● Dorsal aspect of the left hand.

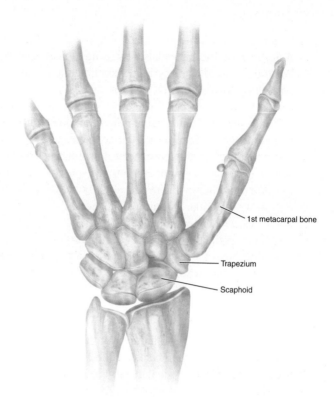

1st metacarpal bone

Trapezium

Scaphoid

3. Mark the injection point directly over the CMC joint.
4. At that site, press firmly on the skin with the retracted tip of a ballpoint pen. This indention represents the entry point for the needle.
5. After the landmarks are identified, the patient should not move the hand or thumb.

ANESTHESIA

• Local anesthesia of the skin using topical vapocoolant spray.

EQUIPMENT

• Topical vapocoolant spray
• 3-mL syringe
• 25-gauge, 5/8-in. needle
• 0.25 mL of 1% mepivacaine without epinephrine
• 0.25 to 0.5 mL of the steroid solution (10 to 20 mg of triamcinolone acetonide)
• One alcohol prep pad
• Two povidone–iodine prep pads
• Sterile gauze pads
• Sterile adhesive bandage
• Nonsterile, clean chucks pad

TECHNIQUE

1. Prep the insertion site with alcohol followed by the povidone–iodine pads.
2. Achieve good local anesthesia by using topical vapocoolant spray.
3. Position the needle and syringe perpendicular to the skin with the needle tip directed posteriorly toward the first CMC joint.
4. Using the no-touch technique, introduce the needle at the insertion site (Fig. 10.44).
5. Advance the needle in a palmar direction down into the joint.
6. Withdraw the plunger of the syringe to ensure that there is no blood return.
7. Inject the mepivacaine/corticosteroid solution as a bolus into the joint. The injected solution should flow smoothly into the space. If increased resistance is encountered, advance or withdraw the needle slightly before attempting further injection.
8. Following injection, withdraw the needle.
9. Apply a sterile adhesive bandage.
10. Instruct the patient to move his or her thumb through its full range of motion. This movement distributes the mepivacaine/corticosteroid solution throughout the CMC joint.
11. Reexamine the CMC joint in 5 min to assess pain relief.

AFTERCARE

- Avoid excessive use of the thumb over the next 2 weeks.
- Consider the use of a thumb spica splint.
- NSAIDs, ice, and/or physical therapy as indicated.
- Consider follow-up examination in 2 weeks.

CPT codes:
- 20600—Arthrocentesis, aspiration and/or injection, small joint or bursa; without ultrasound guidance
- 20604—With ultrasound guidance, with permanent recording and reporting

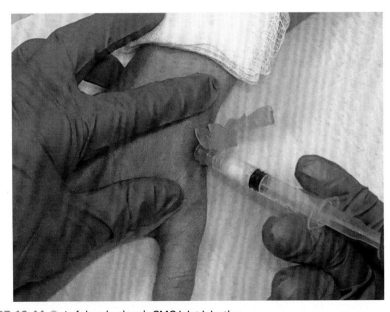

FIGURE 10.44 ● Left hand—thumb CMC joint injection.

PEARLS

- Care should be taken to differentiate this condition from de Quervain's tenosynovitis.
- Applying traction to the thumb in a distal direction will help open up the joint to accommodate the needle.

 A video of a thumb CMC joint injection can be found in the companion eBook.

REFERENCES

1. Maarse W, Watts AC, Bain GI. Medium-term outcome following intra-articular corticosteroid injection in first CMC joint arthritis using fluoroscopy. *Hand Surg.* 2009;14(2–3):99–104.
2. Joshi R. Intraarticular corticosteroid injection for first carpometacarpal osteoarthritis. *J Rheumatol.* 2005;32(7):1305–1306.
3. Swindells MG, Logan AJ, Armstrong DJ, et al. The benefit of radiologically-guided steroid injections for trapeziometacarpal osteoarthritis. *Ann R Coll Surg Engl.* 2010;92(8):680–684.
4. Bahadir C, Onal B, Dayan VY, et al. Comparison of therapeutic effects of sodium hyaluronate and corticosteroid injections on trapeziometacarpal joint osteoarthritis. *Clin Rheumatol.* 2009;28(5):529–533.
5. Meenagh GK, Patton J, Kynes C, et al. A randomised controlled trial of intra-articular corticosteroid injection of the carpometacarpal joint of the thumb in osteoarthritis. *Ann Rheum Dis.* 2004;63(10):1260–1263.
6. Day CS, Gelberman R, Patel AA, et al. Basal joint osteoarthritis of the thumb: A prospective trial of steroid injection and splinting. *J Hand Surg Am.* 2004;29(2):247–251.
7. Bahadir C, Onal B, Dayan VY, et al. Comparison of therapeutic effects of sodium hyaluronate and corticosteroid injections on trapeziometacarpal joint osteoarthritis. *Clin Rheumatol.* 2009;28(5):529–533.
8. Koh SH, Lee SC, Lee WY, et al. Ultrasound-guided intra-articular injection of hyaluronic acid and ketorolac for osteoarthritis of the carpometacarpal joint of the thumb: A retrospective comparative study. *Medicine (Baltimore).* 2019;98(19):e15506.
9. Herold C, Rennekampff HO, Groddeck R, et al. Autologous fat transfer for thumb carpometacarpal joint osteoarthritis: A prospective study. *Plast Reconstr Surg.* 2017;140(2):327–335.
10. To P, McClary KN, Sinclair MK, et al. The accuracy of common hand injections with and without ultrasound: An anatomical study. *Hand (N Y).* 2017;12(6):591–596.

Metacarpophalangeal Joint

Metacarpophalangeal (MCP) joints of the hand are uncommon injection sites for most primary care providers. An MCP joint may become inflamed with osteoarthritis, inflammatory arthritis, or septic arthritis. Intra-articular injections of corticosteroid have shown effectiveness in the short and medium term.[1,2]

A small-diameter needle is employed since this technique is generally only used to inject steroid solution into the MCP joint. There should not be a significant joint effusion to remove.

Indications	ICD-10 Code
MCP joint pain	M25.549
MCP joint arthritis, unspecified	M19.049
MCP joint osteoarthritis, primary	M19.049
MCP joint osteoarthritis, posttraumatic	M19.149
MCP joint osteoarthritis, secondary	M19.249

Relevant Anatomy: (Fig. 10.45)

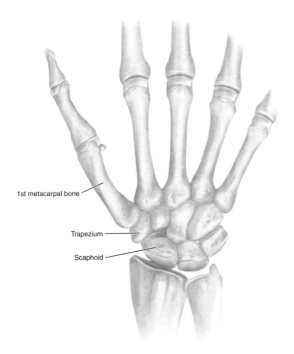

FIGURE 10.45 ● Dorsal aspect of the right hand.

1st metacarpal bone

Trapezium

Scaphoid

PATIENT POSITION

- Supine on the examination table with the head of the bed elevated 30 degrees.
- The affected wrist is held in a neutral position. The wrist is pronated, and the patient is asked to gently flex the MCP joints to make a "loose fist".
- The hand is supported with the placement of chucks pads or towels.
- Rotate the patient's head away from the side that is being injected. This minimizes anxiety and pain perception.

LANDMARKS

1. With the patient supine on the examination table, the clinician stands lateral to the affected hand.
2. Locate the affected MCP joint.
3. The point of entry is located directly over the MCP joint, just radial or ulnar to the extensor tendon.
4. At that site, press firmly on the skin with the retracted tip of a ballpoint pen. This indention represents the entry point for the needle.
5. After the landmarks are identified, the patient should not move the hand or fingers.

ANESTHESIA

- Local anesthesia of the skin using topical vapocoolant spray.

EQUIPMENT

- Topical vapocoolant spray
- 3-mL syringe
- 25-gauge, 5/8-in. needle
- 0.25 mL of 1% mepivacaine without epinephrine
- 0.25 mL of the steroid solution (10 mg of triamcinolone acetonide)
- One alcohol prep pad
- Two povidone–iodine prep pads
- Sterile gauze pads
- Sterile adhesive bandage
- Nonsterile, clean chucks pad

TECHNIQUE

1. Prep the insertion site with alcohol followed by the povidone–iodine pads.
2. Achieve good local anesthesia by using topical vapocoolant spray.
3. Position the needle and syringe perpendicular to the skin with the needle tip directed in a palmar direction toward the MCP joint.
4. Using the no-touch technique, introduce the needle at the insertion site (Fig. 10.46).
5. Advance the needle down into the joint.
6. Withdraw the plunger of the syringe to ensure that there is no blood return.
7. Inject the mepivacaine/corticosteroid solution as a bolus into the joint. The injected solution should flow smoothly into the space. If increased resistance is encountered, advance or withdraw the needle slightly before attempting further injection.

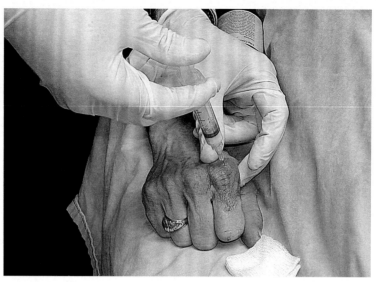

FIGURE 10.46 ● Metacarpophalangeal joint injection.

8. Following injection, withdraw the needle.
9. Apply a sterile adhesive bandage.
10. Instruct the patient to move his or her MCP joint through its full range of motion. This movement distributes the mepivacaine/corticosteroid solution throughout the joint.
11. Reexamine the MCP joint in 5 min to assess pain relief.

AFTERCARE

- Avoid excessive use of the affected hand and finger over the next 2 weeks.
- Consider the use of a volar wrist splint.
- NSAIDs, ice, and/or physical therapy as indicated.
- Consider follow-up examination in 2 weeks.

CPT codes:
- 20600—Arthrocentesis, aspiration and/or injection, small joint or bursa; without ultrasound guidance
- 20604—With ultrasound guidance, with permanent recording and reporting

PEARLS

- Approach the MCP joint dorsally, but avoid inserting the needle through the extensor tendon.
- Applying traction to the affected finger in a distal direction will help open up the joint to accommodate the needle.
- Avoid the development of a subdermal wheal during injection. This indicates the deposition of steroid solution that may cause localized skin atrophy and hypopigmentation.

 A video showing an MCP joint injection can be found in the companion eBook.

REFERENCES

1. Wang S, Wang X, Liu Y, et al. Ultrasound-guided intra-articular triamcinolone acetonide injection for treating refractory small joints arthritis of rheumatoid arthritis patients. *Medicine (Baltimore).* 2019;98(33):e16714.
2. Furtado RNV, Machado FS, Luz KRD, et al. Intra-articular injection with triamcinolone hexacetonide in patients with rheumatoid arthritis: Prospective assessment of goniometry and joint inflammation parameters. *Rev Bras Reumatol Engl Ed.* 2017;57(2):115–121.

Trigger Finger

Stenosing tenosynovitis, or trigger finger, is the term given for tendinosis of the flexor tendons of the digits. This tendinopathy with nodule formation usually occurs as a result of repetitive compression injury. It is more common in patients with diabetes and rheumatoid arthritis. In this disorder, the nodule forms where the flexor tendon passes over the metacarpal head of a finger or, less commonly, the MCP joint of the thumb. Ultrasound studies show associated thickening of the A1 pulley and the volar plate.[3] With flexion of the digit, the nodule passes over the proximal edge of the thickened first annular (A-1) pulley of the tendon sheath and becomes entrapped.

Trigger finger corticosteroid injection is a very common procedure performed by primary care providers. A discrete injection at the site of the palpable, painful nodule offers an effective nonsurgical first-line treatment of this condition.[4,5] A study by Dala-Ali and colleagues showed 66% success rate with a single injection.[6] Dardas further demonstrated 39% long-term response to 2nd and 3rd injections.[7] Ultrasound-guided extra-sheath injection at the level of A1 pulley is as effective as an intra-sheath administration.[8] Therefore, ultrasound is not necessary to conduct this injection. Schultz showed a greater treatment response in patients with mild to moderate symptoms vs. those with moderate to severe disease.[9] Prognostic indicators for recurrence include younger age, insulin-dependent diabetes mellitus,[10] involvement of multiple digits, and a history of other tendinopathies of the upper extremity.[11]

Corticosteroid injection is a viable first-line option for patients presenting with mild to moderate triggering. Initial and repeat injections of trigger fingers should be considered in patients who prefer nonsurgical treatment. For more severe triggering or in patients with poor prognostic indicators, the success of steroid injection is lower and an early referral for surgery should be considered.

Indications	ICD-10 Code
Trigger finger	M65.30
Trigger thumb	M65.319

Relevant Anatomy: (Fig. 10.47)

PATIENT POSITION

- Supine on the examination table with the head of the bed elevated 30 degrees.
- The affected wrist is held in a neutral position and fully supinated.
- The hand is supported with the placement of chucks pads or towels.
- Rotate the patient's head away from the side that is being injected. This minimizes anxiety and pain perception.

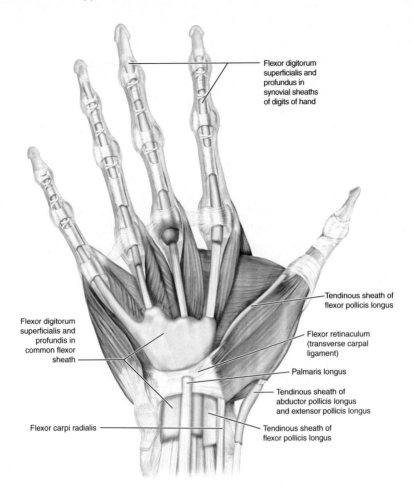

Flexor digitorum
superficialis and
profundus in
synovial sheaths
of digits of hand

Tendinous sheath of
flexor pollicis longus

Flexor digitorum
superficialis and
profundis in
common flexor
sheath

Flexor retinaculum
(transverse carpal
ligament)

Palmaris longus

Tendinous sheath of
abductor pollicis longus
and extensor pollicis longus

Flexor carpi radialis

Tendinous sheath of
flexor pollicis longus

FIGURE 10.47 ● Tendinous (synovial) sheaths of long flexor tendons of the digits. An inflamed nodule is shown in the flexor tendon of the long finger.

LANDMARKS

1. With the patient supine on the examination table, the clinician stands anterior to the affected hand.
2. Identify and mark the tender nodule located in the finger's flexor tendon and its sheath. This should be located over the metatarsal heads.
3. Mark a point 1 cm distal to the nodule.
4. At that site, press firmly on the skin with the retracted tip of a ballpoint pen. This indention represents the entry point for the needle.
5. After the landmarks are identified, the patient should not move the hand or the fingers.

ANESTHESIA

• Local anesthesia of the skin using topical vapocoolant spray.

EQUIPMENT

• Topical vapocoolant spray
• 3-mL syringe

- 25-gauge, 5/8-in. needle
- 0.5 mL of 1% lidocaine without epinephrine
- 0.5 mL of the steroid solution (20 mg of triamcinolone acetonide)[12]
- One alcohol prep pad
- Two povidone–iodine prep pads
- Sterile gauze pads
- Sterile adhesive bandage
- Nonsterile, clean chucks pad

TECHNIQUE

1. Prep the insertion site with alcohol followed by the povidone–iodine pads.
2. Achieve good local anesthesia by using topical vapocoolant spray.
3. Position the needle and syringe at a 45-degree angle to the skin with the needle tip directed proximally at the nodule.
4. Using the no-touch technique, introduce the needle at the insertion site (Fig. 10.48).
5. Advance the needle until the needle tip is located at the tendon nodule. Back up the needle 1 mm.
6. Withdraw the plunger of the syringe to ensure that there is no blood return.
7. Slowly inject the lidocaine/corticosteroid solution around the nodule into the tendon sheath. A subtle bulge in the shape of a sausage may develop in the tendon sheath.
8. If increased resistance is encountered, advance or withdraw the needle slightly before attempting further injection.
9. Following injection, withdraw the needle.
10. Apply a sterile adhesive bandage.
11. Instruct the patient to move his or her finger through its full range of motion. This movement distributes the lidocaine/corticosteroid solution throughout the tenosynovial sheath.
12. Reexamine the hand in 5 min to assess pain relief.

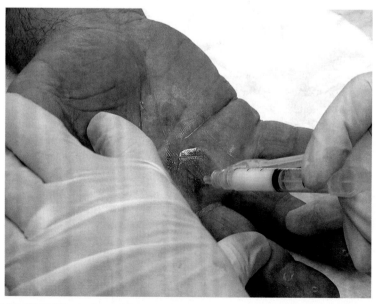

FIGURE 10.48 ● Trigger finger injection.

AFTERCARE

- Avoid excessive repetitive handgrip activities over the next 2 weeks.
- NSAIDs, ice, heat, and/or physical therapy as indicated.
- Consider follow-up examination in 2 weeks.

CPT codes:
- 20550—Injection(s); single tendon sheath, or ligament, aponeurosis
- 76942 (optional)—Ultrasonic guidance for needle placement with imaging supervision and interpretation with permanent recording

PEARLS

- The flexor tendon nodule may be approached from either a distal or a proximal direction. It, however, is easier to perform this injection in a distal-to-proximal direction.

 A video showing a trigger finger injection can be found in the companion eBook.

REFERENCES

1. Tanaka Y, Gotani H, Yano K, et al. Sonographic evaluation of effects of the volar plate on trigger finger. *J Orthop Sci*. 2015;20(6):999–1004.
2. Ma S, Wang C, Li J, et al. Efficacy of corticosteroid injection for treatment of trigger finger: A meta-analysis of randomized controlled trials. *J Invest Surg*. 2019;32(5):433–441.
3. Peters-Veluthamaningal C, van der Windt DA, Winters JC, et al. Corticosteroid injection for trigger finger in adults. *Cochrane Database Syst Rev*. 2009;(1):CD005617.
4. Dala-Ali BM, Nakhdjevani A, Lloyd MA, et al. The efficacy of steroid injection in the treatment of trigger finger. *Clin Orthop Surg*. 2012;4(4):263–268.
5. Dardas AZ, VandenBerg J, Shen T, et al. Long-term effectiveness of repeat corticosteroid injections for trigger finger. *J Hand Surg Am*. 2017;42(4):227–235.
6. Mardani-Kivi M, Karimi-Mobarakeh M, Babaei Jandaghi A, et al. Intra-sheath versus extra-sheath ultrasound guided corticosteroid injection for trigger finger: A triple blinded randomized clinical trial. *Phys Sportsmed*. 2018;46(1):93–97.
7. Shultz KJ, Kittinger JL, Czerwinski WL, et al. Outcomes of corticosteroid treatment for trigger finger by stage. *Plast Reconstr Surg*. 2018;142(4):983–990.
8. Chang CJ, Chang SP, Kao LT, et al. A meta-analysis of corticosteroid injection for trigger digits among patients with diabetes. *Orthopedics*. 2018;41(1):e8–e14.
9. Rozental TD, Zurakowski D, Blazar PE. Trigger finger: prognostic indicators of recurrence following corticosteroid injection. *J Bone Joint Surg Am*. 2008;90(8):1665–1672.
10. Kosiyatrakul A, Loketkrawee W, Luenam S. Different dosages of triamcinolone acetonide injection for the treatment of trigger finger and thumb: A randomized controlled trial. *J Hand Surg Asian Pac Vol*. 2018;23(2):163–169.

Digital Mucous Cyst

Patients frequently present to their primary care providers with digital mucous cysts (a.k.a. digital myxoid cysts). These cysts, which have either a ganglion or myxomatous origin,[1] are located over the dorsal aspect of terminal digits adjacent to the fingernail. They contain clear mucinous fluid. Typically, there is underlying osteoarthritis of the DIP joint. It is believed that a dorsal osteophyte weakens the joint capsule and allows the fluid to track distally. This pedicle terminates at the proximal nailfold where the fluid accumulates in a cystic structure. Over time, the cyst enlarges, applies pressure on the nail matrix, and produces an indention in the fingernail.[2]

Digital mucous cysts are commonly treated similarly to ganglion cysts with recurrent aspiration or needling. Unfortunately, the recurrence rate is high.[3] In a recent review, surgery yielded the highest cure rate among all treatment modalities (95%) compared to sclerotherapy (77%), cryotherapy (72%), corticosteroid injection (61%), and expression of cyst content (39%).[4] If recurrent, they are best managed with surgical excision of the cyst that includes a rotation advancement skin flap.[5]

Indication	ICD-10 Code
Digital mucous cyst	M67.449

Relevant Anatomy: (Figs. 10.49 and 10.50)

PATIENT POSITION

- Supine on the examination table with the head of the bed elevated 30 degrees.
- The wrist is held in pronation.
- The hand is supported with the placement of chucks pads or towels.
- Rotate the patient's head away from the side that is being injected. This minimizes anxiety and pain perception.

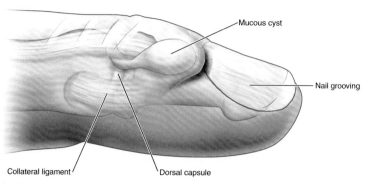

Mucous cyst

Nail grooving

Collateral ligament

Dorsal capsule

FIGURE 10.49 ● Digital mucous cyst.

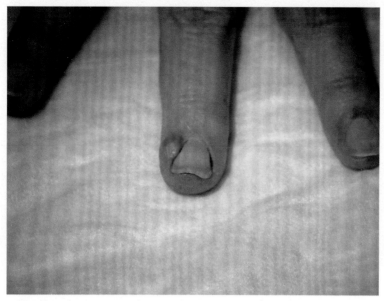

FIGURE 10.50 ● Digital mucous cyst.

LANDMARKS

1. With the patient supine on the examination table, the clinician stands lateral to the affected hand.
2. Identify the cystic structure over the dorsal aspect of the finger, just proximal to the nailfold.
3. The injection point is located directly over the cyst.
4. The patient should not move the hand.

ANESTHESIA

- Digital block anesthesia of the finger using injected 1% lidocaine with epinephrine, as described in Chapter 7.

EQUIPMENT

- Topical vapocoolant spray
- 3-mL syringe
- 18-gauge, 1½-in. needle
- One alcohol prep pad
- Two povidone–iodine prep pads
- Sterile gauze pads
- Sterile adhesive bandage
- Nonsterile, clean chucks pad

TECHNIQUE

1. Achieve good digital block anesthesia.
2. Prep the insertion site with alcohol followed by the povidone–iodine pads.
3. Position the needle and syringe perpendicular to the skin with the needle tip directed to the center of the cyst.

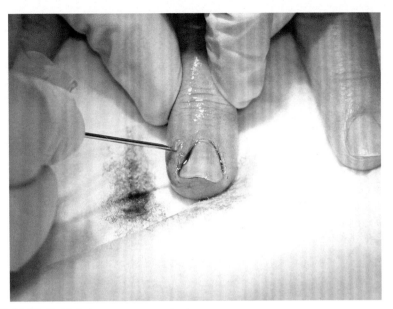

FIGURE 10.51 ● Digital mucous cyst aspiration.

4. Using the no-touch technique, introduce the needle at the insertion site (Fig. 10.51).
5. Advance the needle quickly but carefully into the cyst.
6. Apply suction with the syringe and withdraw the expected small amount of a clear gel.
7. Following aspiration, withdraw the needle.
8. With either the shaft of the needle or gloved fingers, apply firm pressure to the tissues surrounding the punctured cyst. Remove all extruded clear gel with sterile gauze pads (Fig. 10.52).

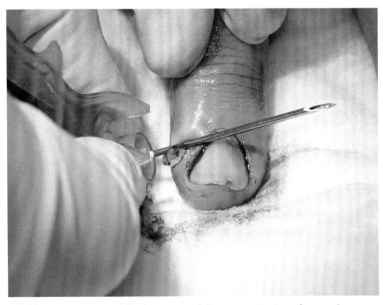

FIGURE 10.52 ● Expression of fluid remaining following aspiration of a ganglion cyst with direct pressure to the surrounding tissues.

9. Injection of steroid solution is often not helpful.
10. Apply a sterile adhesive bandage.

AFTERCARE

- Consider follow-up examination in 2 weeks.

CPT codes:
- 20612—Aspiration and/or injection of ganglion cyst(s) any location
- 76942 (optional)—Ultrasonic guidance for needle placement with imaging supervision and interpretation with permanent recording

PEARLS

- Initial treatment of a symptomatic digital mucous cyst usually requires only cyst aspiration with manual extrusion of remaining contents.
- Cysts that recur despite repeated aspirations/needling have not been found to respond to injections of corticosteroid.
- Even with proficient technique, digital mucous cysts frequently recur and may require early surgical treatment.

 A video showing a digital mucous cyst aspiration can be found in the companion eBook.

REFERENCES

1. Lin YC, Wu YH, Scher RK. Nail changes and association of osteoarthritis in digital myxoid cyst. *Dermatol Surg*. 2008;34(3):364–369.
2. Gofeld M, Hurdle MF, Agur A. Biceps tendon sheath injection: An anatomical conundrum. *Pain Med*. 2019;20(1):138–142.
3. Epstein E. A simple technique for managing digital mucous cysts. *Arch Dermatol*. 1979;115(11):1315–1316.
4. Jabbour S, Kechichian E, Haber R, et al. Management of digital mucous cysts: A systematic review and treatment algorithm. *Int J Dermatol*. 2017;56(7):701–708.
5. Johnson SM, et al. A reliable surgical treatment for digital mucous cysts. *J Hand Surg Eur Vol*. 2014;39(8):856–860.

Hip Joint—Preferred Lateral Approach

James W. McNabb

Hip joint pain from arthritis or capsulitis is a common condition seen in primary care medical practice. This often occurs as a result of osteoarthrosis, posttraumatic arthritis, and rheumatoid arthritis. Patients typically represent the middle-aged and older population. Septic arthritis in children is fortunately now a rare occurrence since the development of the *Haemophilus influenzae* and pneumococcal vaccines. Diagnostic injections using anesthetic (mepivacaine) and therapeutic injections into and around the hip have become an important part of the treatment algorithm for hip pain.

The selection of therapeutic agent and clinical circumstances are of utmost importance. In the case of diagnostic injections, mepivacaine can be used alone. Although corticosteroids have been used for many years, it appears that there may be substantial risk involved. Four main adverse joint findings have been structurally observed in patients after intra-articular corticosteroid injections: accelerated OA progression, subchondral insufficiency fracture, complications of osteonecrosis, and rapid joint destruction, including bone loss.[1,2] Considering these potential risks, it may be preferable to reserve corticosteroid injections for use in patients who present with severe pain,[3] those pending total hip arthroplasty,[4] or patients with malignant hip pain.[5] Promising treatment options for patients with osteoarthritis of the hip include tanezumab,[6] platelet-rich plasma,[7] and hyaluronic acid.[8] More research will be needed to identify the treatment efficacy and safety of these and other therapeutic options.

Because of the joint's perceived inaccessibility, fear of vascular puncture, and the remote risk of avascular necrosis of the head of the femur, primary care providers rarely perform aspiration and corticosteroid injections of the hip joint. In fact, access to this joint is straightforward. Anterior and lateral approaches have been described. The landmark-guided anterior approach has success rates of 60% to 93%.[9,10] The lateral approach also has good success rates of about 80%.[1,11] However, the anterior approach is associated with significantly more risk to the femoral artery and femoral nerve than is the lateral approach.[1,3] For this reason, the lateral approach is preferred in the setting where image guidance is not available. In both cases, the use of ultrasound to guide needle placement significantly improves the safety and success rates of hip injections.[12,13] Guidance is particularly important in obese patients, patients with advanced osteoarthritis with no joint space, and those with flexion deformity.[14]

Indications	ICD-10 Code
Hip joint pain	M25.559
Hip capsulitis	M76.899
Hip arthritis, unspecified	M16.10
Hip osteoarthritis, primary	M16.10
Hip osteoarthritis, posttraumatic	M16.50
Hip osteoarthritis, secondary	M16.7

Relevant Anatomy: (Fig. 11.1)

PATIENT POSITION

- Lying on the examination table in the lateral decubitus position on the unaffected hip

LANDMARKS

1. With the patient lying on the examination table in the lateral decubitus position on the unaffected hip, the clinician stands posterior to the affected hip.
2. Identify the trochanter of the femur.
3. Mark a point 1 cm proximal to the tip of the greater trochanter.

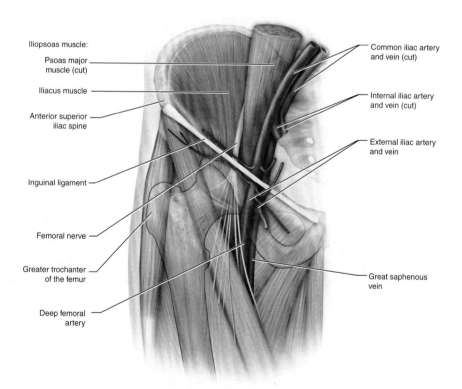

Iliopsoas muscle:
Psoas major muscle (cut)
Iliacus muscle
Anterior superior iliac spine
Inguinal ligament
Femoral nerve
Greater trochanter of the femur
Deep femoral artery

Common iliac artery and vein (cut)
Internal iliac artery and vein (cut)
External iliac artery and vein
Great saphenous vein

FIGURE 11.1 ● Right lateral hip and femoral triangle. (Modified from Gest TR. *Lippincott Atlas of Anatomy*, 2nd Ed. Philadelphia, PA: Wolters Kluwer, 2019.)

4. (Optional) Use ultrasound to image the hip joint.
5. At that site, press firmly on the skin with the retracted tip of a ballpoint pen. This indention represents the entry point for the needle.
6. After the landmarks are identified, the patient should not move the hip.

ANESTHESIA

- Local anesthesia of the skin using topical vapocoolant spray

EQUIPMENT

- Topical vapocoolant spray
- 20-mL syringe—for aspiration
- 3-mL syringe—for the injection of corticosteroid/local anesthetic mixture
- 25-gauge, 2-in. needle in thin individuals. Otherwise, use a 25-gauge, 3½ in. spinal needle (for injections only)
- 20-gauge, 2-in. needle in thin individuals. Otherwise, use a 20-gauge, 3½-in. spinal needle (for aspirations and injections)
- 1 mL of 1% mepivacaine without epinephrine
- 1 mL of the steroid solution (40 mg of triamcinolone acetonide)
- One alcohol prep pad
- Two povidone–iodine prep pads
- Sterile gauze pads
- Sterile adhesive bandage
- Nonsterile, clean chucks pad

TECHNIQUE

1. (Optional) Use an ultrasound to image the hip joint using an adjacent but separate acoustic window. This allows imaging separate from the injection site so that there is no contamination from the ultrasound gel. Alternatively, the entire site may be prepped in an aseptic manner and sterile ultrasound gel utilized.
2. Prep the insertion site with alcohol followed by the povidone–iodine pads.
3. Achieve good local anesthesia by using topical vapocoolant spray.
4. Position the needle and syringe perpendicular to the skin with the tip of the needle directed medially toward the hip joint.
5. Using the no-touch technique, introduce the needle at the insertion site (Fig. 11.2).
6. Advance the needle toward the hip joint until the needle tip contacts the femoral neck/head. Back up the needle 1 to 2 mm.
7. Withdraw the plunger of the syringe to ensure that there is no blood return.
8. Inject the mepivacaine/corticosteroid solution as a bolus into the hip joint capsule. The injected solution should flow smoothly into the space. If increased resistance is encountered, advance or withdraw the needle slightly before attempting further injection.
9. Following injection, withdraw the needle.
10. Apply a sterile adhesive bandage.
11. Instruct the patient to move his or her hip through its full range of motion. This movement distributes the mepivacaine/corticosteroid solution throughout the hip joint capsule.
12. Reexamine the hip in 5 min to assess pain relief.

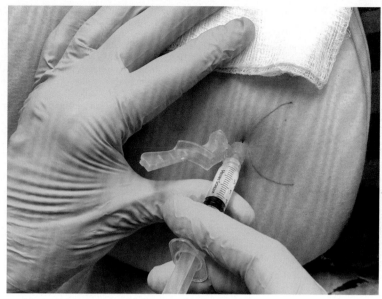

FIGURE 11.2 ● Hip joint injection—preferred lateral approach.

AFTERCARE

- Avoid excessive weight bearing and hip movement over the next 2 weeks.
- Nonsteroidal anti-inflammatory drugs (NSAIDs), and/or physical therapy as indicated.
- Consider follow-up examination in 2 weeks.

CPT codes:
- 20610—Arthrocentesis, aspiration and/or injection, major joint or bursa; without ultrasound guidance
- 20611—With ultrasound guidance, with permanent recording and reporting

PEARLS

- Guidance is particularly important in obese patients, patients with advanced osteoarthritis with no joint space, and those with flexion deformity.[14]

 A video showing a hip joint injection can be found in the companion eBook.

REFERENCES

1. Kompel AJ, Roemer FW, Murakami AM, et al. Intra-articular corticosteroid injections in the hip and knee: perhaps not as safe as we thought? *Radiology*. 2019;293(3):656–663.
2. Simeone FJ, Vicentini JRT, Bredella MA, et al. Are patients more likely to have hip osteoarthritis progression and femoral head collapse after hip steroid/anesthetic injections? A retrospective observational study. *Skeletal Radiol*. 2019;48(9):1417–1426.
3. van Middelkoop M, Arden NK, Atchia I, et al. The OA Trial Bank: meta-analysis of individual patient data from knee and hip osteoarthritis trials show that patients with severe pain exhibit greater benefit from intra-articular glucocorticoids. *Osteoarthritis Cartilage*. 2016;24(7):1143–1152.
4. Pereira LC, Kerr J, Jolles BM. Intra-articular steroid injection for osteoarthritis of the hip prior to total hip arthroplasty: is it safe? a systematic review. *Bone Joint J*. 2016;98-B(8):1027–1035.
5. Rakesh N, Magram YC, Shah JM, et al. Localized corticosteroid injections for malignant joint pain in the oncologic population: a case series. *A A Pract*. 2019;13(1):27–30.

6. Schnitzer TJ, Easton R, Pang S, et al. Effect of Tanezumab on joint pain, physical function, and patient global assessment of osteoarthritis among patients with osteoarthritis of the hip or knee: a randomized clinical trial. *JAMA*. 2019;322(1):37–48.

7. De Luigi AJ, Blatz D, Karam C, et al. Use of platelet-rich plasma for the treatment of acetabular labral tear of the hip: a Pilot study. *Am J Phys Med Rehabil*. 2019;98(11):1010–1017.

8. Clementi D, D'Ambrosi R, Bertocco P, et al. Efficacy of a single intra-articular injection of ultra-high molecular weight hyaluronic acid for hip osteoarthritis: a randomized controlled study. *Eur J Orthop Surg Traumatol*. 2018;28(5):915–922.

9. Leopold SS, Battista V, Oliverio JA. Safety and efficacy of intraarticular hip injection using anatomic landmarks. *Clin Orthop Relat Res*. 2001;(391):192–197.

10. Mei-Dan O, McConkey MO, Petersen B, et al. The anterior approach for a non-image-guided intra-articular hip injection. *Arthroscopy*. 2013;29(6):1025–1033.

11. Ziv YB, Kardosh R, Debi R, et al. An inexpensive and accurate method for hip injections without the use of imaging. *J Clin Rheumatol*. 2009;15(3):103–105.

12. Gilliland CA, Salazar LD, Borchers JR. Ultrasound versus anatomic guidance for intra-articular and peri-articular injection: a systematic review. *Phys Sportsmed*. 2011;39(3):121–131.

13. Lynch TS, Oshlag BL, Bottiglieri TS, et al. Ultrasound-guided hip injections. *J Am Acad Orthop Surg*. 2019;27(10):e451–e461.

14. Kurup H, Ward P. Do we need radiological guidance for hip joint injections? *Acta Orthop Belg*. 2010;76(2):205–207.

Hip Joint—Anterior Approach

Hip joint pain from arthritis or capsulitis is a common condition seen in primary care medical practice. This often occurs as a result of osteoarthrosis, posttraumatic arthritis, and rheumatoid arthritis. Patients typically represent the middle-aged and older population. Septic arthritis in children is fortunately now a rare occurrence since the development of the *H. influenzae* and pneumococcal vaccines. Diagnostic injections using anesthetic (mepivacaine) and therapeutic injections into and around the hip have become an important part of the treatment algorithm for hip pain.

Because of the joint's perceived inaccessibility, fear of vascular puncture, and the remote risk of avascular necrosis of the head of the femur, primary care providers rarely perform aspiration and corticosteroid injections of the hip joint. In fact, access to this joint is straightforward. Anterior and lateral approaches have been described. The landmark-guided anterior approach has success rates of 60% to 93%.[1,2] The lateral approach also has good success rates of about 80%.[3,4] However, the anterior approach is associated with significantly more risk to the femoral artery and femoral nerve than is the lateral approach.[3,5] For this reason, the lateral approach is preferred in the setting where image guidance is not available. In both cases, the use of ultrasound to guide needle placement significantly improves the safety and success rates of hip injections.[6,7] Guidance is particularly important in obese patients, patients with advanced osteoarthritis with no joint space, and those with flexion deformity.[8]

Please read additional details concerning hip joint injection that are presented in the preceding chapter.

Indications	ICD-10 Code
Hip joint pain	M25.559
Hip capsulitis	M76.899
Hip arthritis, unspecified	M16.10
Hip osteoarthritis, primary	M16.10
Hip osteoarthritis, posttraumatic	M16.50
Hip osteoarthritis, secondary	M16.7

Relevant Anatomy: (Fig. 11.3)

PATIENT POSITION

- Supine on the examination table with the head of the bed slightly elevated

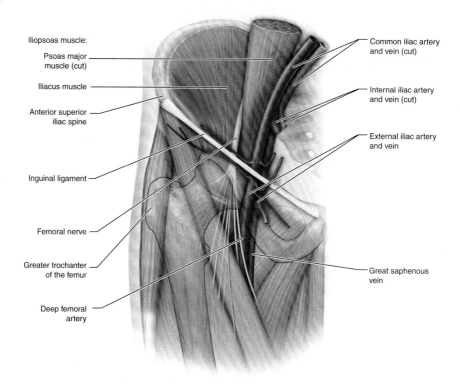

FIGURE 11.3 ● Right anterior hip and femoral triangle. (Modified from Gest TR. *Lippincott Atlas of Anatomy*, 2nd Ed. Philadelphia, PA: Wolters Kluwer, 2019.)

LANDMARKS

1. With the patient supine on the examination table, the clinician stands lateral to the affected hip.
2. Over the anterior aspect of the hip, identify the point at the intersection of two perpendicular lines. The first is distal and sagittal from the anterior superior iliac spine, and the second line is transverse from the proximal tip of the greater trochanter. This point will be located about 3 cm lateral to the femoral artery. Mark that spot, which is directly over the hip joint.
3. (Optional) Use ultrasound to image the hip joint.
4. At that site, press firmly on the skin with the retracted tip of a ballpoint pen. This indention represents the entry point for the needle.
5. After the landmarks are identified, the patient should not move the hip.

ANESTHESIA

- Local anesthesia of the skin using topical vapocoolant spray

EQUIPMENT

- Topical vapocoolant spray
- 20-mL syringe—for aspiration
- 3-mL syringe—for the injection of corticosteroid/local anesthetic mixture

- 25-gauge, 1½-in. needle in thin individuals. Otherwise, use a 25-gauge, 3½-in. needle (for injections only)
- 20-gauge, 1½-in. needle in thin individuals. Otherwise, use a 20-gauge, 3½-in. needle (for aspirations and injections)
- 1 mL of 1% mepivacaine without epinephrine
- 1 mL of the steroid solution (40 mg of triamcinolone acetonide)
- One alcohol prep pad
- Two povidone–iodine prep pads
- Sterile gauze pads
- Sterile adhesive bandage
- Nonsterile, clean chucks pad

TECHNIQUE

1. (Optional) Use an ultrasound to image the hip joint using an adjacent but separate acoustic window. This allows imaging separate from the injection site so that there is no contamination from the ultrasound gel. Alternatively, the entire site may be prepped in an aseptic manner and sterile ultrasound gel utilized.
2. Prep the insertion site with alcohol followed by the povidone–iodine pads.
3. Achieve good local anesthesia by using topical vapocoolant spray.
4. Position the needle and syringe perpendicular to the skin with the tip of the needle directed posteriorly toward the hip joint.
5. Using the no-touch technique, introduce the needle at the insertion site (Fig. 11.4).
6. Advance the needle toward the hip joint until the needle tip contacts the junction of the femoral neck and femoral head. Back up the needle 1 to 2 mm.
7. Withdraw the plunger of the syringe to ensure that there is no blood return.
8. Inject the mepivacaine/corticosteroid solution as a bolus into the hip joint capsule. The injected solution should flow smoothly into the space. If increased resistance is encountered, advance or withdraw the needle slightly before attempting further injection.

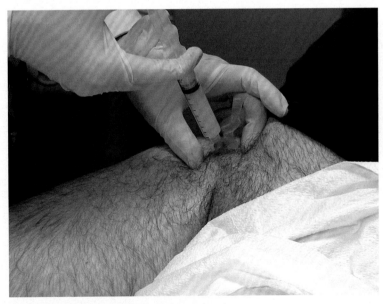

FIGURE 11.4 ● Hip joint injection—anterior approach.

9. Following injection, withdraw the needle.
10. Apply a sterile adhesive bandage.
11. Instruct the patient to move his or her hip through its full range of motion. This movement distributes the mepivacaine/corticosteroid solution throughout the hip joint capsule.
12. Reexamine the hip in 5 min to assess pain relief.

AFTERCARE

- Avoid excessive weight bearing and hip movement over the next 2 weeks.
- NSAIDs and/or physical therapy as indicated.
- Consider follow-up examination in 2 weeks.

CPT codes:
- 20610—Arthrocentesis, aspiration and/or injection, major joint or bursa; without ultrasound guidance
- 20611—With ultrasound guidance, with permanent recording and reporting

PEARLS

- Guidance is particularly important in obese patients, patients with advanced osteoarthritis with no joint space, and those with flexion deformity.[9]

 A video showing a hip joint injection can be found in the companion eBook.

REFERENCES

1. Leopold SS, Battista V, Oliverio JA. Safety and efficacy of intraarticular hip injection using anatomic landmarks. *Clin Orthop Relat Res.* 2001;(391):192–197.
2. Mei-Dan O, McConkey MO, Petersen B, et al. The anterior approach for a non-image-guided intra-articular hip injection. *Arthroscopy.* 2013;29(6):1025–1033.
3. Kompel AJ, Roemer FW, Murakami AM, et al. Intra-articular corticosteroid injections in the hip and knee: perhaps not as safe as we thought? *Radiology.* 2019;293(3):656–663.
4. Ziv YB, Kardosh R, Debi R, et al. An inexpensive and accurate method for hip injections without the use of imaging. *J Clin Rheumatol.* 2009;15(3):103–105.
5. van Middelkoop M, Arden NK, Atchia I, et al. The OA Trial Bank: meta-analysis of individual patient data from knee and hip osteoarthritis trials show that patients with severe pain exhibit greater benefit from intra-articular glucocorticoids. *Osteoarthritis Cartilage.* 2016;24(7):1143–1152.
6. Gilliland CA, Salazar LD, Borchers JR. Ultrasound versus anatomic guidance for intra-articular and peri-articular injection: a systematic review. *Phys Sportsmed.* 2011;39(3):121–131.
7. Lynch TS, Oshlag BL, Bottiglieri TS, et al. Ultrasound-guided hip injections. *J Am Acad Orthop Surg.* 2019;27(10):e451–e461.
8. Kurup H, Ward P. Do we need radiological guidance for hip joint injections? *Acta Orthop Belg.* 2010;76(2):205–207.
9. Schnitzer TJ, Easton R, Pang S, et al. Effect of Tanezumab on joint pain, physical function, and patient global assessment of osteoarthritis among patients with osteoarthritis of the hip or knee: a randomized clinical trial. *JAMA.* 2019;322(1):37–48.

Piriformis Syndrome

Patients uncommonly present to the primary care office for the evaluation of piriformis syndrome. This is an often overlooked disorder attributed to 6% to 8% of patients presenting with low back and leg pain. It is presumed to be a compression neuropathy that occurs when an abnormally tight piriformis muscle compresses the sciatic nerve. Piriformis syndrome may occur following trauma, vigorous physical activity, developmental abnormalities, or tumor or after total hip arthroplasty. There is a common pathological end pathway involving hypertrophy, spasm, contracture, inflammation, and scarring of the piriformis muscle, leading to impingement of the sciatic nerve. The diagnosis may be made by excluding other causes of sciatica, palpating an abnormally tight and tender piriformis muscle, and the demonstration of a positive figure-four test. Treatment consists of stretching, physical therapy, local corticosteroid injection,[1,2] botulinum toxin injection,[3,4] or hydrodissection.[5] Image guidance improves injection success rates.[6,7] Recalcitrant lesions require surgical release.

Indication	ICD-10 Code
Piriformis syndrome	G57.00

Relevant Anatomy: (Fig. 11.5)

PATIENT POSITION

- Standing up with the back in forward flexion and hands/arms supported by the examination table.
- Alternatively, this injection may be performed with the patient lying in the lateral decubitus position on the examination table.

LANDMARKS

1. With the patient standing up with the back in forward flexion and hands/arms supported by the examination table, the clinician stands directly behind the patient.
2. Locate the S2 median sacral crest and the lateral aspect of the femoral trochanter.
3. Identify the point of maximal tenderness over the piriformis muscle. This will be one-third to one-half of the distance from the sacral crest.
4. At that site, press firmly on the skin with the retracted tip of a ballpoint pen. This indention represents the entry point for the needle.
5. After the landmarks are identified, the patient should not move.

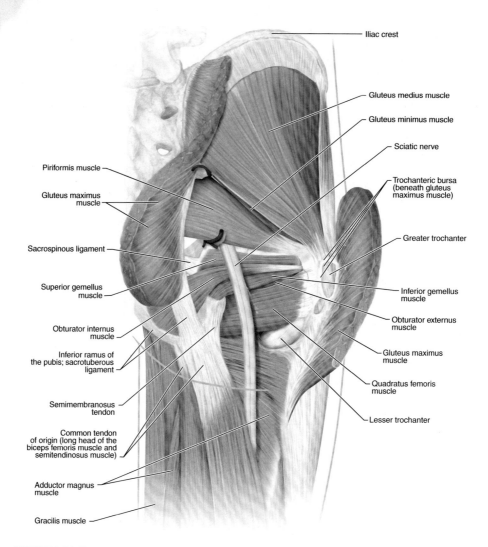

FIGURE 11.5 ● Middle and deep gluteal muscles and sciatic nerve. (Modified from Gest TR. *Lippincott Atlas of Anatomy*, 2nd Ed. Philadelphia, PA: Wolters Kluwer, 2019.)

ANESTHESIA

- Local anesthesia of the skin with a topical vapocoolant spray may be used, but it is not necessary in most patients.

EQUIPMENT

- Topical vapocoolant spray
- 3-mL syringe
- 25-gauge, 2-in. needle
- 1 mL of 1% lidocaine without epinephrine
- 1 mL of the steroid solution (40 mg of triamcinolone acetonide)
- One alcohol prep pad
- Two povidone–iodine prep pads
- Sterile gauze pads
- Sterile adhesive bandage

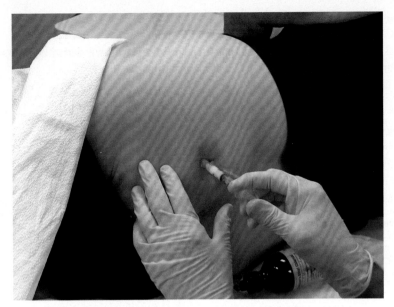

FIGURE 11.6 ● Piriformis muscle injection.

TECHNIQUE

1. Prep the insertion site with alcohol followed by the povidone–iodine pads.
2. Achieve good local anesthesia by using a topical vapocoolant spray.
3. Position the needle and syringe perpendicular to the skin with the tip of the needle directed anteriorly.
4. Using the no-touch technique, introduce the needle at the insertion site (Fig. 11.6).
5. Advance the needle until you feel that there is an increase in resistance in the muscle due to spasm and/or fibrosis. If the patient experiences sudden shooting pain down the leg, the sciatic nerve has been contacted. Back up the needle a few millimeters until there is no pain.
6. Withdraw the plunger of the syringe to ensure that there is no blood return.
7. Inject the lidocaine/corticosteroid solution into the soft tissues. The injected solution should flow smoothly. If increased resistance is encountered, advance or withdraw the needle slightly before attempting further injection.
8. Following injection, withdraw the needle.
9. Apply a sterile adhesive bandage.
10. Instruct the patient to move his or her hip through its full range of motion. This movement distributes the lidocaine/corticosteroid solution throughout the course of the piriformis muscle.
11. Reexamine the piriformis muscle in 5 min to assess pain relief.

AFTERCARE

- Avoid excessive use of the affected hip over the next 2 weeks.
- NSAIDs, ice, and/or physical therapy as indicated.
- Consider follow-up examination in 2 weeks.

CPT codes:

- 20552—Injection of single or multiple trigger point(s), 1 or 2 muscles
- 76942 (optional)—Ultrasonic guidance for needle placement with imaging supervision and interpretation with permanent recording

 A video showing a piriformis injection can be found in the companion eBook.

REFERENCES

1. Terlemez R, Erçalık T. Effect of piriformis injection on neuropathic pain. *Agri.* 2019;31(4):178–182.
2. Masala S, Crusco S, Meschini A, et al. Piriformis syndrome: long-term follow-up in patients treated with percutaneous injection of anesthetic and corticosteroid under CT guidance. *Cardiovasc Intervent Radiol.* 2012;35(2):375–382.
3. Waseem Z, Boulias C, Gordon A, et al. Botulinum toxin injections for low-back pain and sciatica. *Cochrane Database Syst Rev.* 2011;(1):CD008257.
4. Santamato A, Micello MF, Valeno G, et al. Ultrasound-guided injection of botulinum toxin type A for piriformis muscle syndrome: a case report and review of the literature. *Toxins (Basel).* 2015;7(8):3045–3056.
5. Burke CJ, Walter WR, Adler RS. Targeted ultrasound-guided perineural hydrodissection of the sciatic nerve for the treatment of piriformis syndrome. *Ultrasound Q.* 2019;35(2):125–129.
6. Kompel AJ, Roemer FW, Murakami AM, et al. Intra-articular corticosteroid injections in the hip and knee: perhaps not as safe as we thought? *Radiology.* 2019;293(3):656–663.
7. Chang KV, Wu WT, Lew HL, et al. Ultrasound imaging and guided injection for the lateral and posterior hip. *Am J Phys Med Rehabil.* 2018;97(4):285–291.

Hamstring Tendon and Ischial Bursa

Patients occasionally present to the primary care office for the evaluation and treatment of pain over the buttock and posterior thigh upon extension of the hip and flexion of the lower leg. The semimembranosus, semitendinosus, and biceps femoris muscles/tendons span between the ischial tuberosity to the proximal aspect of the tibia and fibula. Hamstring injuries almost always occur at the proximal myotendinous junction. Acute injury or chronic overuse may cause tendonitis, tendinopathy, or disruption of the hamstring tendons. The biceps femoris is most commonly injured. The main presenting complaint is pain in the lower gluteal or ischial region that usually radiates along the hamstrings in the posterior thigh. The pain increases with direct palpation over the ischial tuberosity and proximal tendons, passive stretching, and resistance to contraction. Proximal hamstring tendinopathy pain and dysfunction are often long-standing and limit athletic and daily activities. Imaging with either ultrasound or MRI may be required to delineate the anatomic pathology and extent of injury.

In chronic tendinopathy, treatment is often lengthy and difficult. Physical therapy is the cornerstone of treatment. Zissen showed that 50% of patients receiving corticosteroid injections had symptomatic improvement lasting longer than 1 month and 24% of patients had symptom relief for more than 6 months.[1] Ultrasound guidance improves the accuracy and efficacy of this injection.[2] Intratendinous injections of platelet-rich plasma[3,4] and percutaneous needle fenestration[5] demonstrate improvement in pain and function. When refractory to conservative management, hamstring injuries may be treated with surgical débridement and reattachment.[6]

Indications	ICD-10 Code
Hamstring tendonitis	M76.899
Enthesopathy of the hip	M76.899
Ischial bursitis	M70.70

Relevant Anatomy: (Fig. 11.7)

PATIENT POSITION

- Lying prone on the examination table.
- The hip will be in a position of extension.

LANDMARKS

1. With the patient lying prone on the examination table, the clinician stands lateral to the opposite hip.

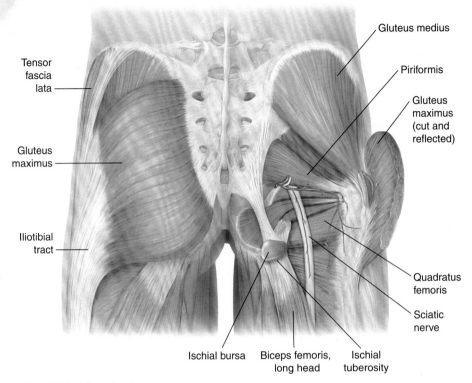

FIGURE 11.7 ● Ischial bursa.

2. Locate the ischial tuberosity and firmly palpate it with the patient extending the hip until determining the origin of the hamstring tendons.
3. Determine the site of maximal tenderness over the ischial tuberosity and origin of the hamstring tendons, and mark it with an ink pen.
4. At that site, press firmly on the skin with the retracted tip of a ballpoint pen. This indention represents the entry point for the area.
5. After the landmarks are identified, the patient should not move the hip.

ANESTHESIA

• Local anesthesia of the skin using a topical vapocoolant spray

EQUIPMENT

• Topical vapocoolant spray
• 3-mL syringe
• 25-gauge, 2-in. needle
• 1 mL of 1% lidocaine without epinephrine
• 1 mL of the steroid solution (40 mg of triamcinolone acetonide)
• One alcohol prep pad
• Two povidone–iodine prep pads
• Sterile gauze pads
• Sterile adhesive bandage

TECHNIQUE

1. Prep the insertion site with alcohol followed by the povidone–iodine pads.
2. Achieve good local anesthesia by using a topical vapocoolant spray.
3. Position the needle and syringe perpendicular to the skin with the tip of the needle directed anteriorly.
4. Using the no-touch technique, introduce the needle at the insertion site (Fig. 11.8).
5. Advance the needle so that it is positioned at the junction of the ischial tuberosity and tendons, but not in the substance of the tendons.
6. Withdraw the plunger of the syringe to ensure that there is no blood return.
7. Inject the lidocaine/corticosteroid solution as a bolus around the hamstring tendons and the bursa. The injected solution should flow smoothly into the space. If increased resistance is encountered, advance or withdraw the needle slightly before attempting further injection.
8. Following injection, withdraw the needle.
9. Apply a sterile adhesive bandage.
10. Instruct the patient to massage the area and flex/extend the hip. This movement distributes the lidocaine/corticosteroid solution along the hamstring tendons and ischial bursa.
11. Reexamine the affected area in 5 min to assess pain relief.

AFTERCARE

- Avoid excessive use of the hip and thigh—hip extension and lower leg flexion (especially running/sprinting) over the next 2 weeks.
- Begin a program of physical therapy.
- NSAIDs, ice, and heat as indicated.
- Consider follow-up examination in 2 weeks.

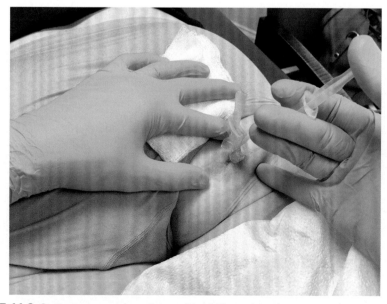

FIGURE 11.8 ● Hamstring tendon origin and ischial bursa injection.

CPT codes:

- 20551—Injection; single tendon origin/insertion—for hamstring tendonitis.
- 20610—Arthrocentesis, aspiration and/or injection, major joint or bursa; without ultrasound guidance—for ischial bursitis
- 76942 (optional)—Ultrasonic guidance for needle placement with imaging supervision and interpretation with permanent recording

 A video showing a hamstring tendon—ischial bursa injection can be found in the companion eBook.

REFERENCES

1. Zissen MH, Wallace G, Stevens KJ, et al. High hamstring tendinopathy: MRI and ultrasound imaging and therapeutic efficacy of percutaneous corticosteroid injection. *AJR Am J Roentgenol.* 2010;195(4):993–998.
2. Chang KV, Wu WT, Lew HL, et al. Ultrasound imaging and guided injection for the lateral and posterior hip. *Am J Phys Med Rehabil.* 2018;97(4):285–291.
3. Davenport KL, Campos JS, Nguyen J, et al. Ultrasound-guided intratendinous injections with platelet-rich plasma or autologous whole blood for treatment of proximal hamstring tendinopathy: a double-blind randomized controlled trial. *J Ultrasound Med.* 2015;34(8):1455–1463.
4. Wetzel RJ, Patel RM, Terry MA. Platelet-rich plasma as an effective treatment for proximal hamstring injuries. *Orthopedics.* 2013;36(1):e64–e70.
5. Jacobson JA, Rubin J, Yablon CM, et al. Ultrasound-guided fenestration of tendons about the hip and pelvis: clinical outcomes. *J Ultrasound Med.* 2015;34(11):2029–2035.
6. Startzman AN, Fowler O, Carreira D. Proximal hamstring tendinosis and partial ruptures. *Orthopedics.* 2017;40(4):e574–e582.

Meralgia Paresthetica

Patients occasionally present to their primary care provider with burning pain, numbness, or paresthesias over the lateral aspect of the thigh. Meralgia paresthetica is most commonly caused by a compression neuropathy of the lateral femoral cutaneous nerve (a pure sensory nerve) as it passes through a tunnel formed by the lateral attachment of the inguinal ligament and the anterior superior iliac spine. It is more common in patients with diabetes and those who are obese. Percussion of the nerve over this tunnel just anterior to the anterior iliac spine or extending the thigh posteriorly may reproduce or worsen the symptoms. Conservative management includes relieving chronic pressure over the nerve, weight loss, and antineuropathic medications. Corticosteroid injections at the site of nerve compression demonstrate high success rates when guided by ultrasound.[1,2] Other treatment options include ultrasound-guided hydrodissection of the nerve,[3] and surgical decompression[4] or nerve transection.

Indication	ICD-10 Code
Meralgia paresthetica	G57.10

Relevant Anatomy: (Figs. 11.9 and 11.10)

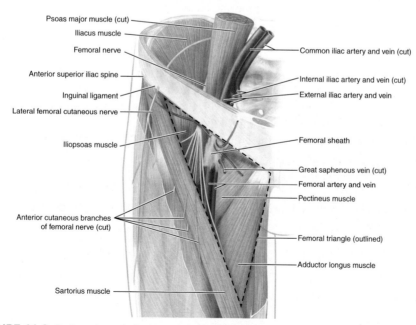

FIGURE 11.9 ● Anterior right hip neurovascular structures. (Modified from Gest TR. *Lippincott Atlas of Anatomy*, 2nd Ed. Philadelphia, PA: Wolters Kluwer, 2019.)

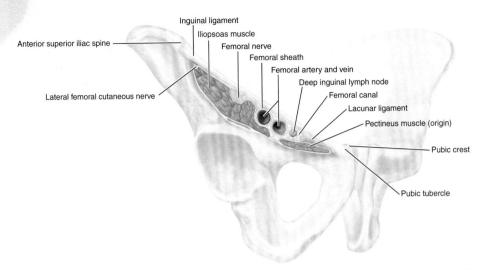

FIGURE 11.10 ● Section through the right femoral sheath. (From Gest TR. *Lippincott Atlas of Anatomy*, 2nd Ed. Philadelphia, PA: Wolters Kluwer, 2019.)

PATIENT POSITION

- Lying supine on the examination table.
- Rotate the patient's head away from the side that is being injected. This minimizes anxiety and pain perception.

LANDMARKS

1. With the patient supine on the examination table, the clinician stands lateral to the affected hip.
2. Find the anterior superior iliac spine and the pubic bone.
3. Firmly palpate the inguinal ligament that connects these two structures.
4. The lateral femoral cutaneous nerve of the thigh traverses the inguinal ligament about 2 cm inferior and medial to the anterior superior iliac spine under the inguinal ligament. Tap over this area or press firmly until discomfort is elicited. Mark that spot with ink.
5. At that site, press firmly on the skin with the retracted tip of a ballpoint pen. This indention represents the entry point for the needle.
6. After the landmarks are identified, the patient should not move the hip or leg.

ANESTHESIA

- Local anesthesia of the skin with a topical vapocoolant spray may be used, but it is not necessary in most patients.

EQUIPMENT

- Topical vapocoolant spray
- 3-mL syringe
- 25-gauge, 1½-in. needle
- 2 mL of 1% lidocaine without epinephrine

- 1 mL of the steroid solution (40 mg of triamcinolone acetonide)
- One alcohol prep pad
- Two povidone–iodine prep pads
- Sterile gauze pads
- Sterile adhesive bandage

TECHNIQUE

1. Prep the insertion site with alcohol followed by the povidone–iodine pads.
2. Achieve good local anesthesia by using a topical vapocoolant spray.
3. Position the needle and syringe perpendicular to the skin with the tip of the needle directed posteriorly.
4. Using the no-touch technique, introduce the needle at the insertion site (Fig. 11.11).
5. Advance the needle 2 to 3 cm until the needle tip is located under the inguinal ligament.
6. Withdraw the plunger to ensure that there is no blood return.
7. Inject the lidocaine/corticosteroid solution as a bolus into the area. The injected solution should flow smoothly into the space. If increased resistance is encountered, advance or withdraw the needle slightly before attempting further injection.
8. Following injection, withdraw the needle.
9. Apply a sterile adhesive bandage.
10. Instruct the patient to move his or her hip through its full range of motion. This movement distributes the lidocaine/corticosteroid solution throughout the area.

AFTERCARE

- Treatment is directed at relieving the compression and usually consists of wearing looser clothing or losing weight.
- Consider follow-up examination in 2 weeks.

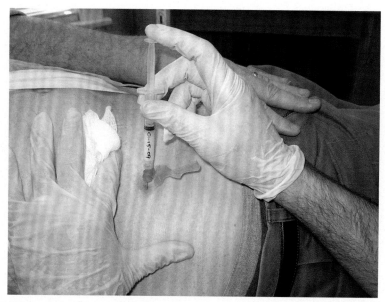

FIGURE 11.11 ● Meralgia paresthetica injection.

CPT codes:
- 64450—Injection, nerve block, therapeutic, other peripheral nerve or branch
- 76942 (optional)—Ultrasonic guidance for needle placement with imaging supervision and interpretation with permanent recording

 A video showing a meralgia paresthetica injection can be found in the companion eBook.

REFERENCES

1. Hurdle MF, Weingarten TN, Crisostomo RA, et al. Ultrasound-guided blockade of the lateral femoral cutaneous nerve: technical description and review of 10 cases. *Arch Phys Med Rehabil.* 2007;88(10):1362–1364.
2. Tagliafico A, Serafini G, Lacelli F, et al. Ultrasound-guided treatment of meralgia paresthetica (lateral femoral cutaneous neuropathy): technical description and results of treatment in 20 consecutive patients. *J Ultrasound Med.* 2011;30(10):1341–1346.
3. Mulvaney SW. Ultrasound-guided percutaneous neuroplasty of the lateral femoral cutaneous nerve for the treatment of meralgia paresthetica: a case report and description of a new ultrasound-guided technique. *Curr Sports Med Rep.* 2011;10(2):99–104.
4. Siu TL, Chandran KN. Neurolysis for meralgia paresthetica: an operative series of 45 cases. *Surg Neurol.* 2005;63(1):19–23.

Greater Trochanteric Pain Syndrome

Greater trochanteric pain syndrome is a term used to describe pain involving the lateral aspect of the hip. This regional pain syndrome includes pain from trochanteric bursitis but also often mimics pain from other sources including myofascial pain, degenerative joint disease, sciatica, and spinal pathology. There is overlap of symptoms due to gluteus medius and minimus disorders including tendinosis and tendon tears. The prevalence is higher in women, and patients with coexisting low back pain, osteoarthritis, iliotibial band tenderness, and obesity. Symptoms include persistent pain over the lateral hip that may radiate along the lateral aspect of the thigh to the knee and occasionally to the buttock. Physical examination reveals point tenderness over the lateral aspect of the greater trochanter.[1]

Conservative therapy includes stretching, therapeutic exercise, and physical modalities focused on the low back/pelvic core and sacroiliac joints. Local corticosteroid injection into the area of maximal tenderness has demonstrated effectiveness and safety.[2–4] Alternative therapies include injections of platelet-rich plasma,[5] percutaneous needle tendon fenestration,[6] and dry-needling.[7] In most cases, ultrasound guidance is not necessary, more expensive, and less cost-effective. Landmark-based injection remains the method of choice. Ultrasound guidance should be reserved for extreme obesity or injection failure.[8] Recalcitrant cases may be treated with shockwave therapy[9] or require surgical referral to consider iliotibial band release, subgluteal bursectomy, or trochanteric reduction osteotomy.

Indications	ICD-10 Code
Greater trochanteric pain syndrome	M25.559
Trochanteric bursitis	M70.60

Relevant Anatomy: (Fig. 11.12)

PATIENT POSITION

• Lying on the examination table in the lateral decubitus position on the unaffected hip

LANDMARKS

1. With the patient lying on the examination table in the lateral decubitus position on the unaffected hip, the clinician stands behind the patient.
2. Identify and mark the area(s) of maximal tenderness over the greater trochanter.
3. At that area, press firmly on the skin with the retracted tip of a ballpoint pen. This indention represents the entry point(s) for the needle.
4. After the landmarks are identified, the patient should not move the hip.

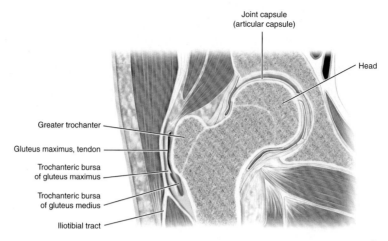

FIGURE 11.12 ● Right anterior hip joint and trochanteric structures.

ANESTHESIA

- Local anesthesia of the skin with topical vapocoolant spray may be used.

EQUIPMENT

- Topical vapocoolant spray
- 5-mL syringe
- 25-gauge, 2-in. needle
- 3 mL of 1% lidocaine without epinephrine
- 1 mL of the steroid solution (40 mg of triamcinolone acetonide)
- One alcohol prep pad
- Two povidone–iodine prep pads
- Sterile gauze pads
- Sterile adhesive bandage

TECHNIQUE

1. Prep the insertion site(s) with alcohol followed by the povidone–iodine pads.
2. Achieve good local anesthesia by using topical vapocoolant spray.
3. Position the needle and syringe perpendicular to the skin with the tip of the needle directed medially.
4. Using the no-touch technique, introduce the needle at the insertion site(s).
5. Advance the needle toward the femoral trochanter until the needle tip touches the bone. Back up the needle 1 to 2 mm.
6. Withdraw the plunger of the syringe to ensure that there is no blood return.
7. Inject the steroid solution as a bolus steadily in the area of the trochanteric bursa. The injected solution should flow smoothly into the space. If increased resistance is encountered, advance or withdraw the needle slightly before attempting further injection.
8. Repeat the injection at other adjacent painful areas if needed.
9. Following injection(s), withdraw the needle.

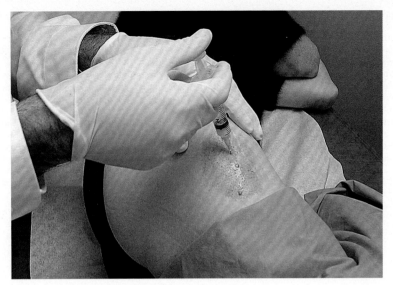

FIGURE 11.13 ● Greater trochanteric pain syndrome injection.

10. Apply a sterile adhesive bandage(s).
11. Instruct the patient to massage the area and move his or her hip through its full range of motion. This movement distributes the steroid solution throughout the trochanteric bursa.
12. Reexamine the area of the trochanteric bursa in 5 min to confirm pain relief (Fig. 11.13).

AFTERCARE

- Avoid excessive hip movement over the next 2 weeks.
- NSAIDs, ice, heat, and/or physical therapy as indicated.
- Consider follow-up examination in 2 weeks.

CPT codes:

- 20610—Arthrocentesis, aspiration and/or injection, major joint or bursa; without ultrasound guidance
- 20611—With ultrasound guidance, with permanent recording and reporting

PEARLS

- Consider fanning this injection to disperse the corticosteroid solution over a wider area.

 A video showing a trochanteric pain syndrome injection can be found in the companion eBook.

REFERENCES

1. Williams BS, Cohen SP. Greater trochanteric pain syndrome: a review of anatomy, diagnosis and treatment. *Anesth Analg*. 2009;108(5):1662–1670.
2. Torres A, Fernández-Fairen M, Sueiro-Fernández J. Greater trochanteric pain syndrome and gluteus medius and minimus tendinosis: nonsurgical treatment. *Pain Manag*. 2018;8(1):45–55.

3. Brinks A, van Rijn RM, Willemsen SP, et al. Corticosteroid injections for greater trochanteric pain syndrome: a randomized controlled trial in primary care. *Ann Fam Med.* 2011;9(3):226–234.
4. McEvoy JR, Lee KS, Blankenbaker DG, et al. Ultrasound-guided corticosteroid injections for treatment of greater trochanteric pain syndrome: greater trochanter bursa versus subgluteus medius bursa. *AJR Am J Roentgenol.* 2013;201(2):W313–W317.
5. Fitzpatrick J, Bulsara MK, O'Donnell J, et al. The effectiveness of platelet-rich plasma injections in gluteal tendinopathy: a randomized, double-blind controlled trial comparing a single platelet-rich plasma injection with a single corticosteroid injection. *Am J Sports Med.* 2018;46(4):933–939.
6. Jacobson JA, Yablon CM, Henning PT, et al. Greater trochanteric pain syndrome: percutaneous tendon fenestration versus platelet-rich plasma injection for treatment of gluteal tendinosis. *J Ultrasound Med.* 2016;35(11):2413–2420.
7. Brennan KL, Allen BC, Maldonado YM. Dry needling versus cortisone injection in the treatment of greater trochanteric pain syndrome: a noninferiority randomized clinical trial. *J Orthop Sports Phys Ther.* 2017;47(4):232–239.
8. Mitchell WG, Kettwich SC, Sibbitt WL, et al. Outcomes and cost-effectiveness of ultrasound-guided injection of the trochanteric bursa. *Rheumatol Int.* 2018;38(3):393–401.
9. Simeone FJ, Vicentini JRT, Bredella MA, et al. Are patients more likely to have hip osteoarthritis progression and femoral head collapse after hip steroid/anesthetic injections? A retrospective observational study. *Skeletal Radiol.* 2019;48(9):1417–1426.

Gluteal Pain Syndrome

The gluteus medius and minimus muscles function as primary hip abductors. They originate at the external surface of the ilium and insert onto the superior, posterior lateral surface of the greater trochanter. Gluteal pain syndrome, a term used to describe pain involving tendinopathy and gluteus bursitis, is now recognized as a primary local source of lateral hip pain.[1] This disorder may occur secondary to acute direct trauma, changes in activity with a repetitive motion injury, chronic excessive hip adduction, or abnormal biomechanics due to conditions involving distal structures. It is frequently seen in middle-aged women who start a vigorous exercise program. Pain typically occurs with hip flexion such as walking, climbing stairs, or getting out of a car or a chair. Night pain while lying on the affected side is classic. Occasionally, snapping may be present over the lateral hip with hip flexion or extension. On examination, pain is palpated over the superior, posterolateral aspect of the femoral trochanter and increases with resisted hip abduction. Diagnostic ultrasound may be performed to determine the presence of gluteal bursa fluid, echogenic features of tendinopathy, or tears of the gluteus medius tendon.

Management includes education, activity modification, ice, heat, therapeutic ultrasound, physical therapy, and NSAIDs. Corticosteroid injections given with or without ultrasound guidance have been traditionally employed, but effectiveness past the short to medium term has not been demonstrated.[2] Ultrasound-guided platelet-rich plasma injections have shown greater clinical improvement at 12 weeks than corticosteroid injections.[3] A recent well-designed study revealed 2-year sustained improvement in pain following ultrasound-guided leukocyte-rich platelet-rich plasma (PRP).[4] Ultrasound-guided gluteal tendon fenestration compared to injections of platelet-rich plasma showed no statistically significant difference in pain scores at 90 days.[5] Patients who do not respond to these measures may be candidates for open or arthroscopic repair of gluteus medius tears.[6]

Indications	ICD-10 Code
Tendinopathy of left gluteus medius	M67.952
Tendinopathy of right gluteus medius	M67.98

Relevant Anatomy: (Fig. 11.14)

PATIENT POSITION

• Lying on the examination table in the lateral decubitus position on the unaffected hip

LANDMARKS

1. With the patient lying on the examination table in the lateral decubitus position on the unaffected hip, the clinician stands behind the patient.

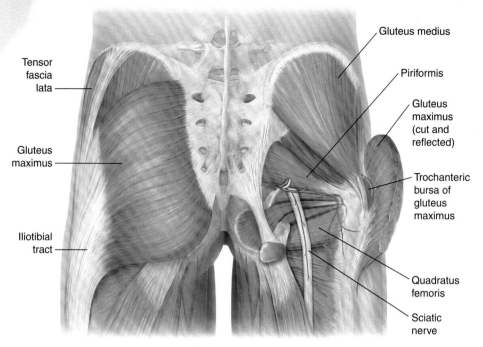

FIGURE 11.14 ● Muscles of gluteal region.

2. Identify and mark the area(s) of maximal tenderness over the superior, posterior, lateral aspect of the greater trochanter.
3. At that area, press firmly on the skin with the retracted tip of a ballpoint pen. This indention represents the entry point(s) for the needle.
4. After the landmarks are identified, the patient should not move the hip.

ANESTHESIA

- Local anesthesia of the skin with topical vapocoolant spray may be used.

EQUIPMENT

- Topical vapocoolant spray
- 5-mL syringe
- 25-gauge, 2-in. needle
- 3 mL of 1% lidocaine without epinephrine
- 1 mL of the steroid solution (40 mg of triamcinolone acetonide)
- One alcohol prep pad
- Two povidone–iodine prep pads
- Sterile gauze pads
- Sterile adhesive bandage

TECHNIQUE

1. Prep the insertion site(s) with alcohol followed by the povidone–iodine pads.
2. Achieve good local anesthesia by using topical vapocoolant spray.

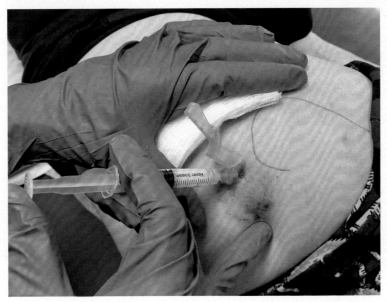

FIGURE 11.15 ● Injection for gluteal pain syndrome - superior and posterior to the right trochanter.

3. Position the needle and syringe perpendicular to the skin with the tip of the needle directed medially.
4. Using the no-touch technique, introduce the needle at the insertion site(s) (Fig. 11.15).
5. Advance the needle toward the femoral trochanter until the needle tip touches the bone. Back up the needle 1 to 2 mm.
6. Withdraw the plunger of the syringe to ensure that there is no blood return.
7. Inject the lidocaine/corticosteroid solution as a bolus steadily in the area of the gluteus medius and minimus tendons. The injected solution should flow smoothly into the space. If increased resistance is encountered, advance or withdraw the needle slightly before attempting further injection.
8. Repeat the injection at other adjacent painful areas if needed.
9. Following injection(s), withdraw the needle.
10. Apply a sterile adhesive bandage(s).
11. Instruct the patient to massage the area and move his or her hip through its full range of motion. This movement distributes the lidocaine/corticosteroid solution throughout the gluteal tendons and bursa.
12. Reexamine the area of the gluteal tendons/bursa in 5 min to assess pain relief.

AFTERCARE

- Avoid excessive hip movement over the next 2 weeks.
- NSAIDs, ice, heat, and/or physical therapy as indicated.
- Consider follow-up examination in 2 weeks.

CPT codes:
- 20551—Injection; single tendon origin/insertion
- 76942 (optional)—Ultrasonic guidance for needle placement with imaging supervision and interpretation with permanent recording

PEARLS

- Consider fanning this injection to disperse the corticosteroid solution along the course of the gluteus medius and minimus tendons.

 A video showing a gluteal pain syndrome injection can be found in the companion eBook.

REFERENCES

1. Grimaldi A, Mellor R, Hodges P, et al. Gluteal tendinopathy: a review of mechanisms, assessment and management. *Sports Med.* 2015;45(8):1107–1119.
2. Bolton WS, Kidanu D, Dube B, et al. Do ultrasound guided trochanteric bursa injections of corticosteroid for greater trochanteric pain syndrome provide sustained benefit and are imaging features associated with treatment response? *Clin Radiol.* 2018;73(5):505.e9–505.e15.
3. Fitzpatrick J, Bulsara MK, O'Donnell J, et al. The effectiveness of platelet-rich plasma injections in gluteal tendinopathy: a randomized, double-blind controlled trial comparing a single platelet-rich plasma injection with a single corticosteroid injection. *Am J Sports Med.* 2018;46(4):933–939.
4. Fitzpatrick J, Bulsara MK, O'Donnell J, et al. Leucocyte-rich platelet-rich plasma treatment of gluteus medius and minimus tendinopathy: a double-blind randomized controlled trial with 2-year follow-up. *Am J Sports Med.* 2019;47(5):1130–1137.
5. Jacobson JA, Yablon CM, Henning PT, et al. Greater trochanteric pain syndrome: percutaneous tendon fenestration versus platelet-rich plasma injection for treatment of gluteal tendinosis. *J Ultrasound Med.* 2016;35(11):2413–2420.
6. LaPorte C, Vasaris M, Gossett L, et al. Gluteus medius tears of the hip: a comprehensive approach. *Phys Sportsmed.* 2019;47(1):15–20.

Hip Adductor Tendon

Patients uncommonly present to the primary care office for the evaluation and treatment of pain upon adduction of the hip. The pectineus, adductor longus, magnus, and medius muscles connect the medial aspect of the femur to the pubic bone. Acute injury or chronic overuse may cause tendonitis or tendinopathy of the hip adductors. The adductor longus is most commonly injured, and patients classically present with pain upon palpation of the muscle belly and insertion, passive stretching, and resistance to contraction. In chronic tendinopathy, treatment is often lengthy and difficult. Physical therapy is the cornerstone of treatment. It may be facilitated by the judicious use of corticosteroid injections given around the affected tendon(s).

Indications	ICD-10 Code
Hip adductor tendonitis	M76.899
Enthesopathy of the hip	M76.899

Relevant Anatomy: (Fig. 11.16)

PATIENT POSITION

- Lying supine on the examination table.
- Place the hip in a position of combined flexion abduction and external rotation.
- Rotate the patient's head away from the side that is being injected. This minimizes anxiety and pain perception.

LANDMARKS

1. With the patient lying supine on the examination table, the clinician stands lateral and posterior to the affected hip.
2. Locate the symphysis pubis and firmly palpate the pubic bone laterally until meeting the origin of the hip adductor muscles.
3. Determine the site of maximal tenderness over the tendons, and mark it with an ink pen.
4. At that site, press firmly on the skin with the retracted tip of a ballpoint pen. This indention represents the entry point for the needle.
5. After the landmarks are identified, the patient should not move the hip.

ANESTHESIA

- Local anesthesia of the skin using a topical vapocoolant spray

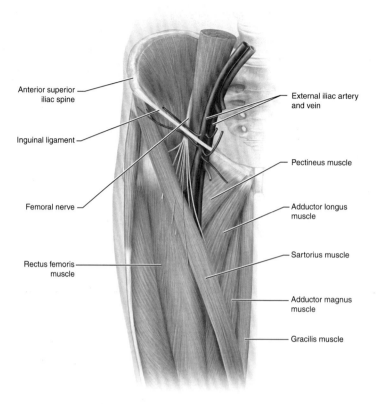

FIGURE 11.16 ● Right thigh and femoral triangle structures. (Modified from Gest TR. *Lippincott Atlas of Anatomy*, 2nd Ed. Philadelphia, PA: Wolters Kluwer, 2019.)

EQUIPMENT

- Topical vapocoolant spray
- 3-mL syringe
- 25-gauge, 2-in. needle
- 1 mL of 1% lidocaine without epinephrine
- 1 mL of the steroid solution (40 mg of triamcinolone acetonide)
- One alcohol prep pad
- Two povidone–iodine prep pads
- Sterile gauze pads
- Sterile adhesive bandage

TECHNIQUE

1. Prep the insertion site with alcohol followed by the povidone–iodine pads.
2. Achieve good local anesthesia by using a topical vapocoolant spray.
3. Position the needle and syringe at an angle of 30 degrees to the skin with the tip of the needle directed proximally toward the pubic bone.
4. Using the no-touch technique, introduce the needle at the insertion site (Fig. 11.17).

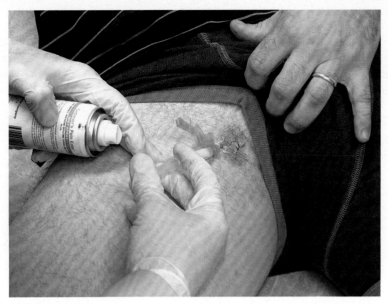

FIGURE 11.17 • Hip adductor tendonitis injection.

5. Advance the needle so that it is positioned around the affected tendon, but not in the substance of the tendon.
6. Withdraw the plunger of the syringe to ensure that there is no blood return.
7. Inject the lidocaine/corticosteroid solution as a bolus around the adductor tendon(s). The injected solution should flow smoothly into the space. If increased resistance is encountered, advance or withdraw the needle slightly before attempting further injection.
8. Following injection, withdraw the needle.
9. Apply a sterile adhesive bandage.
10. Instruct the patient to massage the area and move his or her hip through its full range of motion. This movement distributes the lidocaine/corticosteroid solution along the adductor tendon(s).
11. Reexamine the medial aspect of the hip in 5 min to assess pain relief.

AFTERCARE

- Avoid excessive use of the hip—especially hip abduction and adduction over the next 2 weeks.
- Begin a program of physical therapy.
- NSAIDs, ice, and heat as indicated.
- Consider follow-up examination in 2 weeks.

CPT codes:
- 20551—Injection; single tendon origin/insertion
- 76942 (optional)—Ultrasonic guidance for needle placement with imaging supervision and interpretation with permanent recording

PEARLS

- This injection can be superficial—especially in thin persons. Depositing corticosteroid in the subcutaneous tissues can result in the complication of skin atrophy and hypopigmentation. Avoid the development of a subdermal wheal while performing all injections of corticosteroid solutions.

 A video showing a hip adductor tendonitis injection can be found in the companion eBook.

Knee Joint Injections

The need for aspiration and injection of the knee joint is frequently encountered by primary care providers. The most common indications for this procedure include evaluation and treatment of monoarthritis, osteoarthritis, and inflammatory arthritis; ruling out septic arthritis; and removal of blood or reactive fluid following trauma. Arthrocentesis (aspiration) is employed to remove fluid from a joint for diagnostic synovial fluid analysis, to enhance comfort, to improve proprioception,[1] and to minimize dilution of injected substances. Injections of various products are also employed including corticosteroids,[2] hyaluronic acid viscosupplements,[3,4] platelet-rich plasma,[5] dextrose (prolotherapy),[6] etaneracept,[7] botulinum toxin,[8] and others.

Most practitioners use one of four palpation-based, anatomic landmark-guided approaches to perform aspirations and injections of the knee joint. Figure 11.18A and B shows the most common knee joint approaches—the extended-knee lateral suprapatellar, extended-knee lateral midpatellar, flexed-knee anteromedial, and flexed-knee anterolateral portals. The author avoids the medial suprapatellar and medial midpatellar approaches because of the limited operating space on the medial aspect of the knee/leg, to preserve patient modesty, and due to the lack of demonstrated accuracy and effectiveness in the medical literature. There is a general lack of consensus among experts regarding the best technique for knee joint injection and aspiration. An examination of the current medical literature (below), however, gives us some guidance. Although it appears that the lateral suprapatellar and lateral midpatellar approaches have an advantage over the others, the individual provider will ultimately determine the desired portal based on the scientific data, their expertise, history of success, and other patient-specific factors.

A comprehensive review of intra-articular knee joint injection accuracy was published in 2013 by Maricar et al.[9] Data from 23 publications were pooled and revealed that injections at the lateral suprapatellar portal were most accurate (87%), while medial midpatellar (64%) and anterolateral joint line sites (70%) were least accurate. Furthermore, lateral suprapatellar, medial midpatellar, and medial suprapatellar sites were more accurate when using image guidance than when using anatomic landmarks. Another systematic review of nine studies by Hermans and associates[10] found the extended-leg lateral suprapatellar approach (91%) to be the most accurate, as compared with the lateral midpatellar (85%), anteromedial (72%), and anterolateral (67%) approaches. This success makes sense when the location of synovial fluid in the knee joint is considered. Hirsch and colleagues[11] demonstrated that small effusions were more commonly detected in the lateral suprapatellar pouch than elsewhere. In patients with painful knee arthritis, fluid distributes maximally to the lateral suprapatellar pouch in the extended knee. Furthermore, Zhang et al.[12] found a "dry tap" rate of 10% in the extended leg supine position and 25% in the sitting position.

In an individual study by Jackson and colleagues[13] using a 1½-in., 21-gauge needle, the landmark-based, lateral midpatellar approach was significantly more accurate (93%) than were the anteromedial (75%) and anterolateral (71%) approaches. Toda and

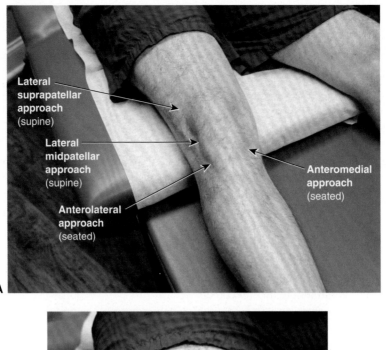

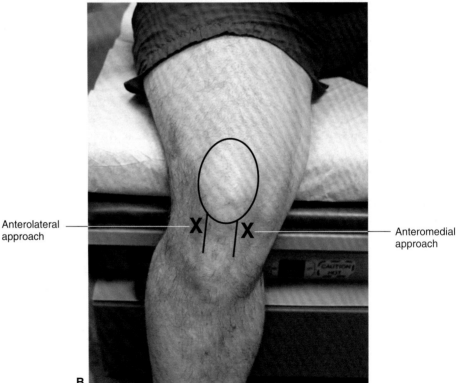

FIGURE 11.18 ● A: Right knee—the most common knee joint approaches. B: Flexed knee showing landmarks.

Tsukimura[14] reported that a modified 30-degree flexed-knee approach incorporating distal knee traction was significantly more accurate (86%) than were seated anteromedial (62%) and extended-leg lateral suprapatellar (70%) approaches using a 1½ in., 25-gauge needle. Accuracy rates increased with the presence of severe osteoarthritis. In another investigation by Chavez-Chiang,[15] an anterolateral knee portal with 90-degree flexion targeting the synovial membrane of the medial femoral condyle with a 2-in., 21-gauge needle yielded an accuracy rate of 97%. This approach might be useful for patients who cannot lie down, transfer to an examination table, or extend the knee or those with flexion contractures.

The use of musculoskeletal ultrasound dramatically increases the accuracy of knee injections. A number of studies now demonstrate significantly increased accuracy rates of injections when using ultrasound-guided techniques. The use of ultrasound increases the success rate to nearly 100%, even when performed by less experienced practitioners.[16] A study of ultrasound-guided injections in patients with moderate osteoarthritis using a 1½-in., 25-gauge needle showed success rates of 100% for the lateral suprapatellar, 95% for the lateral midpatellar, and 75% for the anteromedial approaches.[17] A review of 13 studies of the knee showed that imaging guidance with ultrasound improved the accuracy of intra-articular injections of the knee to 95.8% versus 77.8%, $P < 0.001$.[18] Employing a joint cupping maneuver from an inferior approach also improves the detection and removal of knee joint effusion by improving ultrasound visualization of the effusion.[19] The use of image-guided techniques is particularly important in patients without joint effusion and especially when injecting intra-articular viscosupplements to treat osteoarthritis of the knee.[20] Most importantly, there is statistically significant improvement in short-term (2 weeks) patient outcomes of pain and function with a reduction in adverse events when ultrasound-guided injections are compared to those guided by palpation of landmarks. These image-guided techniques also cause significantly less procedural pain, take no additional time to perform, lead to greater provider confidence with the procedure, and improve cost-effectiveness.[21,22,23]

The extended-knee, lateral suprapatellar approach to a knee joint intra-articular injection is a relatively easy procedure to perform, easily lends itself to ultrasound guidance without bony obstruction, and is well accepted by patients. Additionally, because of supine positioning, patients may not see the approaching needle and anxiety is diminished. For these reasons and based on the published studies, this approach is the author's preferred technique and is highly recommended to others.

REFERENCES

1. Cho YR, Hong BY, Lim SH, et al. Effects of joint effusion on proprioception in patients with knee osteoarthritis: a single-blind, randomized controlled clinical trial. *Osteoarthritis Cartilage.* 2011;19(1):22–28.
2. Leung A, Liew D, Lim J, et al. The effect of joint aspiration and corticosteroid injections in osteoarthritis of the knee. *Int J Rheum Dis.* 2011;14(4):384–389.
3. Saito S, Kotake S. Is there evidence in support of the use of intra-articular hyaluronate in treating rheumatoid arthritis of the knee? A meta-analysis of the published literature. *Mod Rheumatol.* 2009;19(5):493–501.
4. Foti C, Cisari C, Carda S, et al. A prospective observational study of the clinical efficacy and safety of intra-articular sodium hyaluronate in synovial joints with osteoarthritis. *Eur J Phys Rehabil Med.* 2011;47(3):407–415.
5. Spaková T, Rosocha J, Lacko M, et al. Treatment of knee joint osteoarthritis with autologous platelet-rich plasma in comparison with hyaluronic acid. *Am J Phys Med Rehabil.* 2012;91(5):411–417.
6. Rabago D, Patterson JJ, Mundt M, et al. Dextrose prolotherapy for knee osteoarthritis: a randomized controlled trial. *Ann Fam Med.* 2013;11(3):229–237.
7. Liang DF, Huang F, Zhang JL, et al. A randomized, single-blind, parallel, controlled clinical study on single intra-articular injection of etanercept in treatment of inflammatory knee arthritis. *Zhonghua Nei Ke Za Zhi.* 2010;49(11):930–934.
8. Chou CL, Lee SH, Lu SY, et al. Therapeutic effects of intra-articular botulinum neurotoxin in advanced knee osteoarthritis. *J Chin Med Assoc.* 2010;73(11):573–580.
9. Maricar N, Parkes MJ, Callaghan MJ, et al. Where and how to inject the knee—a systematic review. *Semin Arthritis Rheum.* 2013;43(2):195–203.

10. Hermans J, Bierma-Zeinstra SM, Bos PK, et al. The most accurate approach for intra-articular needle placement in the knee joint: a systematic review. *Semin Arthritis Rheum.* 2011;41(2):106–115.
11. Hirsch G, O'Neill T, Kitas G, et al. Distribution of effusion in knee arthritis as measured by high-resolution ultrasound. *Clin Rheumatol.* 2012;31(8):1243–1246.
12. Zhang Q, Zhang T, Lv H, et al. Comparison of two positions of knee arthrocentesis: how to obtain complete drainage. *Am J Phys Med Rehabil.* 2012;91(7):611–615.
13. Jackson DW, Evans NA, Thomas BM. Accuracy of needle placement into the intra-articular space of the knee. *J Bone Joint Surg Am.* 2002;84-A(9):1522–1527.
14. Toda Y, Tsukimura N. A comparison of intra-articular hyaluronan injection accuracy rates between three approaches based on radiographic severity of knee osteoarthritis. *Osteoarthritis Cartilage.* 2008;16(9):980–985.
15. Chavez-Chiang CE, Sibbitt WL Jr, Band PA, et al. The highly accurate anteriolateral portal for injecting the knee. *Sports Med Arthrosc Rehabil Ther Technol.* 2011;3(1):6.
16. Curtiss HM, Finnoff JT, Peck E, et al. Accuracy of ultrasound-guided and palpation-guided knee injections by an experienced and less-experienced injector using a superolateral approach: a cadaveric study. *PM R.* 2011;3(6):507–515.
17. Park Y, Lee SC, Nam HS, et al. Comparison of sonographically guided intra-articular injections at 3 different sites of the knee. *J Ultrasound Med.* 2011;30(12):1669–1676.
18. Berkoff DJ, Miller LE, Block JE. Clinical utility of ultrasound guidance for intra-articular knee injections: a review. *Clin Interv Aging.* 2012;7:89–95.
19. Uryasev O, Joseph OC, McNamara JP, et al. Novel joint cupping clinical maneuver for ultrasonographic detection of knee joint effusions. *Am J Emerg Med.* 2013;31(11):1598–1600.
20. Gilliland CA, Salazar LD, Borchers JR. Ultrasound versus anatomic guidance for intra-articular and peri-articular injection: a systematic review. *Phys Sportsmed.* 2011;39(3):121–131.
21. Punzi L, Oliviero F. Arthrocentesis and synovial fluid analysis in clinical practice: value of sonography in difficult cases. *Ann N Y Acad Sci.* 2009;1154:152–158.
22. Wiler JL, Costantino TG, et al. Comparison of ultrasound-guided and standard landmark techniques for knee arthrocentesis. *J Emerg Med.* 2010;39(1):76–82.
23. Sibbitt WL Jr, Kettwich LG, Band PA, et al. Does ultrasound guidance improve the outcomes of arthrocentesis and corticosteroid injection of the knee? *Scand J Rheumatol.* 2012;41(1):66–72.

Knee Joint—Preferred Lateral Suprapatellar Approach

The supine, extended-leg, lateral suprapatellar approach to the knee joint is relatively easy to perform and is well accepted by patients. Because of supine positioning, patients may not see the approaching needle and anxiety is diminished. This approach is considered a safe procedure since there are no major arteries or nerves in the immediate path of the needle. Also, since the injection is done using the suprapatellar approach, it is extra-articular but still within the joint capsule. As a result, joint fluid can be removed and injections performed without direct, large-needle injury to articular cartilage. With the use of local anesthetic, this injection can help the clinician differentiate the etiology of knee pain. After pain has been eliminated as a confounding factor, the knee can be reexamined to assess structural integrity of the ligaments and menisci. For the reasons previously noted, the extended-leg, lateral suprapatellar approach is the preferred technique to perform knee joint aspirations and injections.

Indications	ICD-10 Code
Knee joint pain	M25.569
Knee arthritis, unspecified	M17.10
Knee osteoarthritis, primary	M17.10
Knee osteoarthritis, posttraumatic	M17.30
Knee osteoarthritis, secondary	M17.5

Relevant Anatomy: (Fig. 11.19)

PATIENT POSITION

- Lying supine on the examination table with the knee extended, or slightly flexed and supported with a pillow or folded chucks pads as needed for patient comfort.
- Rotate the patient's head away from the side that is being injected. This minimizes anxiety and pain perception.

LANDMARKS

1. With the patient lying supine on the examination table, the clinician stands lateral to the affected knee.
2. Locate the superior aspect of the patella.
3. Draw a line vertically 1 cm superior to the proximal margin of the patella (Fig. 11.20).

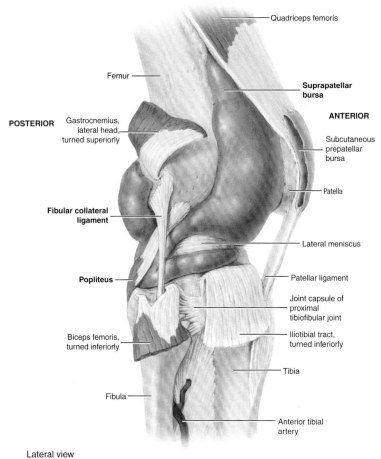

Quadriceps femoris

Femur

Suprapatellar bursa

ANTERIOR

POSTERIOR   Gastrocnemius, lateral head, turned superiorly

Subcutaneous prepatellar bursa

Patella

Fibular collateral ligament

Lateral meniscus

Popliteus

Patellar ligament

Joint capsule of proximal tibiofibular joint

Biceps femoris, turned inferiorly

Iliotibial tract, turned inferiorly

Tibia

Fibula

Anterior tibial artery

Lateral view

FIGURE 11.19 ● Lateral aspect of the right knee showing the extent of the knee joint capsule (in *purple*). (From Agur AM, Dalley AF. *Grant's Atlas of Anatomy*, 14th Ed. Philadelphia, PA: Wolters Kluwer, 2016.)

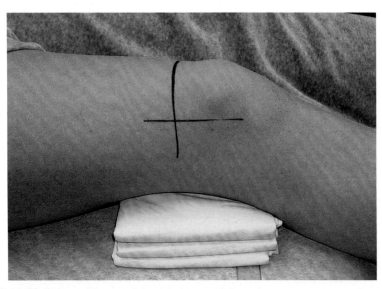

FIGURE 11.20 ● Lateral aspect of the right knee with lines drawn.

4. Next, draw a line horizontally along the posterior edge of the patella.
5. Identify the point where these two lines intersect. Make sure that this intersection lies underneath the quadriceps tendon.
6. At that site, press firmly on the skin with the retracted tip of a ballpoint pen. This indention represents the entry point for the needle.
7. After the landmarks are identified, the patient should not move the knee.

ANESTHESIA

- Local anesthesia of the skin using topical vapocoolant spray.
- (Optional) Local anesthesia and vasoconstriction of the skin and soft tissues may be augmented using an injection of 2 to 4 mL of 1% lidocaine with epinephrine (see "Pearls").

EQUIPMENT

- Topical vapocoolant spray
- 3-mL syringe—for injection of the mepivacaine/corticosteroid mixture
- 25-gauge, 2-in. needle—for direct injection of the mepivacaine/corticosteroid mixture
- (Optional) 10- to 60-mL syringe(s) —for aspiration
- (Optional) 5-mL syringe—for injection of 1% lidocaine with epinephrine to provide augmented local tissue anesthesia
- (Optional) 25-gauge, 1½-in. needle—for injection of 1% lidocaine with epinephrine to provide local tissue anesthesia—in preparation for an 18-gauge needle.
- (Optional) 18-gauge, 1½-in. needle—for aspiration
- (Optional) 2 to 4 mL of 1% lidocaine with epinephrine—for local tissue anesthesia of skin and knee joint capsule—in preparation for an 18-gauge needle
- 1 mL of 1% mepivacaine without epinephrine—to dilute the corticosteroid
- 1 mL of the corticosteroid solution (40 mg of triamcinolone acetonide)
- (Optional) Viscosupplementation agent of choice—if indicated
- One alcohol prep pad
- Two povidone–iodine prep pads
- Sterile gauze pads
- Sterile adhesive bandage
- Nonsterile, clean chucks pad

TECHNIQUE

1. (Optional) Use ultrasound to image the knee joint structures using an adjacent, but separate, acoustic window (Fig. 11.21). This allows separate imaging from the injection site so that there is no contamination from the ultrasound gel. Alternatively, the entire site may be prepped in an aseptic manner and sterile ultrasound gel utilized (Fig. 11.22).
2. Create an aseptic insertion site by wiping with a single alcohol prep pad followed by two 10% povidone–iodine prep pads. Allow this site to completely dry by evaporation.
3. If significant intra-articular fluid accumulation is not suspected, or not seen on ultrasound examination, then proceed with direct injection of the mepivacaine/corticosteroid solution (Step 4). If fluid is suspected or confirmed on ultrasound, proceed to Step 9.

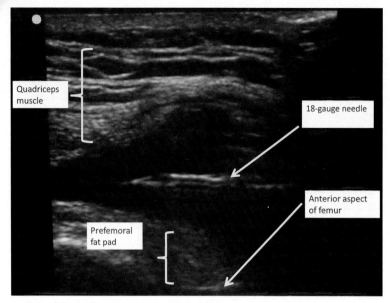

FIGURE 11.21 ● Ultrasound imaging of knee joint.

4. Achieve good local anesthesia by using topical vapocoolant spray.
5. Position the 25-gauge, 2-in. needle and syringe perpendicularly to the skin, parallel to the floor, at a right angle to the other two previously drawn skin lines and with the tip of the needle directed medially.
6. Using the aseptic, no-touch technique, quickly introduce that needle at the insertion site.
7. Advance the 25-gauge, 2-in. needle under the quadriceps tendon and toward the anterior surface of the distal femur until the needle tip is located within the joint capsule.

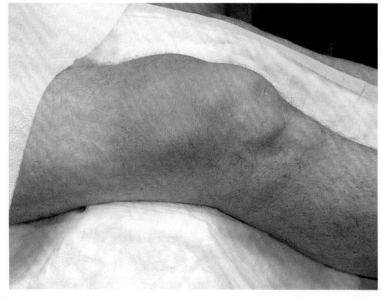

FIGURE 11.22 ● Right knee joint—distended with a large amount of intra-articular fluid. Note bulging of the joint capsule (suprapatellar bursa) proximal to the patella.

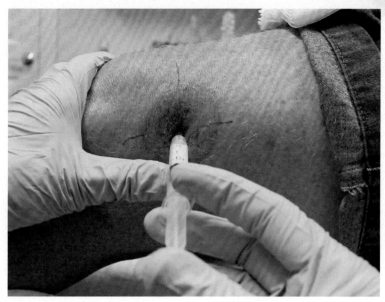

FIGURE 11.23 ● Landmark-based left knee corticosteroid injection.

The needle may contact the distal femur itself. Should that happen, withdraw the needle a few centimeters and advance the needle as needed to "walk" it over the anterior aspect of the femur.

8. Withdraw the plunger of the syringe to ensure that there is no blood return.
9. Inject the mepivacaine/corticosteroid solution as a bolus into the knee joint. The injected solution should flow smoothly into the joint space. If increased resistance is encountered, advance or withdraw the needle slightly before attempting further injection (Fig. 11.23).
10. (Optional) Achieve good local anesthesia by using topical vapocoolant spray.
11. Using the no-touch technique, introduce the 25-gauge, 1½-in. needle for local anesthesia at the insertion site. Inject 2 to 4 mL of 1% lidocaine with epinephrine to provide adequate local anesthesia. Infuse the anesthetic under the skin and at the joint capsule.
12. Position the 18-gauge, 1½-in. needle and syringe perpendicularly to the skin, parallel to the floor, at a right angle to the other two previously drawn skin lines and with the tip of the needle directed medially.
13. Using the aseptic, no-touch technique, quickly introduce that needle at the insertion site.
14. Advance the 18-gauge 1½-in. needle under the quadriceps tendon and toward the anterior surface of the distal femur until the needle tip is located in the joint capsule. (This may occur after advancing only 1 to 2 cm if the lateral pocket of a distended knee joint capsule is present.) Apply suction to the syringe while advancing the needle. The appearance of fluid in the syringe confirms that the joint capsule has been entered (Fig. 11.24). If fluid is aspirated, stop advancing the needle. The needle may contact the distal femur itself. Should that happen, withdraw the needle a few centimeters and advance the needle as needed to "walk" it over the femur and into the joint capsule.
15. Multiple syringes may be required in order to drain all of the synovial fluid if a large effusion is present.

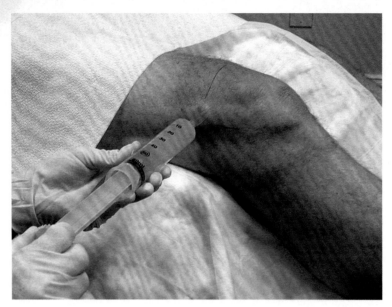

FIGURE 11.24 ● Right knee aspiration of distended joint using the preferred lateral suprapatellar approach.

16. If injection following aspiration is elected, remove the large syringe from the 18-gauge needle and then attach the 3-mL syringe filled with the mepivacaine/corticosteroid solution (Fig. 11.23) or a proprietary glass syringe prefilled with viscosupplement (Fig. 11.25).
17. Inject the mepivacaine/corticosteroid solution or viscosupplement as a bolus into the knee joint. The injected solution should flow smoothly into the joint space. If increased resistance is encountered, advance or withdraw the needle slightly, and confirm aspiration of a small amount of joint fluid before attempting further injection (Fig. 11.23).
18. Following injection, withdraw the needle.

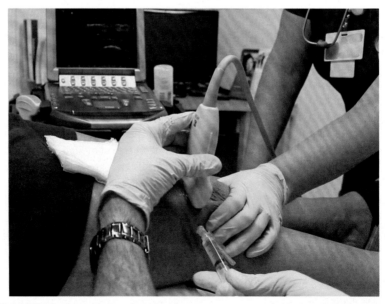

FIGURE 11.25 ● Ultrasound-guided right knee aspiration, immediately preceding corticosteroid injection.

19. Apply a sterile adhesive bandage.
20. Instruct the patient to move his or her knee through its full range of motion. This movement distributes the mepivacaine/corticosteroid solution or viscosupplement throughout the knee joint.
21. Reexamine the knee in 5 min to assess pain relief.

AFTERCARE

- Avoid more than light use of the affected knee over the next 2 weeks.
- Use other complementary treatment modalities including physical therapy as indicated.
- Consider follow-up examination in 2 weeks.

CPT codes:

- 20610—Arthrocentesis, aspiration and/or injection, major joint or bursa; without ultrasound guidance
- 20611—With ultrasound guidance, with permanent recording and reporting

PEARLS

- Although both the lateral and medial suprapatellar approaches may be used, the preferred approach is from the lateral aspect. This approach affords the operator more room, avoids inadvertent kicking of the clinician by the patient with the uninvolved leg, and preserves patient modesty.
- Usually, this procedure can be conducted in a pain-free manner with the use of topical vapocoolant spray. However, an occasional patient may complain of pain when the 18-gauge needle is advanced into contact with the joint capsule. In this case, that needle should be withdrawn and a 1½-in., 25-gauge needle advanced in the same direction. A total of 2 to 4 mL of 1% lidocaine with epinephrine is deposited under the skin and at the margin of the joint capsule. In almost all such cases where pain is reported, it is the author's experience that an ultrasound examination often shows that the synovial capsule is thickened and presumably inflamed.
- If the clinician encounters the unusual situation of experiencing difficulty finding the joint capsule, then either of the following maneuvers can be attempted.
  - Firmly squeeze the anterodistal aspect of the patella and displace it posteriorly and proximally (the "cupping" maneuver) thereby shifting the joint fluid and filling the suprapatellar pouch (See Figure 11.25).[1]
  - Redirect the needle in a distal direction to target the undersurface of the patella. However, this technique may potentially result in injury to the patellar cartilage.
- Ultrasound-guided aspiration and injection is indicated when an effusion is not detected, or in a very obese patient. Ultrasound is also very useful in locating fluid in the knee joint to ensure placement accuracy when injecting expensive viscosupplement products.

 A video showing a knee joint aspiration and injection utilizing the preferred lateral suprapatellar approach can be found in the companion eBook.

REFERENCE

1. Uryasev O, Joseph OC, McNamara JP, et al. Novel joint cupping clinical maneuver for ultrasonographic detection of knee joint effusions. *Am J Emerg Med.* 2013;31(11):1598–1600.

Knee Joint—Lateral Midpatellar Approach

The supine, extended-leg lateral midpatellar approach to the knee joint is relatively easy to perform and is well accepted by patients. As noted previously, injection through this portal has a high likelihood of success. Because of supine positioning, patients may not see the approaching needle and anxiety is diminished. This approach is considered a safe procedure since there are no major arteries or nerves in the immediate path of the needle. Since the needle tip may come into contact with the lateral aspect of the patellar cartilage, direct trauma may result, but this is usually lateral to the appositional joint surface and should not be clinically significant. With the use of local anesthetic, this injection can help the clinician differentiate the etiology of knee pain. After pain has been eliminated as a confounding factor, the knee can be reexamined to assess structural integrity of the ligaments and menisci.

Indications	ICD-10 Code
Knee joint pain	M25.569
Knee arthritis, unspecified	M17.10
Knee osteoarthritis, primary	M17.10
Knee osteoarthritis, posttraumatic	M17.30
Knee osteoarthritis, secondary	M17.5

Relevant Anatomy: (see Fig. 11.19)

PATIENT POSITION

- Lying supine on the examination table with the knee extended, or slightly flexed and supported with a pillow or folded chucks pads as needed for patient comfort.
- Rotate the patient's head away from the side that is being injected. This minimizes anxiety and pain perception.

LANDMARKS

1. With the patient lying supine on the examination table, the clinician stands lateral to the affected knee.
2. Locate the lateral aspect of the patella.
3. Have the patient relax the quadriceps muscles; then, apply pressure to the medial aspect of the patella in order to displace it laterally.

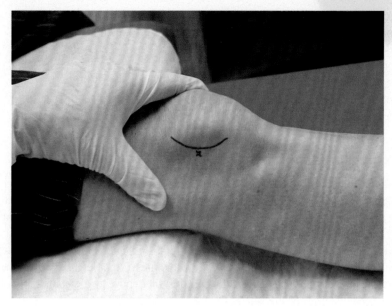

FIGURE 11.26 ● Lateral aspect of the right knee with patella outlined and injection site drawn.

4. Identify the sulcus at the midpatella that develops between the lateral undersurface of the patella and the lateral femoral condyle (Fig. 11.26).
5. At that site, press firmly on the skin with the retracted tip of a ballpoint pen. This indention represents the entry point for the needle.
6. After this landmark is identified, the patient should not move the knee.

ANESTHESIA

- Local anesthesia of the skin using topical vapocoolant spray.
- (Optional) Local anesthesia and vasoconstriction of the skin and soft tissues may be augmented using an injection of 2 to 4 mL of 1% lidocaine with epinephrine (see Pearls).

EQUIPMENT

- Topical vapocoolant spray
- 3-mL syringe—for injection of the mepivacaine/corticosteroid mixture
- 25-gauge, 1½-in. needle—for direct injection of the mepivacaine/corticosteroid mixture
- (Optional) 10- to 60-mL syringe(s) —for aspiration
- (Optional) 5-mL syringe—for injection of 1% lidocaine with epinephrine to provide augmented local tissue anesthesia
- (Optional) 25-gauge, 1-in. needle—for injection of 1% lidocaine with epinephrine to provide local tissue anesthesia—in preparation for an 18-gauge needle.
- (Optional) 18-gauge, 1½-in. needle—for aspiration
- (Optional) 2 to 4 mL of 1% lidocaine with epinephrine—for local tissue anesthesia of skin and knee joint capsule—in preparation for an 18-gauge needle.
- 1 mL of 1% mepivacaine without epinephrine—to dilute the corticosteroid

- 1 mL of the corticosteroid solution (40 mg of triamcinolone acetonide)
- (Optional) Viscosupplementation agent of choice—if indicated
- One alcohol prep pad
- Two povidone–iodine prep pads
- Sterile gauze pads
- Sterile adhesive bandage
- Nonsterile, clean chucks pad

TECHNIQUE

1. (Optional) Use ultrasound to image the knee joint structures using an adjacent, but separate, acoustic window. This allows separate imaging from the injection site so that there is no contamination from the ultrasound gel. Alternatively, the entire site may be prepped in an aseptic manner and sterile ultrasound gel utilized.
2. Create an aseptic insertion site by wiping with a single alcohol prep pad followed by two 10% povidone–iodine prep pads. Allow this site to completely dry by evaporation.
3. Have the patient relax the quadriceps muscles; then, have an assistant apply pressure to the medial aspect of the patella in order to displace it laterally.
4. If significant intra-articular fluid accumulation is not suspected, or not seen on ultrasound examination, then proceed with direct injection of the mepivacaine/corticosteroid solution (Step 6). If fluid is suspected or confirmed on ultrasound, proceed to Step 10.
5. Achieve good local anesthesia by using topical vapocoolant spray.
6. Position the 25-gauge, 1½-in. needle and syringe perpendicularly to the skin, parallel to the floor, at a right angle to the other two previously drawn skin lines, and with the tip of the needle directed medially.
7. Using the aseptic, no-touch technique, quickly introduce that needle at the insertion site.
8. Advance the 25-gauge, 1½-in. needle medially underneath the patella and over the lateral femoral condyle until the needle tip is located within the joint capsule in the patellofemoral articulation (Fig. 11.27).
9. Withdraw the plunger of the syringe to ensure that there is no blood return.
10. Inject the mepivacaine/corticosteroid solution as a bolus into the knee joint. The injected solution should flow smoothly into the joint space. If increased resistance is encountered, advance or withdraw the needle slightly before attempting further injection.
11. (Optional) Achieve good local anesthesia by using topical vapocoolant spray.
12. Using the no-touch technique, introduce the 25-gauge, 1 in. needle for local anesthesia at the insertion site. Inject 2 to 4 mL of 1% lidocaine with epinephrine to provide adequate local anesthesia. Infuse the anesthetic under the skin and at the joint capsule.
13. Position the 18-gauge, 1½ in. needle and syringe perpendicularly to the skin, parallel to the floor, at a right angle to the other two previously drawn skin lines and with the tip of the needle directed medially.
14. Using the aseptic, no-touch technique, quickly introduce that needle at the insertion site.
15. Advance the 18-gauge, 1½-in. needle medially underneath the patella and over the lateral femoral condyle until the needle tip is located within the joint capsule in the patellofemoral articulation (Fig. 11.27). Apply suction to the syringe while

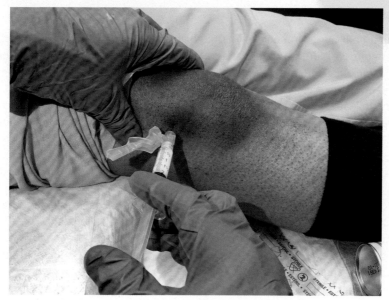

FIGURE 11.27 ● Right knee injection using the lateral midpatellar approach.

advancing the needle. The appearance of fluid in the syringe confirms that the joint capsule has been entered. If fluid is aspirated, stop advancing the needle.

16. Multiple syringes may be required in order to drain all of the synovial fluid if a large effusion is present.

17. If injection following aspiration is elected, remove the large syringe from the 18-gauge needle and then attach the 3-mL syringe filled with the mepivacaine/corticosteroid solution or a proprietary glass syringe prefilled with viscosupplement.

18. Inject the mepivacaine/corticosteroid solution or viscosupplement as a bolus into the knee joint. The injected solution should flow smoothly into the joint space. If increased resistance is encountered, advance or withdraw the needle slightly, and confirm aspiration of a small amount of joint fluid before attempting further injection.

19. Following injection, withdraw the needle.

20. Apply a sterile adhesive bandage.

21. Instruct the patient to move his or her knee through its full range of motion. This movement distributes the mepivacaine/corticosteroid solution or viscosupplement throughout the knee joint.

22. Reexamine the knee in 5 min to assess pain relief.

AFTERCARE

- Avoid more than light use of the affected knee over the next 2 weeks.
- Use other complementary treatment modalities including physical therapy as indicated.
- Consider follow-up examination in 2 weeks.

CPT codes:

- 20610—Arthrocentesis, aspiration and/or injection, major joint or bursa; without ultrasound guidance
- 20611—With ultrasound guidance, with permanent recording and reporting

PEARLS

- Although both the lateral and medial midpatellar approaches may be used, the preferred approach is from the lateral aspect. This approach affords the operator more room, avoids inadvertent kicking of the clinician by the patient with the uninvolved leg, and preserves patient modesty.
- Usually, this procedure can be conducted in a pain-free manner with the use of topical vapocoolant spray. However, an occasional patient may complain of pain when the 18-gauge needle is advanced into contact with the joint capsule. In this case, that needle should be withdrawn and a 1-in., 25-gauge needle advanced in the same direction. A total of 2 to 4 mL of 1% lidocaine with epinephrine is deposited under the skin and in the soft tissue at the joint capsule.
- If the clinician encounters the unusual situation of experiencing difficulty finding the joint capsule, then either of the following maneuvers can be attempted.
  - Firmly squeeze the anterodistal aspect of the patella and displace it posteriorly and proximally (the "cupping" maneuver) thereby shifting the joint fluid and filling the suprapatellar pouch.[1]
  - Abandon this approach and use the lateral suprapatellar portal. Alternatively, ultrasound imaging may be utilized.
- Ultrasound-guided aspiration and injection are indicated when an effusion is not detected or in a very obese patient. Ultrasound is also very useful in locating fluid in the knee joint to ensure placement accuracy when injecting expensive viscosupplement products.

 A video showing a knee joint aspiration and injection utilizing the lateral midpatellar approach can be found in the companion eBook.

REFERENCE

1. Uryasev O, Joseph OC, McNamara JP, et al. Novel joint cupping clinical maneuver for ultrasonographic detection of knee joint effusions. *Am J Emerg Med.* 2013;31(11):1598–1600.

Knee Joint—Anteromedial and Anterolateral Approaches

The infrapatellar anteromedial and anterolateral approaches to the knee joint are more difficult to perform than the extended-leg lateral approaches. They are also less well accepted by patients since they are usually performed with patients sitting where they can see the approaching needle. There is increased anxiety with these procedures, and the patients are at increased risk of injury if they develop a vasovagal reaction and fall from the examination table. Alternatively, the patient may be placed supine with hip and knee flexion so the plantar aspect of the foot contacts the exam tabletop. Since these injections are intra-articular, the knee cartilage over the distal femur may suffer direct damage from gouging by an aggressively placed 18-gauge needle. For these reasons, and documented lower success rates as compared to the extended-leg approaches, the anteromedial and anterolateral techniques are considered secondary options. However, they represent a valuable alternative technique in patients who are confined to a wheelchair and in those who cannot be easily moved up onto an examination table.

Indications	ICD-10 Code
Knee joint pain	M25.569
Knee arthritis, unspecified	M17.10
Knee osteoarthritis, primary	M17.10
Knee osteoarthritis, posttraumatic	M17.30
Knee osteoarthritis, secondary	M17.5

Relevant Anatomy: (see Fig. 11.19)

PATIENT POSITION

- Sitting on the examination table with the affected knee flexed at an angle of 90 degrees.
- Alternatively, the patient may be sitting in a wheelchair or side chair, or even lying supine on the examination table with both knees flexed at 90 degrees.
- Rotate the patient's head away from the side that is being injected. This may minimize anxiety and pain perception.

LANDMARKS

1. With the patient sitting up on the examination table or in a chair, the clinician sits on an examination stool in front of the affected knee.
2. With the patient lying supine on the examination table, the clinician stands medial or lateral to the affected knee.

3. Palpate the anterior aspect of the knee to locate the patellar tendon.
4. At the midpoint of the tendon, move about 2 cm medially or laterally. There is usually a soft depression at that spot. Mark it with ink.
5. At that site, press firmly on the skin with the retracted tip of a ballpoint pen. This indention represents the entry point for the needle.
6. After the landmarks are identified, the patient should not move the knee (Fig. 11.28A and B).

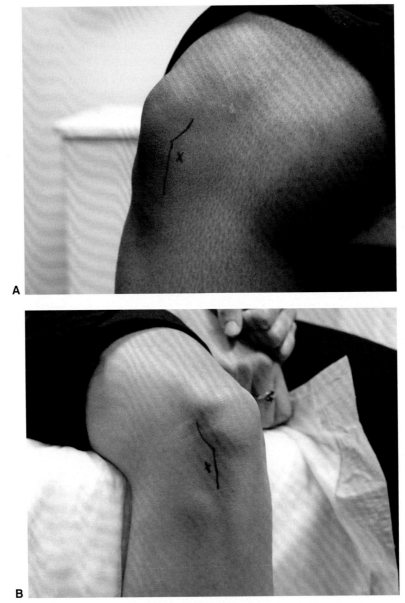

FIGURE 11.28 ● **A:** Anteromedial aspect of the right knee with injection sites drawn. **B:** Antero-lateral aspect of the right knee with injection sites drawn.

ANESTHESIA

- Local anesthesia of the skin using topical vapocoolant spray.
- (Optional) Local anesthesia and vasoconstriction of the skin and soft tissues may be augmented using an injection of 2 to 4 mL of 1% lidocaine with epinephrine (see "Pearls").

EQUIPMENT

- Topical vapocoolant spray
- 3-mL syringe—for injection of the mepivacaine/corticosteroid mixture
- 25-gauge, 2-in. needle—for direct injection of the mepivacaine/corticosteroid mixture
- (Optional) 10- to 60-mL syringe(s)—for aspiration
- (Optional) 5-mL syringe—for injection of 1% lidocaine with epinephrine to provide augmented local tissue anesthesia
- (Optional) 25-gauge, 1½-in. needle—for injection of 1% lidocaine with epinephrine to provide local tissue anesthesia—in preparation for an 18-gauge needle.
- (Optional) 18-gauge, 1½-in. needle—for aspiration
- (Optional) 2 to 4 mL of 1% lidocaine with epinephrine—for local tissue anesthesia of skin and knee joint capsule—in preparation for an 18-gauge needle
- 1 mL of 1% mepivacaine without epinephrine—to dilute the corticosteroid
- 1 mL of the corticosteroid solution (40 mg of triamcinolone acetonide)
- (Optional) Viscosupplementation agent of choice—if indicated
- One alcohol prep pad
- Two povidone–iodine prep pads
- Sterile gauze pads
- Sterile adhesive bandage
- Nonsterile, clean chucks pad

TECHNIQUE

1. (Optional) Use ultrasound to image the knee joint structures using an adjacent, but separate, acoustic window. This allows separate imaging from the injection site so that there is no contamination from the ultrasound gel. Alternatively, the entire site may be prepped in an aseptic manner and sterile ultrasound gel utilized.
2. Create an aseptic insertion site by wiping with a single alcohol prep pad followed by two 10% povidone–iodine prep pads. Allow this site to completely dry by evaporation.
3. If significant intra-articular fluid accumulation is not suspected, or not seen on ultrasound examination, then proceed with direct injection of the mepivacaine/corticosteroid solution (Step 4). If fluid is suspected or confirmed on ultrasound, proceed to Step 9.
4. Achieve good local anesthesia by using topical vapocoolant spray.
5. Position the 25-gauge, 2-in. needle and syringe perpendicularly to the skin, parallel to the floor, with the tip of the needle directed at a 45-degree angle into the center of the knee.
6. Using the aseptic, no-touch technique, quickly introduce that needle at the insertion site.

7. Advance the 25-gauge, 2-in. needle toward the center of the knee until the needle tip is located in the joint capsule or contacts the cartilage over the distal femur deep in center of the knee joint.

8. Withdraw the plunger of the syringe to ensure that there is no blood return.

9. Inject the mepivacaine/corticosteroid solution as a bolus into the knee joint. The injected solution should flow smoothly into the joint space. If increased resistance is encountered, advance or withdraw the needle slightly before attempting further injection

10. (Optional) Achieve good local anesthesia by using topical vapocoolant spray.

11. Using the no-touch technique, introduce the 25-gauge, 1½-in. needle for local anesthesia at the insertion site (Fig. 11.29). Inject 2 to 4 mL of 1% lidocaine with epinephrine to provide adequate local anesthesia. Infuse the anesthetic under the skin and at the joint capsule.

12. Position the 18-gauge, 1½-in. needle and syringe perpendicularly to the skin, parallel to the floor, with the tip of the needle directed at a 45-degree angle into the center of the knee.

13. Using the aseptic, no-touch technique, quickly introduce that needle at the insertion site.

14. Advance the 18-gauge 1½-in. needle toward the center of the knee until the needle tip is located in the joint capsule or contacts the cartilage over the distal femur deep in center of the knee joint. Apply suction to the syringe while advancing the needle. The appearance of fluid in the syringe confirms that the joint capsule has been entered. If fluid is aspirated, stop advancing the needle.

15. Multiple syringes may be required in order to drain all of the synovial fluid if a large effusion is present.

16. If injection following aspiration is elected, remove the large syringe from the 18-gauge needle and then attach the 3-mL syringe filled with the mepivacaine/corticosteroid solution or a proprietary glass syringe prefilled with viscosupplement.

17. Inject the mepivacaine/corticosteroid solution or viscosupplement as a bolus into the knee joint. The injected solution should flow smoothly into the joint space. If increased resistance is encountered, advance or withdraw the needle slightly, and confirm aspiration of a small amount of joint fluid before attempting further injection.

18. Following injection, withdraw the needle.

19. Apply a sterile adhesive bandage.

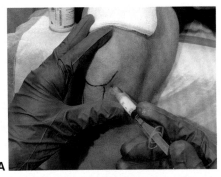 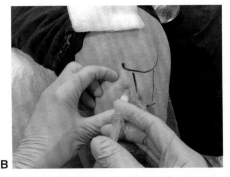

FIGURE 11.29 ● **A:** Right knee injection using the anteromedial approach. **B:** Right knee injection using the anterolateral approach.

20. Instruct the patient to move his or her knee through its full range of motion. This movement distributes the mepivacaine/corticosteroid solution throughout the knee joint.
21. Reexamine the knee in 5 min to assess pain relief.

AFTERCARE

- Avoid more than light use of the affected knee over the next 2 weeks.
- Use other complementary treatment modalities including physical therapy as indicated.
- Consider follow-up examination in 2 weeks.

CPT codes:
- 20610—Arthrocentesis, aspiration and/or injection, major joint or bursa; without ultrasound guidance
- 20611—With ultrasound guidance, with permanent recording and reporting

PEARLS

- Because of potential direct needle injury to articular cartilage and documented decreased success rates, the medial and lateral infrapatellar approaches should only be used in special circumstances where the suprapatellar and midpatellar approaches cannot be performed. This may occur in patients with local cellulitis or soft tissue injury, or in a patient confined to a wheelchair who cannot be easily moved onto an examination table.
- Ultrasound-assisted aspiration and injection using an indirect technique is useful in ensuring the accuracy of injecting expensive viscosupplementation products.

 Videos showing knee joint aspirations and injections utilizing the antero-medial and anterolateral approaches can be found in the companion eBook.

Knee Joint—Popliteal Synovial (Baker's) Cyst

A popliteal synovial (Baker's) cyst is a fluid- and fibrin-filled structure over the posterior aspect of the knee. It is not an uncommon presentation in a primary care medical office. This structure forms when an excessive amount of synovial fluid is produced in the knee joint, usually as a result of osteoarthritis. Other associated conditions include inflammatory synovitis and meniscal tears. Fluid pressure causes the gradual formation of a synovial outpouching in the medial inferior aspect of the popliteal fossa in an area of relative weakness located in the gastrocnemiosemimembranosus bursa.[1] The cyst communicates with the knee joint via a slender neck that functions as a one-way valve. Baker's cysts typically present as an enlarging cystic structure over the posterior aspect of the knee that may be tender, cause lower leg swelling, or limit full flexion of the knee.

Popliteal synovial cysts may be effectively treated with aspiration and corticosteroid injection. Caution is advised when performing large-diameter needle–based procedures in the popliteal area due to the presence of the popliteal artery, popliteal vein, and the tibial nerve running longitudinally in the center of this area. Care must be taken to direct the needle anteromedially and away from these critical structures.

Treatment of symptomatic cysts can be done by aspiration of the fluid contents combined with corticosteroid injection either directly into the cyst[2,3] or separately into the knee joint.[4] Needle fenestration has also shown benefit.[5] The aspiration and injection procedures are augmented when combined with physical therapy.[6] Ultrasound guidance enhances safety and accuracy and favorably affects the treatment outcomes of pain and disability.[7] Patients who fail injection management (usually because of the presence of a complex vs. simple cyst), may be referred for surgical excision.

Indication	ICD-10 Code
Popliteal synovial cyst	M71.20

Relevant Anatomy: (Fig. 11.30)

PATIENT POSITION

- Lying prone on the examination table with the knee extended

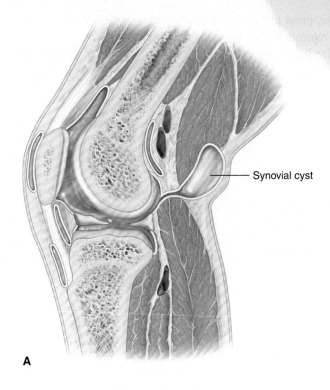

A

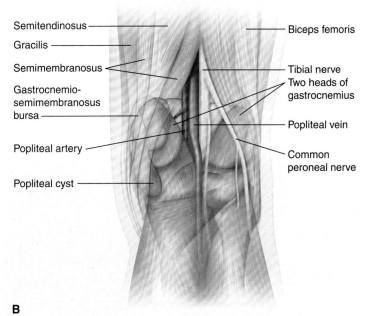

Semitendinosus

Gracilis

Semimembranosus

Gastrocnemio-
semimembranosus
bursa

Popliteal artery

Popliteal cyst

Biceps femoris

Tibial nerve

Two heads of
gastrocnemius

Popliteal vein

Common
peroneal nerve

B

FIGURE 11.30 ● **A:** Popliteal anatomy—sagittal. **B:** Popliteal anatomy—coronal—with location of the gastrocnemiosemimembranosus bursa marked.

LANDMARKS

1. With the patient lying prone on the examination table, the clinician stands lateral to the affected knee.
2. Locate the most prominent aspect of the popliteal cyst that is located over the medial inferior aspect of the popliteal space.

3. At that site, press firmly on the skin with the retracted tip of a ballpoint pen. This
   indention represents the entry point for the needle.
4. After the landmarks are identified, the patient should not move the knee.

ANESTHESIA

• Local anesthesia of the skin using topical vapocoolant spray

EQUIPMENT

• Topical vapocoolant spray
• 10- to 20-mL syringe—for aspiration
• 18-gauge, 1½-in. needle—for aspiration of the Baker's cyst
• 3 mL syringe—for injection of the mepivacaine/corticosteroid mixture
• 1 mL of 1% mepivacaine without epinephrine—to dilute the corticosteroid
• 1 mL of the corticosteroid solution (40 mg of triamcinolone acetonide)
• One alcohol prep pad
• Two povidone–iodine prep pads
• Sterile gauze pads
• Sterile adhesive bandage
• Nonsterile, clean chucks pad

TECHNIQUE

1. (Optional) Use ultrasound to image the posterior knee joint structures using an adjacent, but separate, acoustic window (Fig. 11.31). This allows separate imaging from
   the injection site so that there is no contamination from the ultrasound gel. Alternatively, the entire site may be prepped in an aseptic manner and sterile ultrasound gel
   utilized.
2. Create an aseptic insertion site by wiping with a single alcohol prep pad followed by
   two 10% povidone–iodine prep pads. Allow this site to completely dry by evaporation.

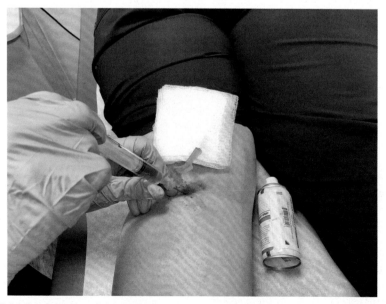

FIGURE 11.31 ● Baker's cyst aspiration.

3. Achieve good local anesthesia by using topical vapocoolant spray.
4. Position the 18-gauge, 1½-in. needle and syringe perpendicularly to the skin and with the tip of the needle directed anteromedially.
5. Using the aseptic, no-touch technique, quickly introduce that needle at the insertion site.
6. While withdrawing the plunger of the syringe, advance the needle into the popliteal synovial cyst.
7. Stop the advancement when clear fluid is aspirated. Then completely aspirate the cyst contents.
8. Next, remove the large syringe from the 18-gauge needle and then attach the 3-mL syringe filled with the mepivacaine/corticosteroid solution
9. Inject the mepivacaine/corticosteroid solution as a bolus into the cyst. The injected solution should flow smoothly into the joint space. If increased resistance is encountered, advance or withdraw the needle slightly.
10. Following injection, withdraw the needle.
11. Apply a sterile adhesive bandage.
12. Instruct the patient to move his or her knee through its full range of motion. This movement distributes the mepivacaine/corticosteroid solution throughout the synovial cyst.
13. Reexamine the knee in 5 min to assess pain relief.

AFTERCARE

- Avoid more than light use of the affected knee over the next 2 weeks.
- Use other complementary treatment modalities including physical therapy as indicated.
- Consider follow-up examination in 2 weeks.

CPT codes:
- 20610—Arthrocentesis, aspiration and/or injection, major joint or bursa; without ultrasound guidance
- 20611—With ultrasound guidance, with permanent recording and reporting

PEARLS

- Be very careful to avoid inadvertent injury to the popliteal artery, popliteal vein, and the tibial nerve running longitudinally in the center of the popliteal space.
- Direct the needle anteromedially and away from these critical structures.
- Ultrasound-guided aspiration and injection is usually not necessary, but is useful to guide needle placement and ensure safety of this procedure.

 A video showing a Baker's cyst aspiration and injection can be found in the companion eBook.

REFERENCES

1. Herman AM, Marzo JM. Popliteal cysts: a current review. *Orthopedics*. 2014;37(8):e678–e684.
2. Köroğlu M, Callıoğlu M, Eriş HN, et al. Ultrasound guided percutaneous treatment and follow-up of Baker's cyst in knee osteoarthritis. *Eur J Radiol*. 2012;81(11):3466–3471.

3. Bandinelli F, Fedi R, Generini S, et al. Longitudinal ultrasound and clinical follow-up of Baker's cysts injection with steroids in knee osteoarthritis. *Clin Rheumatol*. 2012;31(4):727–731.

4. Di Sante L, Paoloni M, Ioppolo F, et al. Ultrasound-guided aspiration and corticosteroid injection of Baker's cysts in knee osteoarthritis: a prospective observational study. *Am J Phys Med Rehabil*. 2010;89(12):970–975.

5. Smith MK, Lesniak B, Baraga MG, et al. Treatment of Popliteal (Baker) cysts with ultrasound-guided aspiration, fenestration, and injection: long-term follow-up. *Sports Health*. 2015;7(5):409–414.

6. Di Sante L, Paoloni M, Dimaggio M, et al. Ultrasound-guided aspiration and corticosteroid injection compared to horizontal therapy for treatment of knee osteoarthritis complicated with Baker's cyst: a randomized, controlled trial. *Eur J Phys Rehabil Med*. 2012;48(4):561–567.

7. Çağlayan G, Özçakar L, Kaymak SU, et al. Effects of Sono-feedback during aspiration of Baker's cysts: A controlled clinical trial. *J Rehabil Med*. 2016;48(4):386–389.

Prepatellar Bursitis

Prepatellar bursitis is a fairly common condition encountered by primary care practitioners. Approximately one-third of cases are septic, and two-thirds of cases are nonseptic. General conservative treatment measures consist of bursal aspiration, NSAIDs, and a combination of protection, rest, ice, compression, and elevation. Analysis of the fluid from the bursa is critical to distinguish septic from nonseptic cases. Successful aspiration is usually easily accomplished because the location of bursa is readily evident. The subcutaneous prepatellar bursa may become inflamed and accumulate fluid when subjected to repeated excessive pressure or friction. A large-diameter needle is selected since the fluid collection may consist of blood in acute trauma, thick proteinaceous mucoid fluid after repetitive injury, or purulence if infected. For patients with confirmed nonseptic bursitis and high athletic or occupational demands, intrabursal corticosteroid injection may be performed. In the case of septic bursitis, antibiotic therapy should be initiated. Surgical treatment with incision and drainage, or bursectomy, should be restricted to severe, refractory, or chronic/recurrent cases.[1] Unfortunately, there are no studies found in the peer-reviewed medical literature that address injection treatment.

Indication	ICD-10 Code
Prepatellar bursitis	M70.40

Relevant Anatomy: (Fig. 11.32)

PATIENT POSITION

- Lying supine on the examination table with the knee extended, or slightly flexed and supported with a pillow or folded chucks pads as needed for patient comfort.
- Rotate the patient's head away from the side that is being injected. This minimizes anxiety and pain perception.

LANDMARKS

1. With the patient lying supine on the examination table, the clinician stands lateral to the affected knee.
2. The point of maximal fluctuance is identified.
3. At that site, press firmly on the skin with the retracted tip of a ballpoint pen. This indention represents the entry point for the needle.
4. After the landmarks are identified, the patient should not move the knee.

ANESTHESIA

- Local anesthesia of the skin using topical vapocoolant spray

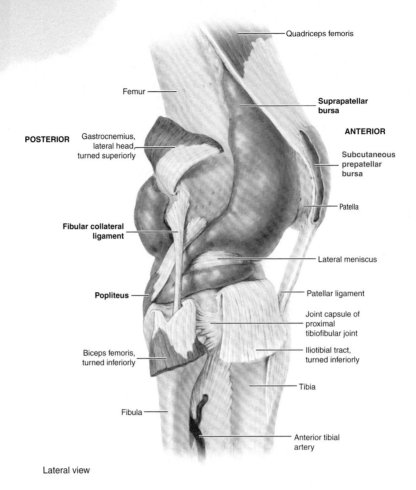

Lateral view

FIGURE 11.32 Lateral aspect of the right knee showing the extent of the knee joint capsule (in *purple*). (From Agur AM, Dalley AF. *Grant's Atlas of Anatomy*, 14th Ed. Philadelphia, PA: Wolters Kluwer, 2016.)

EQUIPMENT

- Topical vapocoolant spray
- 20-mL syringe
- 3-mL syringe—for optional injection
- 18-gauge, 1½-in. needle
- 1 mL of 1% lidocaine without epinephrine—for optional injection
- 1 mL of the steroid solution (40 mg of triamcinolone acetonide)—for optional injection
- One alcohol prep pad
- Two povidone–iodine prep pads
- Sterile gauze pads
- Sterile adhesive bandage
- Nonsterile, clean chucks pad

TECHNIQUE

1. Prep the insertion site with alcohol followed by the povidone–iodine pads.
2. Achieve good local anesthesia by using topical vapocoolant spray.

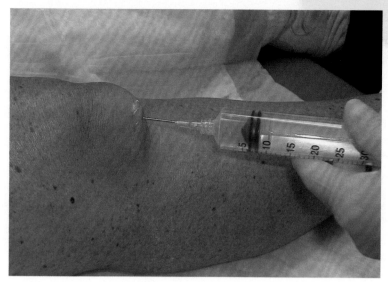

FIGURE 11.33 ● Prepatellar bursitis aspiration.

3. Stabilize the soft tissues by grasping the bursa firmly with your nondominant hand thumb and index finger. Then, squeeze to compress the fluid accumulation.
4. Position the 18-gauge needle and syringe with the tip of the needle directed toward the center of maximal fluid collection.
5. Using the no-touch technique, quickly introduce the needle at the insertion site (Fig. 11.33).
6. Advance the needle into the center of the bursa.
7. Aspiration should be easily accomplished. Use multiple syringes if the effusion is large.
8. (Optional) If a corticosteroid injection following aspiration is elected, do not remove the needle. Grasp the hub of the 18-gauge needle, remove the large syringe, and then attach the 3-mL syringe filled with the lidocaine/corticosteroid solution.
9. The injected solution should flow smoothly into the space. If increased resistance is encountered, advance or withdraw the needle slightly before attempting further injection.
10. Following completed aspiration, and possible injection, withdraw the needle.
11. Apply a sterile adhesive bandage followed by a compressive elastic bandage.
12. Reexamine the knee in 5 min to assess pain relief.

AFTERCARE

- Avoid excessive use of the affected knee over the next 2 weeks.
- Consider the use of a knee compression wrap.
- NSAIDs, and a combination of protection, rest, ice, compression, and elevation as indicated.
- Consider follow-up examination in 2 weeks.

CPT codes:
- 20610—Arthrocentesis, aspiration and/or injection, major joint or bursa; without ultrasound guidance
- 20611—With ultrasound guidance, with permanent recording and reporting

PEARLS

- If the prepatellar bursitis is due to an infection or acute hemorrhagic event, do not follow aspiration with corticosteroid injection.
- Injection of corticosteroid solution is usually reserved for recurrent bursitis.

 A video showing a prepatellar bursitis aspiration and injection can be found in the companion eBook.

REFERENCE

1. Baumbach SF, Lobo CM, Badyine I, et al. Prepatellar and olecranon bursitis: literature review and development of a treatment algorithm. *Arch Orthop Trauma Surg.* 2014;134(3):359–370.

Patellar Tendon

Patients occasionally present to the primary care office for the evaluation and treatment of pain over the patellar tendon. This tendon connects the patella and therefore the quadriceps muscles to the anterior, proximal tibia at the tibial tubercle. The usual inciting factor is chronic overuse that causes tendonitis, tendinopathy, or disruption of the patellar tendon. Predisposing conditions include older age, diabetes, collagen vascular disease, glucocorticoids, and fluoroquinolone use.[1] The primary presenting complaint is the insidious onset of pain located directly over the patellar tendon. The pain increases with direct palpation over the tendon, passive stretching, and active knee extension—particularly with jumping. Patellar tendinopathy and dysfunction are often long-standing and limit athletic and daily activities. The diagnosis is usually easily made on the basis of clinical examination without imaging.

In chronic tendinopathy, treatment is often lengthy and difficult. Physical therapy utilizing eccentric exercise is the primary treatment. Although Fredberg and colleagues[2] demonstrated efficacy of ultrasound-guided peritendinous steroid injections, corticosteroid injection therapy is traditionally avoided due to the increased risk of devastating tendon rupture. There is currently no evidence in the medical literature that platelet-rich plasma injections are effective for the treatment of patellar tendon disease.[3] When refractory to conservative management, patellar tendon injuries may be treated with arthroscopic or open surgical techniques.[4,5]

Indication	ICD-10 Code
Patellar tendonitis	M76.50

Relevant Anatomy: (Fig. 11.34)

PEARLS

- Corticosteroid injection therapy is traditionally avoided due to the increased risk of devastating tendon rupture.

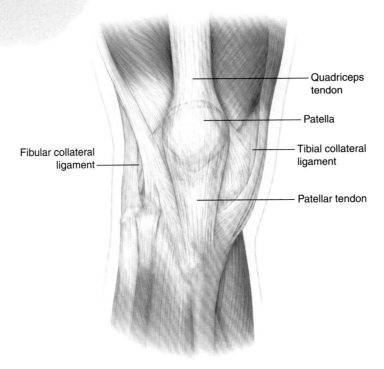

Quadriceps tendon

Patella

Fibular collateral ligament

Tibial collateral ligament

Patellar tendon

FIGURE 11.34 ● Patellar tendon.

REFERENCES

1. Alves C, Mendes D, Marques FB. Fluoroquinolones and the risk of tendon injury: a systematic review and meta-analysis. *Eur J Clin Pharmacol*. 2019;75(10):1431–1443.
2. Fredberg U, Bolvig L, Pfeiffer-Jensen M, et al. Ultrasonography as a tool for diagnosis, guidance of local steroid injection and, together with pressure algometry, monitoring of the treatment of athletes with chronic jumper's knee and Achilles tendinitis: a randomized, double-blind, placebo-controlled study. *Scand J Rheumatol*. 2004;33(2):94–101.
3. Pas HIMFL, Moen MH, Haisma HJ, et al. No evidence for the use of stem cell therapy for tendon disorders: a systematic review. *Br J Sports Med*. 2017;51(13):996–1002.
4. Khan WS, Smart A. Outcome of surgery for chronic patellar tendinopathy: a systematic review. *Acta Orthop Belg*. 2016;82(3):610-326.
5. Stuhlman CR, Stowers K, Stowers L, et al. Current concepts and the role of surgery in the treatment of jumper's knee. *Orthopedics*. 2016;39(6):e1028–e1035.

Pes Anserine Syndrome

Injection of corticosteroids for the treatment of pes anserine syndrome is a fairly common condition encountered in clinical practice. The pes anserinus is the shared insertion for the tendons of the sartorius, gracilis, and semitendinosus muscles. It is located over the medial aspect of the proximal tibia about 2 to 5 cm distal to the anteromedial joint margin of the knee. Since little is known regarding the structural defect responsible for this condition and it presents with features of bursitis, tendinitis, or both, this is usually referred to as pes anserine syndrome.[1] Pain and swelling may occur with overuse or excessive valgus stress on the knee. It is most commonly seen in overweight, middle-aged, and older women with diabetes a frequent risk factor. Pes anserine bursitis is commonly associated with knee osteoarthritis and increases in prevalence with the severity of the osteoarthritis.[2,3] A small-diameter needle is selected since there is rarely a collection of fluid. Corticosteroids may be used to treat this condition, but this is controversial.[4–6]

Indication	ICD-10 Code
Pes anserine bursitis	M70.50

Relevant Anatomy: (Fig. 11.35)

PATIENT POSITION

- Lying supine on the examination table with the affected knee extended or slightly flexed and supported with folded towels or chucks pads as needed for patient comfort.
- Rotate the patient's head away from the side that is being injected. This minimizes anxiety and pain perception.

LANDMARKS

1. With the patient lying supine on the examination table, the clinician stands lateral to the affected knee.
2. The point of maximal tenderness over the proximal medial anterior tibia is identified.
3. At that site, press firmly on the skin with the retracted tip of a ballpoint pen. This indention represents the entry point for the needle.
4. After the landmarks are identified, the patient should not move the knee.

ANESTHESIA

- Local anesthesia of the skin using topical vapocoolant spray

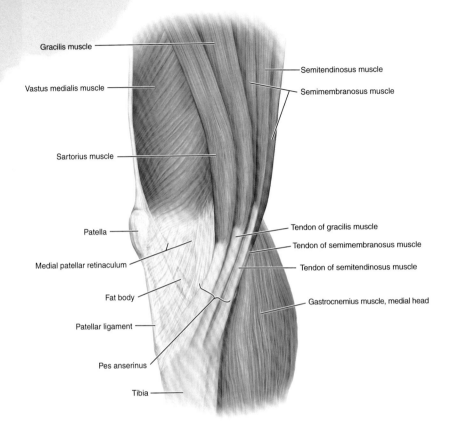

FIGURE 11.35 ● Medial aspect of the right knee/leg.

EQUIPMENT

- Topical vapocoolant spray
- 3-mL syringe
- 25-gauge, 1-in. needle
- 1 mL of 1% lidocaine without epinephrine
- 0.5 to 1 mL of the steroid solution (20 to 40 mg of triamcinolone acetonide)
- One alcohol prep pad
- Two povidone–iodine prep pads
- Sterile gauze pads
- Sterile adhesive bandage
- Nonsterile, clean chucks pad

TECHNIQUE

1. Prep the insertion site with alcohol followed by the povidone–iodine pads.
2. Achieve good local anesthesia by using topical vapocoolant spray.
3. Position the needle and syringe perpendicular to the skin with the tip of the needle directed toward the area of maximal tenderness at the insertion of the tendons.
4. Using the no-touch technique, introduce the needle at the insertion site (Fig. 11.36).

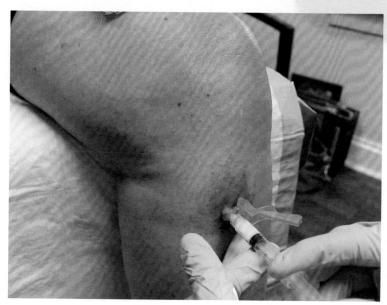

FIGURE 11.36 ● Left knee pes anserine bursitis injection.

5. Advance the needle toward the bone of the proximal medial tibia. Back up the needle 1 to 2 mm.
6. Withdraw the plunger of the syringe to ensure that there is no blood return.
7. Inject the lidocaine/corticosteroid solution as a bolus into this area. The injected solution should flow smoothly into the space. If increased resistance is encountered, advance or withdraw the needle slightly before attempting further injection.
8. Following injection, withdraw the needle.
9. Apply a sterile adhesive bandage.
10. Instruct the patient to massage this area and move his or her knee through its full range of motion. This movement distributes the steroid solution throughout the pes anserine bursa and related tendons.
11. Reexamine the pes anserine bursa in 5 min to assess pain relief.

AFTERCARE

- Avoid excessive knee extension and adduction over the next 2 weeks.
- Consider the use of a compression wrap.
- NSAIDs, ice, heat, and/or physical therapy as indicated.
- Consider follow-up examination in 2 weeks.

CPT codes:

- 20610—Arthrocentesis, aspiration and/or injection, major joint or bursa; without ultrasound guidance
- 20611—With ultrasound guidance, with permanent recording and reporting

PEARLS

- The pes anserine bursa is superficial. As a result, this injection can be complicated by the development of skin atrophy and hypopigmentation. Avoid the development of a subdermal wheal while injecting the corticosteroid solution.

- Since this is an unusual diagnosis, also consider a medial meniscal tear, chondral fracture, or osteonecrosis of the tibia.

 A video showing a pes anserine syndrome injection can be found in the companion eBook.

REFERENCES

1. Helfenstein M Jr, Kuromoto J. Anserine syndrome. *Rev Bras Reumatol.* 2010;50(3):313–327.
2. Uysal F, Akbal A, Gökmen F, et al. Prevalence of pes anserine bursitis in symptomatic osteoarthritis patients: an ultrasonographic prospective study. *Clin Rheumatol.* 2015;34(3):529–533.
3. Kim IJ, Kim DH, Song YW, et al. The prevalence of periarticular lesions detected on magnetic resonance imaging in middle-aged and elderly persons: a cross-sectional study. *BMC Musculoskelet Disord.* 2016;17:186.
4. Vega-Morales D, Esquivel-Valerio JA, Negrete-López R, et al. Safety and efficacy of methylprednisolone infiltration in anserine syndrome treatment. *Reumatol Clin.* 2012;8(2):63–67.
5. Yoon HS, Kim SE, Suh YR, et al. Correlation between ultrasonographic findings and the response to corticosteroid injection in pes anserinus tendinobursitis syndrome in knee osteoarthritis patients. *J Korean Med Sci.* 2005;20(1):109–112.
6. Kang I, Han SW. Anserine bursitis in patients with osteoarthritis of the knee. *South Med J.* 2000;93(2):207–209.

Iliotibial Band Friction Syndrome

Iliotibial band friction syndrome is a common overuse injury typically seen in runners, cyclists, triathletes, and military recruits. Affected patients report lateral knee pain associated with repetitive motion activities. Several etiologies have been proposed for iliotibial band syndrome, including friction of the iliotibial band as it rubs against the lateral femoral epicondyle, compression of the fat and connective tissue deep to the iliotibial band, and chronic inflammation of the iliotibial band bursa.[1] Another factor is a greater strain throughout the support phase of running.[2] In the acute phase of this condition, conservative treatment includes activity modification, ice, and NSAIDS. Corticosteroid injections may be used in cases of severe pain or swelling.[3] However, there is a paucity of research available and only a single, small study to support the use of injected corticosteroids.[4] A small-diameter needle is used since there is no collection of fluid to aspirate. There is a promising study showing that an injection of botulinum toxin into the tensor fascia lata, combined with physical therapy, rendered significant long-term pain relief.[5]

Indication	ICD-10 Code
Iliotibial band syndrome	M76.30

Relevant Anatomy: (Fig. 11.37)

PATIENT POSITION

- Lying supine on the examination table with the knee extended, or slightly flexed and supported with a pillow or folded chucks pads as needed for patient comfort.
- Rotate the patient's head away from the side that is being injected. This minimizes anxiety and pain perception.

LANDMARKS

1. With the patient lying supine on the examination table, the clinician stands lateral to the affected knee.
2. The point of maximal tenderness over the lateral femoral condyle is identified.
3. At that site, press firmly on the skin with the retracted tip of a ballpoint pen. This indention represents the entry point for the needle.
4. After the landmarks are identified, the patient should not move the knee.

ANESTHESIA

- Local anesthesia of the skin using topical vapocoolant spray

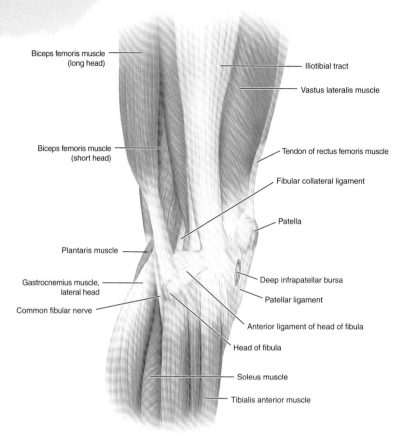

FIGURE 11.37 ● Lateral aspect of the right knee/leg. (Modified from Gest TR. *Lippincott Atlas of Anatomy*, 2nd Ed. Philadelphia, PA: Wolters Kluwer, 2019.)

EQUIPMENT

- Topical vapocoolant spray
- 3-mL syringe
- 25-gauge, 1-in. needle
- 1 mL of 1% lidocaine without epinephrine
- 1 mL of the steroid solution (40 mg of triamcinolone acetonide)
- One alcohol prep pad
- Two povidone–iodine prep pads
- Sterile gauze pads
- Sterile adhesive bandage
- Nonsterile, clean chucks pad

TECHNIQUE

1. Prep the insertion site with alcohol followed by the povidone–iodine pads.
2. Achieve good local anesthesia by using topical vapocoolant spray.
3. Position the needle and syringe perpendicular to the skin with the tip of the needle directed toward the area of maximal tenderness over the lateral femoral condyle.

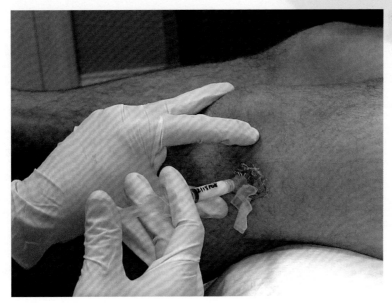

FIGURE 11.38 ● Left leg iliotibial band injection.

4. Using the no-touch technique, introduce the needle at the insertion site (Fig. 11.38).
5. Advance the needle through the iliotibial band and touch the bone of the lateral femoral condyle. Back up the needle 1 to 2 mm.
6. Withdraw the plunger of the syringe to ensure that there is no blood return.
7. Inject the lidocaine/corticosteroid solution as a bolus into this area. The injected solution should flow smoothly into the tissues. If increased resistance is encountered, advance or withdraw the needle slightly before attempting further injection.
8. Following injection, withdraw the needle.
9. Apply a sterile adhesive bandage.
10. Instruct the patient to massage this area and move his or her knee through its full range of motion. This movement distributes the lidocaine/corticosteroid solution throughout the iliotibial tract and related structures.
11. Reexamine the lateral aspect of the knee in 5 min to assess pain relief.

AFTERCARE

- Relative rest with avoidance of the precipitating activity for at least 2 weeks.
- Iliotibial band stretching exercises.
- NSAIDs, ice, heat, and/or physical therapy as indicated.
- Consider follow-up examination in 2 weeks.

CPT codes:
- 20550—Injection(s); single tendon sheath, or ligament, aponeurosis
- 76942 (optional)—Ultrasonic guidance for needle placement with imaging supervision and interpretation with permanent recording

PEARLS

- The iliotibial band can be superficial, especially in thin persons. As a result, this injection can be complicated by the development of skin atrophy and hypopigmentation. Avoid the development of a subdermal wheal while injecting the corticosteroid solution.

A video showing an iliotibial band friction syndrome injection can be found in the companion eBook.

REFERENCES

1. Strauss EJ, Kim S, Calcei JG, et al. Iliotibial band syndrome: evaluation and management. *J Am Acad Orthop Surg*. 2011;19(12):728–736.
2. Hamill J, Miller R, Noehren B, et al. A prospective study of iliotibial band strain in runners. *Clin Biomech (Bristol, Avon)*. 2008;23(8):1018–1025.
3. Fredericson M, Weir A. Practical management of iliotibial band friction syndrome in runners. *Clin J Sport Med*. 2006;16(3):261–268.
4. Gunter P, Schwellnus MP. Local corticosteroid injection in iliotibial band friction syndrome in runners: a randomised controlled trial. *Br J Sports Med*. 2004;38(3):269–272.
5. Stephen JM, Urquhart DW, van Arkel RJ, et al. The use of sonographically guided botulinum toxin type A (Dysport) injections into the tensor fasciae latae for the treatment of lateral patellofemoral overload syndrome. *Am J Sports Med*. 2016;44(5):1195–1202.

Achilles Tendon

Patients occasionally present to the primary care office for the evaluation and treatment of pain over the Achilles tendon. The Achilles tendon connects the gastrocnemius and soleus muscles to the posterior calcaneus. Acute injury or chronic overuse may cause tendonitis, tendinopathy, or disruption of the Achilles tendon. Predisposing conditions include older age, pes cavus, foot hyperpronation, diabetes, collagen vascular disease, glucocorticoids, and flouroquinolone use.[1] The main presenting complaint is pain over the posterior lower leg that increases with direct palpation over the tendon, passive stretching, and active plantar flexion. Achilles tendinopathy and dysfunction are often long-standing and limit athletic and daily activities. Physical examination may be aided with either ultrasound or MRI to delineate the anatomic pathology and extent of injury.

In chronic tendinopathy, treatment is often lengthy and difficult. Physical therapy is the primary treatment. Although Wetke and colleagues[2] demonstrated decreased pain, increased participation in physical therapy, and improved clinical outcomes following corticosteroid injections, corticosteroid injection therapy is traditionally avoided due to the increased risk of devastating tendon rupture. Morath's systematic review of prolotherapy using injected dextrose showed it to be beneficial.[3] Two recent meta-analyses came to the conclusion that platelet-rich plasma injections do not reduce pain, tendon thickness, or color Doppler activity.[4,5] Also, injection of platelet-rich plasma does not improve outcomes after acute Achilles tendon rupture.[6] When refractory to conservative management, Achilles injuries may be treated with surgical débridement and reattachment.

Indications	ICD-10 Code
Achilles tendonitis	M76.60
Achilles tendinosis	M67.88

Relevant Anatomy: (Fig. 11.39)

PEARLS

- Corticosteroid injection therapy is traditionally avoided due to the increased risk of devastating tendon rupture.

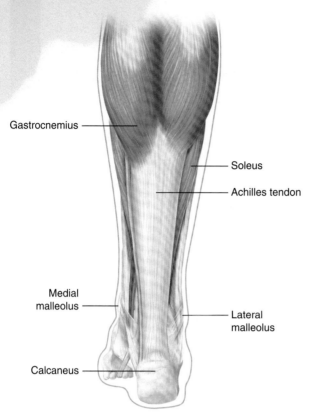

FIGURE 11.39 ● Achilles tendon

Gastrocnemius

Soleus

Achilles tendon

Medial malleolus

Lateral malleolus

Calcaneus

REFERENCES

1. Alves C, Mendes D, Marques FB. Fluoroquinolones and the risk of tendon injury: a systematic review and meta-analysis. *Eur J Clin Pharmacol*. 2019;75(10):1431–1443.
2. Wetke E, Johannsen F, Langberg H. Achilles tendinopathy: a prospective study on the effect of active rehabilitation and steroid injections in a clinical setting. *Scand J Med Sci Sports*. 2015;25(4):e392–e399.
3. Morath O, Kubosch EJ, Taeymans J, et al. The effect of sclerotherapy and prolotherapy on chronic painful Achilles tendinopathy-a systematic review including meta-analysis. *Scand J Med Sci Sports*. 2018;28(1):4-15.
4. Lin MT, Chiang CF, Wu CH, et al. Meta-analysis comparing autologous blood-derived products (including platelet-rich plasma) injection versus placebo in patients with Achilles tendinopathy. *Arthroscopy*. 2018;34(6):1966.e5–1975.e5.
5. Zhang YJ, Xu SZ, Gu PC, et al. Is platelet-rich plasma injection effective for chronic achilles tendinopathy? A meta-analysis. *Clin Orthop Relat Res*. 2018;476(8):1633–1641.
6. Keene DJ, Alsousou J, Harrison P, et al. Platelet rich plasma injection for acute Achilles tendon rupture: PATH-2 randomised, placebo controlled, superiority trial. *BMJ* 2019;367:l6132.

Tibialis Posterior Tendonitis

Tibialis posterior tendonitis is a fairly unusual injection in clinical practice. The tibialis posterior muscle originates from the interosseous membrane and the adjacent posterior surface of the tibia in the proximal third of the lower leg. It courses behind the medial malleolus, passes under the flexor retinaculum, and inserts into the tuberosity of the navicular bone and the medial cuneiform bone. The muscle plantar-flexes the ankle and inverts the foot. Tibialis posterior tendon dysfunction is an often unrecognized disabling cause of progressive flatfoot deformity and is the most frequently ruptured tendon in the rear foot. Tenosynovitis of the tibialis posterior tendon occurs as a result of acute trauma, altered mechanics of the foot, and chronic overuse or with inflammatory conditions such as rheumatoid arthritis. Patients present with pain, difficulty walking, and swelling along the medial malleolus and the arch of the foot. Conservative management includes the use of orthotics, stretching, as well as eccentric and concentric progressive resistive exercises.[1] Discrete injections of corticosteroids may be of some benefit to decrease pain and facilitate physical therapy, but there is little evidence-based support for this recommendation. Surgery is required in the case of tendon rupture or the failure to respond to conservative therapy.

Indications	ICD-10 Code
Tibialis posterior tendonitis	M76.829
Tibialis posterior tendinopathy	M67.979

Relevant Anatomy: (Fig. 11.40)

PATIENT POSITION

- Supine on the examination table with the hip in full external rotation, knee slightly flexed, and the ankle in a neutral position.
- Alternatively, lying on the examination table on the affected side with the knee slightly flexed and the ankle in a neutral position.
- Rotate the patient's head away from the side that is being injected. This minimizes anxiety and pain perception.

LANDMARKS

1. With the patient lying supine on the examination table, the clinician stands or sits medial to the affected ankle.
2. Palpate the medial malleolus of the tibia.
3. Locate the tibialis posterior tendon immediately behind and below the medial malleolus.
4. Determine the location of maximal tenderness along the tendon.

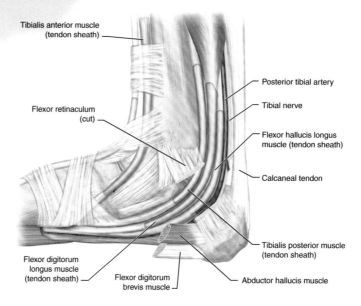

FIGURE 11.40 ● Medial aspect of the right foot.

5. Identify a point along the tendon 1 cm distal to the point of maximal tenderness and mark it in ink.
6. At that site, press firmly on the skin with the retracted tip of a ballpoint pen. This indention represents the entry point for the needle.
7. After the landmarks are identified, the patient should not move the ankle.

ANESTHESIA

- Local anesthesia of the skin with topical vapocoolant spray

EQUIPMENT

- Topical vapocoolant spray
- 3-mL syringe
- 25-gauge, 5/8-in. needle
- 0.5 mL of 1% lidocaine without epinephrine
- 0.5 mL of the steroid solution (20 mg of triamcinolone acetonide)
- One alcohol prep pad
- Two povidone–iodine prep pads
- Sterile gauze pads
- Sterile adhesive bandage
- Nonsterile, clean chucks pad

TECHNIQUE

1. Prep the insertion site with alcohol followed by the povidone–iodine pads.
2. Achieve good local anesthesia by using topical vapocoolant spray.
3. Position the needle and syringe with the needle tip directed proximally at a 30-degree angle to the surface of the skin.

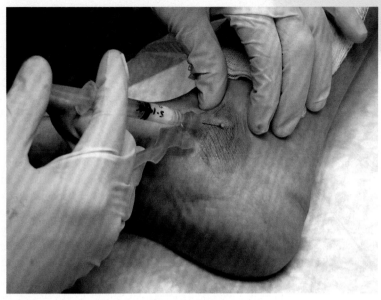

FIGURE 11.41 • Tibialis posterior tendonitis injection.

4. Using the no-touch technique, introduce the needle at the insertion site (Fig. 11.41).
5. Reexamine the tendon in 5 min to assess pain relief.

AFTERCARE

- Avoid excessive use of the foot over the next 2 weeks.
- Begin a program of physical therapy.
- Use orthotics or "motion-control" running shoes if there is excessive foot pronation.
- NSAIDs, ice, and heat as indicated.
- Consider follow-up examination in 2 weeks.

CPT codes:
- 20550—Injection(s); single tendon sheath, or ligament, aponeurosis
- 76942 (optional)—Ultrasonic guidance for needle placement with imaging supervision and interpretation with permanent recording

PEARLS

- This injection can be superficial. Depositing corticosteroid in the subcutaneous tissues can result in the complication of skin atrophy and hypopigmentation. Avoid the development of a subdermal wheal while performing all injections of corticosteroid solutions.

 A video showing a tibialis posterior tendonitis injection can be found in the companion eBook.

REFERENCE

1. Kulig K, Reischl SF, Pomrantz AB, et al. Nonsurgical management of posterior tibial tendon dysfunction with orthoses and resistive exercise: a randomized controlled trial. *Phys Ther.* 2009;89(1):26–37.

Tarsal Tunnel Syndrome

Tarsal tunnel syndrome is a rare condition encountered in primary care. It represents an entrapment neuropathy of the posterior tibial nerve or its branches as it passes underneath the flexor retinaculum at the level of the medial malleolus. It may occur due to trauma from crush injury, stretch injury, fractures, dislocations, and severe ankle sprains. Other causes include overuse in athletes, valgus foot deformity, compression from bony prominences, and systemic conditions such as diabetes, hypothyroidism, rheumatoid arthritis, or amyloidosis. Typical symptoms include pain and paresthesias that radiate from the medial ankle. A positive Tinel's sign may be elicited posterior to the medial malleolus. Electrodiagnostic tests frequently yield false-negative results.[1] Conservative treatment options include relative rest, physical therapy, orthotics, splints, and, perhaps, the injection of corticosteroids. However, there is no literature basis for the use of injections. Complete surgical decompression of the tarsal tunnel is required for patients with persistent symptoms.[2]

Indication	ICD-10 Code
Tarsal tunnel syndrome	G57.50

Relevant Anatomy: (Fig. 11.42)

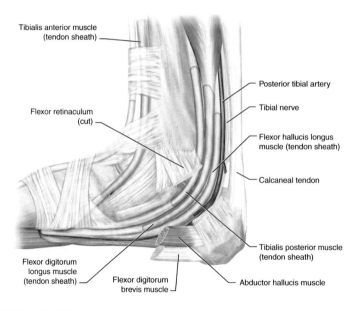

FIGURE 11.42 ● Medial aspect of the right foot.

PATIENT POSITION

- Supine on the examination table with the hip in full external rotation, the knee slightly flexed, and the ankle in a neutral position.
- Alternatively, lying on the examination table on the affected side with the knee slightly flexed and the ankle in a neutral position.
- Rotate the patient's head away from the side that is being injected. This minimizes anxiety and pain perception.

LANDMARKS

1. With the patient lying supine on the examination table, the clinician stands or sits medial to the affected ankle.
2. Locate the medial malleolus of the tibia and then the insertion of the Achilles tendon into the calcaneus.
3. Midway between these two structures, palpate the posterior tibial artery.
4. The posterior tibial nerve is located about 0.5 cm posterior to the posterior tibial artery. Mark the nerve with ink.
5. At that site, press firmly on the skin with the retracted tip of a ballpoint pen. This indention represents the entry point for the needle.
6. After the landmarks are identified, the patient should not move the ankle.

ANESTHESIA

- Local anesthesia of the skin using a topical vapocoolant spray

EQUIPMENT

- Topical vapocoolant spray
- 3-mL syringe
- 25-gauge, 5/8-in. needle
- 1 mL of 1% lidocaine without epinephrine
- 1 mL of the steroid solution (40 mg of triamcinolone acetonide)
- One alcohol prep pad
- Two povidone–iodine prep pads
- Sterile gauze pads
- Sterile adhesive bandage
- Nonsterile, clean chucks pad

TECHNIQUE

1. Prep the insertion site with alcohol followed by the povidone–iodine pads.
2. Achieve good local anesthesia by using a topical vapocoolant spray.
3. Position the needle and syringe with the needle tip directed perpendicularly to the surface of the skin with the tip of the needle directed laterally toward the nerve.
4. Using the no-touch technique, introduce the needle at the insertion site (Fig. 11.43).
5. Advance the needle about 1 cm deep. If any pain, paresthesia, or numbness is encountered, back up the needle 1 to 2 mm.
6. Withdraw the plunger of the syringe to ensure that there is no blood return.

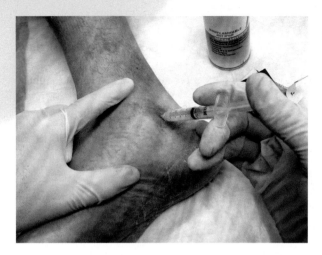

FIGURE 11.43 ● Tarsal tunnel injection.

7. Slowly inject the lidocaine/corticosteroid as a bolus around the posterior tibial nerve and into the tarsal tunnel. If increased resistance is encountered, advance or withdraw the needle slightly before attempting further injection.
8. Following injection, withdraw the needle.
9. Apply a sterile adhesive bandage.
10. Instruct the patient to move his or her ankle through its full range of motion. This movement distributes the lidocaine/corticosteroid solution along the nerve and throughout the tarsal tunnel.
11. Reexamine the foot in 5 min to assess pain relief and/or the development of numbness from the local anesthetic in the distribution of the posterior tibial nerve.

AFTERCARE

- Avoid excessive use of the foot over the next 2 weeks.
- Begin a program of physical therapy.
- Use orthotics or "motion-control" running shoes if there is excessive foot pronation.
- Consider splinting—especially at night.
- NSAIDs, ice, and heat as indicated.
- Consider follow-up examination in 2 weeks.

CPT codes:
- 28899—Unlisted procedure, foot or toes or
- 64450—Injection, nerve block, therapeutic, other peripheral nerve or branch
- 76942 (optional)—Ultrasonic guidance for needle placement with imaging supervision and interpretation with permanent recording

PEARLS

- Warn the patient that the posterior tibial nerve may be contacted when using this approach. Ask him or her to calmly report any pain or electrical shock sensation without jerking his or her foot away.
- This injection can be superficial. Depositing corticosteroid in the subcutaneous tissues can result in the complication of skin atrophy and hypopigmentation. Avoid the development of a subdermal wheal while performing all injections of the corticosteroid solutions.

A video showing a tarsal tunnel syndrome injection can be found in the companion eBook.

REFERENCES

1. Ahmad M, Tsang K, Mackenney PJ, et al. Tarsal tunnel syndrome: a literature review. *Foot Ankle Surg.* 2012;18(3):149–152.
2. Franson J, Baravarian B. Tarsal tunnel syndrome: a compression neuropathy involving four distinct tunnels. *Clin Podiatr Med Surg.* 2006;23(3):597–609.

Ankle Joint—Anterolateral Approach

Although ankle pain is a common presenting complaint in primary care, injection of the ankle joint is fairly uncommon. Ankle joint pain may occur following acute trauma or with osteoarthritis, gout, rheumatoid arthritis, or other inflammatory conditions. Conservative treatment of osteoarthritis includes weight loss, physical therapy, bracing, orthoses, and the use of NSAIDs.[1] The effectiveness of the anterolateral approach to the ankle, especially when combined with imaging guidance has been verified.[2] A small-diameter needle is usually selected as this technique is primarily used to inject steroid solution into a painful ankle joint. Occasionally, joint fluid may need to be aspirated.

There is a growing collection of studies that demonstrate short- to medium-term benefit from corticosteroid injections.[3–5] However, corticosteroids should not be administered immediately following ankle arthroscopy[6] and not within 3 months prior to total ankle arthroplasty.[7] There are increasing favorable data on improvement in pain and function in patients treated with hyaluronic acid viscosupplements.[8,9] However, this treatment is still not approved by the U.S. Food and Drug Administration at the time of publication. Other treatment modalities that appear promising include injections of platelet-rich plasma[10] and mesenchymal stem cells.[11] Those patients who fail conservative interventions may eventually require surgery. The gold standard in end-stage degenerative arthritis remains arthrodesis, but evidence for the superiority in functional outcomes of total ankle arthroplasty is increasing.[12]

Indications	ICD-10 Code
Ankle joint pain	M25.579
Ankle arthritis, unspecified	M19.079
Ankle osteoarthritis, primary	M19.079
Ankle osteoarthritis, posttraumatic	M19.179
Ankle osteoarthritis, secondary	M19.279

Relevant Anatomy: (Fig. 11.44)

PATIENT POSITION

- Supine on the examination table.
- The knee on the affected side is placed in 90 degrees of flexion.
- The ankle is slightly plantar flexed so that the plantar surface is in full contact with the chucks pad covering the exam table.
- Rotate the patient's head away from the side that is being injected. This minimizes anxiety and pain perception.

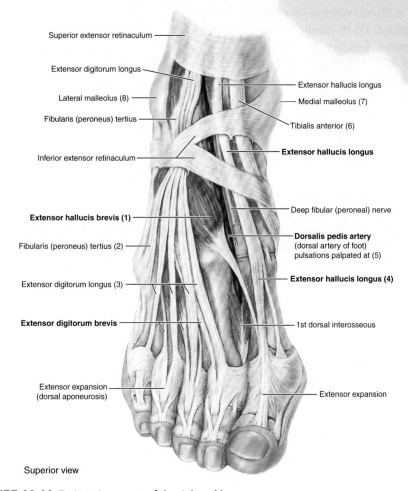

Superior extensor retinaculum

Extensor digitorum longus

Extensor hallucis longus

Lateral malleolus (8)

Medial malleolus (7)

Fibularis (peroneus) tertius

Tibialis anterior (6)

Extensor hallucis longus

Inferior extensor retinaculum

Deep fibular (peroneal) nerve

Extensor hallucis brevis (1)

Dorsalis pedis artery
(dorsal artery of foot)
pulsations palpated at (5)

Fibularis (peroneus) tertius (2)

Extensor digitorum longus (3)

Extensor hallucis longus (4)

Extensor digitorum brevis

1st dorsal interosseous

Extensor expansion
(dorsal aponeurosis)

Extensor expansion

Superior view

FIGURE 11.44 ● Anterior aspect of the right ankle.

LANDMARKS

1. With the patient lying supine on the examination table, the clinician stands or sits lateral to the affected ankle.
2. Identify the junction over the anterolateral aspect of the ankle that is located between the anterior medial aspect of the distal fibula, anterior lateral aspect of the distal tibia, and superior lateral aspect of the talus.
3. Mark a point over this articulation. There is normally a soft depression in that area.
4. At that site, press firmly on the skin with the retracted tip of a ballpoint pen. This indention represents the entry point for the needle.
5. After the landmarks are identified, the patient should not move the ankle.

ANESTHESIA

• Local anesthesia of the skin using topical vapocoolant spray

EQUIPMENT

• Topical vapocoolant spray
• 3-mL syringe—for injection

- 10- or 20-mL syringe—for optional aspiration
- 25-gauge, 1½-in. needle—if not aspirating fluid
- 20-gauge, 1-in. needle—for optional aspiration
- 1 mL of 1% mepivacaine without epinephrine
- 1 mL of the steroid solution (40 mg of triamcinolone acetonide)
- One alcohol prep pad
- Two povidone–iodine prep pads
- Sterile gauze pads
- Sterile adhesive bandage
- Nonsterile, clean chucks pad

TECHNIQUE

1. Prep the insertion site with alcohol followed by the povidone–iodine pads.
2. Achieve good local anesthesia by using topical vapocoolant spray.
3. Position the needle and syringe perpendicular to the skin with the tip of the needle directed both medial and posterior.
4. Using the no-touch technique, introduce the needle at the insertion site (Fig. 11.45).
5. Advance the needle into the ankle joint. This places the needle tip between the distal tibia and fibula within the ankle joint.
6. If only injecting mepivacaine/corticosteroid solution, use a 25-gauge, 1½-in. needle with the 3-mL syringe.
7. If aspirating, withdraw the fluid using a 20-gauge, 1½-in. needle with a 10- or 20-mL syringe.
8. If injection following aspiration is elected, remove the large syringe from the 20-gauge needle and then attach the 3-mL syringe filled with the mepivacaine/corticosteroid solution.
9. Inject the mepivacaine/corticosteroid solution as a bolus into the ankle joint. The injected solution should flow smoothly into the space. If increased resistance is encountered, advance or withdraw the needle slightly before attempting further injection.

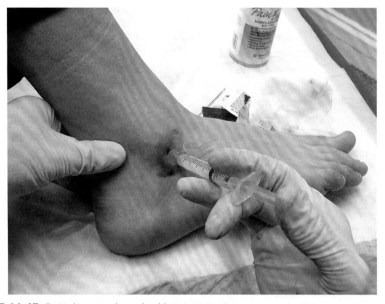

FIGURE 11.45 ● Right anterolateral ankle joint injection.

10. Following injection, withdraw the needle.
11. Apply a sterile adhesive bandage.
12. Instruct the patient to move his or her ankle through its full range of motion. This movement distributes the mepivacaine/corticosteroid solution throughout the ankle joint.
13. Reexamine the ankle in 5 min to assess pain relief.

AFTERCARE

- Consider the use of an ankle brace.
- Avoid vigorous use of the ankle over the next 2 weeks.
- NSAIDs, ice, and/or physical therapy as indicated.
- Consider follow-up examination in 2 weeks.

CPT codes:

- 20605—Arthrocentesis, aspiration and/or injection, intermediate joint or bursa; without ultrasound guidance
- 20606—With ultrasound guidance, with permanent recording and reporting

 A video showing an ankle joint injection can be found in the companion eBook.

REFERENCES

1. Khlopas H, Khlopas A, Samuel LT, et al. Current concepts in osteoarthritis of the ankle: review. *Surg Technol Int.* 2019;35:280–294.
2. Fox MG, Wright PR, Alford B, et al. Lateral mortise approach for therapeutic ankle injection: an alternative to the anteromedial approach. *AJR Am J Roentgenol.* 2013;200(5):1096–1100.
3. Furtado RNV, Machado FS, Luz KRD, et al. Intra-articular injection with triamcinolone hexacetonide in patients with rheumatoid arthritis: prospective assessment of goniometry and joint inflammation parameters. *Rev Bras Reumatol Engl Ed.* 2017;57(2):115–121.
4. Ward ST, Williams PL, Purkayastha S. Intra-articular corticosteroid injections in the foot and ankle: a prospective 1-year follow-up investigation. *J Foot Ankle Surg.* 2008;47(2):138–144.
5. Vannabouathong C, Del Fabbro G, Sales B, et al. Intra-articular injections in the treatment of symptoms from ankle arthritis: a systematic review. *Foot Ankle Int.* 2018;39(10):1141–1150.
6. Brand JC. Editorial commentary: big data suggest that because of a significant increased risk of postoperative infection, steroid injection is not recommended after ankle arthroscopy. *Arthroscopy.* 2016;32(2):355.
7. Uçkay I, Hirose CB, Assal M. Does intra-articular injection of the ankle with corticosteroids increase the risk of subsequent periprosthetic joint infection (PJI) following total ankle arthroplasty (TAA)? If so, how long after a prior intra-articular injection can TAA be safely performed? *Foot Ankle Int.* 2019;40(1_suppl):3S–4S.
8. Papalia R, Albo E, Russo F, et al. The use of hyaluronic acid in the treatment of ankle osteoarthritis: a review of the evidence. *J Biol Regul Homeost Agents.* 2017;31(4 suppl 2):91–102.
9. Lucas Y, Hernandez J, Darcel V, et al. Viscosupplementation of the ankle: a prospective study with an average follow-up of 45.5 months. *Orthop Traumatol Surg Res.* 2013;99(5):593–599.
10. Fukawa T, Yamaguchi S, Akatsu Y, et al. Safety and efficacy of intra-articular injection of platelet-rich plasma in patients with ankle osteoarthritis. *Foot Ankle Int.* 2017;38(6):596–604.
11. McIntyre JA, Jones IA, Han B, et al. Intra-articular Mesenchymal stem cell therapy for the human joint: a systematic review. *Am J Sports Med.* 2018;46(14):3550–3563.
12. Grunfeld R, Aydogan U, Juliano P. Ankle arthritis: review of diagnosis and operative management. *Med Clin North Am.* 2014;98(2):267–289.

Ankle Joint—Anteromedial Approach

Although ankle pain is a common presenting complaint in primary care, injection of the ankle joint is fairly uncommon. Ankle joint pain may occur following acute trauma or with osteoarthritis, gout, rheumatoid arthritis, or other inflammatory conditions. Conservative treatment of osteoarthritis includes weight loss, physical therapy, bracing, orthoses, and the use of NSAIDs.[1] A small-diameter needle is usually selected as this technique is primarily used to inject steroid solution into a painful ankle joint. Occasionally, joint fluid may need to be aspirated.

There is a growing collection of studies that demonstrate short- to medium-term benefit from corticosteroid injections.[2-4] However, corticosteroids should not be administered immediately following ankle arthroscopy[5] and not within 3 months prior to total ankle arthroplasty.[6] There are increasing favorable data on improvement in pain and function in patients treated with hyaluronic acid viscosupplements.[7,8] However, this treatment is still not approved by the U.S. Food and Drug Administration at the time of publication. Other treatment modalities that appear promising include injections of platelet-rich plasma[9] and mesenchymal stem cells.[10] Those patients who fail conservative interventions may eventually require surgery. The gold standard in end-stage degenerative arthritis remains arthrodesis, but evidence for the superiority in functional outcomes of total ankle arthroplasty is increasing.[11]

Indications	ICD-10 Code
Ankle joint pain	M25.579
Ankle arthritis, unspecified	M19.079
Ankle osteoarthritis, primary	M19.079
Ankle osteoarthritis, posttraumatic	M19.179
Ankle osteoarthritis, secondary	M19.279

Relevant Anatomy: (Fig. 11.46)

PATIENT POSITION

- Supine on the examination table.
- The knee on the affected side is placed in 90 degrees of flexion.
- The ankle is slightly plantar flexed so that the plantar surface is in full contact with the chucks pad covering the examination table.
- Rotate the patient's head away from the side that is being injected. This minimizes anxiety and pain perception.

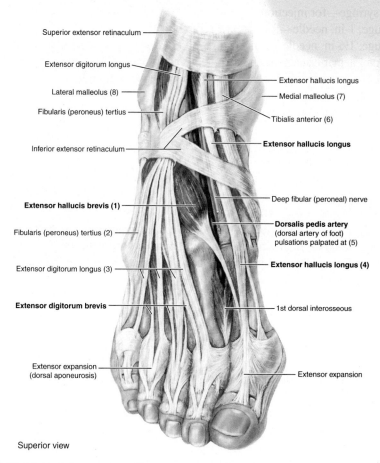

Superior extensor retinaculum

Extensor digitorum longus

Lateral malleolus (8)

Fibularis (peroneus) tertius

Inferior extensor retinaculum

Extensor hallucis longus

Medial malleolus (7)

Tibialis anterior (6)

Extensor hallucis longus

Extensor hallucis brevis (1)

Fibularis (peroneus) tertius (2)

Extensor digitorum longus (3)

Extensor digitorum brevis

Extensor expansion
(dorsal aponeurosis)

Deep fibular (peroneal) nerve

Dorsalis pedis artery
(dorsal artery of foot)
pulsations palpated at (5)

Extensor hallucis longus (4)

1st dorsal interosseous

Extensor expansion

Superior view

FIGURE 11.46 ● Right anterior ankle.

LANDMARKS

1. With the patient lying supine on the examination table, the clinician stands or sits distal to the affected ankle.
2. Locate the junction between the distal tibia and talus over the anteromedial aspect of the ankle.
3. Identify the anterior tibialis tendon by asking the patient to dorsiflex the foot.
4. Mark a point over the ankle joint line that is between the extensor hallucis longus and anterior tibialis tendons. There is normally a soft depression in that area.
5. At that site, press firmly on the skin with the retracted tip of a ballpoint pen. This indention represents the entry point for the needle.
6. After the landmarks are identified, the patient should not move the ankle.

ANESTHESIA

- Local anesthesia of the skin using topical vapocoolant spray

EQUIPMENT

- Topical vapocoolant spray
- 10- or 20-mL syringe—for optional aspiration

- 3-mL syringe—for injection
- 20-gauge, 1-in. needle—for optional aspiration
- 25-gauge, 1½-in. needle—if not aspirating fluid
- 1 mL of 1% mepivacaine without epinephrine
- 1 mL of the steroid solution (40 mg of triamcinolone acetonide)
- One alcohol prep pad
- Two povidone–iodine prep pads
- Sterile gauze pads
- Sterile adhesive bandage
- Nonsterile, clean chucks pad

TECHNIQUE

1. Prep the insertion site with alcohol followed by the povidone–iodine pads.
2. Achieve good local anesthesia by using topical vapocoolant spray.
3. Position the needle and syringe perpendicular to the skin with the tip of the needle directed posteriorly.
4. Using the no-touch technique, introduce the needle at the insertion site (Fig. 11.47).
5. Advance the needle into the ankle joint. This places the needle tip between the distal tibia and talus in the ankle joint.
6. If aspirating, withdraw the fluid using a 20-gauge, 1-in. needle with the 10- or 20-mL syringe.
7. If only injecting mepivacaine/corticosteroid solution, use a 25-gauge, 1½-in. needle with the 3-mL syringe.
8. If injection following aspiration is elected, remove the large syringe from the 20-gauge needle and then attach the 3-mL syringe filled with the mepivacaine/corticosteroid solution.
9. Inject the mepivacaine/corticosteroid solution as a bolus into the ankle joint. The injected solution should flow smoothly into the space. If increased resistance is encountered, advance or withdraw the needle slightly before attempting further injection.

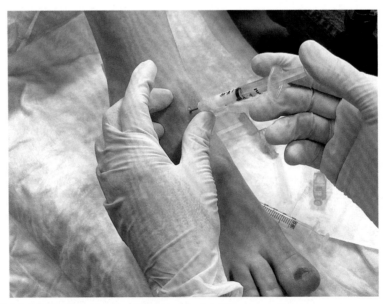

FIGURE 11.47 ● Right anteromedial ankle joint injection.

10. Following injection, withdraw the needle.
11. Apply a sterile adhesive bandage.
12. Instruct the patient to move his or her ankle through its full range of motion. This movement distributes the mepivacaine/corticosteroid solution throughout the ankle joint.
13. Reexamine the ankle in 5 min to assess pain relief.

AFTERCARE

- Consider the use of an ankle brace.
- Avoid vigorous use of the affected ankle over the next 2 weeks.
- NSAIDs, ice, and/or physical therapy as indicated.
- Consider follow-up examination in 2 weeks.

CPT codes:
- 20605—Arthrocentesis, aspiration and/or injection, intermediate joint or bursa; without ultrasound guidance
- 20606—With ultrasound guidance, with permanent recording and reporting

PEARLS

- Insert the needle medially to the anterior tibialis tendon in order to avoid injury to the anterior tibial artery, anterior tibial vein, and deep fibular nerve.

 A video showing an ankle joint injection can be found in the companion eBook.

REFERENCES

1. Khlopas H, Khlopas A, Samuel LT, et al. Current concepts in osteoarthritis of the ankle: review. *Surg Technol Int* 2019;35:280–294.
2. Furtado RNV, Machado FS, Luz KRD, et al. Intra-articular injection with triamcinolone hexacetonide in patients with rheumatoid arthritis: prospective assessment of goniometry and joint inflammation parameters. *Rev Bras Reumatol Engl Ed.* 2017;57(2):115–121.
3. Ward ST, Williams PL, Purkayastha S. Intra-articular corticosteroid injections in the foot and ankle: a prospective 1-year follow-up investigation. *J Foot Ankle Surg.* 2008;47(2):138–144.
4. Vannabouathong C, Del Fabbro G, Sales B, et al. Intra-articular injections in the treatment of symptoms from ankle arthritis: a systematic review. *Foot Ankle Int.* 2018;39(10):1141–1150.
5. Brand JC. Editorial commentary: big data suggest that because of a significant increased risk of postoperative infection, steroid injection is not recommended after ankle arthroscopy. *Arthroscopy.* 2016;32(2):355.
6. Uçkay I, Hirose CB, Assal M. Does intra-articular injection of the ankle with corticosteroids increase the risk of subsequent periprosthetic joint infection (PJI) following total ankle arthroplasty (TAA)? If so, how long after a prior intra-articular injection can TAA be safely performed? *Foot Ankle Int.* 2019;40(1_suppl):3S–4S.
7. Papalia R, Albo E, Russo F, et al. The use of hyaluronic acid in the treatment of ankle osteoarthritis: a review of the evidence. *J Biol Regul Homeost Agents.* 2017;31(4 suppl 2):91–102.
8. Lucas Y, Hernandez J, Darcel V, et al. Viscosupplementation of the ankle: a prospective study with an average follow-up of 45.5 months. *Orthop Traumatol Surg Res.* 2013;99(5):593–599.
9. Fukawa T, Yamaguchi S, Akatsu Y, et al. Safety and efficacy of intra-articular injection of platelet-rich plasma in patients with ankle osteoarthritis. *Foot Ankle Int.* 2017;38(6):596–604.
10. McIntyre JA, Jones IA, Han B, et al. Intra-articular Mesenchymal stem cell therapy for the human joint: a systematic review. *Am J Sports Med.* 2018;46(14):3550–3563.
11. Grunfeld R, Aydogan U, Juliano P. Ankle arthritis: review of diagnosis and operative management. *Med Clin North Am.* 2014;98(2):267–289.

Fibularis Brevis Tendonitis

Injection of corticosteroids for the treatment of tendonitis of the fibularis brevis (formerly known as the peroneus brevis) tendon is a fairly uncommon procedure for primary care physicians. The fibularis longus and brevis tendons are often injured with inversion ankle sprains. This can cause tendinopathy and chronic subluxation of the tendons. Overuse from repeated forceful plantar flexion and resisted foot eversion may also occur. Corticosteroid injections are often provided. Ultrasound-guided tendon sheath injection with steroids has been shown to be a safe intervention with a high technical success rate in patients with juvenile idiopathic arthritis.[1] The most common sonographic finding is peritendinous fluid and sheath thickening. Alternatively, a single case report shows treatment success with application of ultrasound-guided needle tenotomy.[2]

Indication	ICD-10 Code
Peroneus brevis tendonitis	M76.70

Relevant Anatomy: (Fig. 11.48)

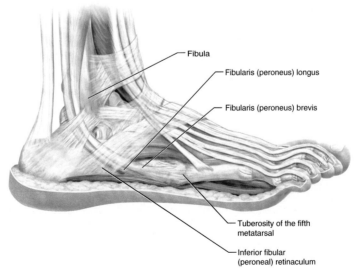

Fibula

Fibularis (peroneus) longus

Fibularis (peroneus) brevis

Tuberosity of the fifth metatarsal

Inferior fibular (peroneal) retinaculum

FIGURE 11.48 ● Lateral aspect of the right foot.

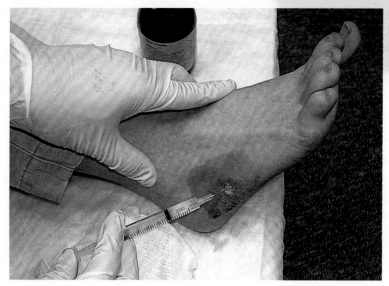

FIGURE 11.49 ● Injection of the right fibularis brevis tendon insertion.

PATIENT POSITION

- Supine on the examination table.
- The ankle and the knee on the affected side are supported by placing rolled towels underneath them.
- The ankle is in a neutral position.
- Rotate the patient's head away from the side that is being injected. This minimizes anxiety and pain perception.

LANDMARKS

1. With the patient lying supine on the examination table, the clinician stands or sits lateral to the affected foot.
2. While the foot is held in a position of active eversion, identify tenderness at and immediately proximal to the head of the fifth metatarsal bone.
3. Palpate the fibularis brevis tendon along its course from posterior and distal to the lateral malleolus to its insertion into the head of the fifth metatarsal bone.
4. Locate the area of maximal tenderness.
5. At that site, press firmly with the retracted tip of a ballpoint pen. This indention represents the entry point for the needle.
6. After the landmarks are identified, the patient should not move the ankle.

ANESTHESIA

- Local anesthesia of the skin using a topical vapocoolant spray

EQUIPMENT

- Topical vapocoolant spray
- 3-mL syringe
- 25-gauge, 5/8-in. needle

- 0.5 mL of 1% lidocaine without epinephrine
- 0.5 mL of the steroid solution (20 mg of triamcinolone acetonide)
- One alcohol prep pad
- Two povidone–iodine prep pads
- Sterile gauze pads
- Sterile adhesive bandage
- Nonsterile, clean chucks pad

TECHNIQUE

1. Prep the insertion site with alcohol followed by the povidone–iodine pads.
2. Achieve good local anesthesia by using a topical vapocoolant spray.
3. If treating tendonitis at the insertion of the fibularis brevis on the fifth metacarpal:
   a. Position the needle and syringe perpendicularly to the skin with the needle tip directed medially.
   b. Using the no-touch technique, introduce the needle at the insertion site.
   c. Advance the needle slowly until the needle tip touches the tendon/bone junction. Back up the needle 1 to 2 mm.
   d. Withdraw the plunger of the syringe to ensure that there is no blood return.
   e. Inject the lidocaine/corticosteroid solution slowly as a bolus around the insertion of the fibularis brevis tendon into the head of the fifth metatarsal. The injected solution should flow smoothly into the space. If increased resistance is encountered, advance or withdraw the needle slightly before attempting further injection.
4. If treating tendonitis along the course of the fibularis brevis tendon proximal to its insertion:
   a. Position the needle and syringe at an angle of 45 degrees to the skin with the needle tip directed proximally.
   b. Using the no-touch technique, introduce the needle at the insertion site (Fig. 11.49).
   c. Advance the needle slowly until the needle tip touches the tendon. Back up the needle 1 to 2 mm.
   d. Withdraw the plunger of the syringe to ensure that there is no blood return.
   e. Inject the lidocaine/corticosteroid solution slowly as a bolus around the fibularis brevis tendon. A small bulge in the shape of a sausage may develop in the tendon sheath. The injected solution should flow smoothly into the tenosynovial space. If increased resistance is encountered, advance or withdraw the needle slightly before attempting further injection.
5. Following injection, withdraw the needle.
6. Apply a sterile adhesive bandage.
7. Instruct the patient to move his or her ankle through its full range of inversion and eversion. This movement distributes the lidocaine/corticosteroid solution throughout the fibularis brevis tenosynovial sheath.
8. Reexamine the foot in 5 min to assess pain relief.

AFTERCARE

- Ensure no excessive plantar flexion over the next 2 weeks by the use of an ankle–foot orthosis or a walking cast boot.

- NSAIDs, ice, heat, and/or physical therapy as indicated.
- Consider follow-up examination in 2 weeks.

CPT codes:
- 20551—Injection; single tendon origin/insertion
- 76942 (optional)—Ultrasonic guidance for needle placement with imaging supervision and interpretation with permanent recording

PEARLS

- The fibularis brevis tendon is superficial. As a result, this injection can be complicated by the development of skin atrophy and hypopigmentation. Avoid the development of a subdermal wheal while injecting the corticosteroid solution.

 A video showing a fibularis brevis tendon injection can be found in the companion eBook.

REFERENCES

1. Peters SE, Laxer RM, Connolly BL, et al. Ultrasound-guided steroid tendon sheath injections in juvenile idiopathic arthritis: a 10-year single-center retrospective study. *Pediatr Rheumatol Online J.* 2017;15(1):22.
2. Sussman WI, Hofmann K. Treatment of insertional peroneus brevis tendinopathy by ultrasound-guided percutaneous ultrasonic needle tenotomy: a case report. *J Foot Ankle Surg.* 2019;58(6):1285–1287.

Plantar Fascia

Plantar fasciitis is a common presenting complaint to primary care offices. Plantar fasciitis is a repetitive motion injury with inflammation in the origin of the plantar aponeurosis at the medial tubercle of the calcaneus. It is usually caused by an excessive pronation of the foot—especially in persons with pes planus. The pain with this condition is worst when bearing weight after a period of rest. To date, there is no definitive treatment guideline for plantar fasciitis. Conservative treatment modalities include relative rest, stretching of the heel cords/plantar fascia, ice massage, and NSAIDs. Many standard treatments such as night splints and orthoses have not shown benefit over placebo.[1]

Corticosteroid injections have been a mainstay of treatment and demonstrate at least short-term symptomatic improvement.[2,3] Efficacy increases with ultrasound guidance.[4,5] In a recent systematic review, corticosteroid injections were shown to be more effective for pain reduction than were noninvasive treatments (physical therapy and shock wave therapy) within 3 months.[6] Furthermore, a combination of both corticosteroid injections and physical therapy provides improved short- and long-term pain and functional outcomes compared with each treatment individually.[7]

Other injection treatment options that demonstrate improvements in both pain and function compared to corticosteroid injections include prolotherapy,[8] platelet-rich plasma,[9,10] and botulinum toxin.[11,12] Surgical procedures should be considered if conservative management fails.

Indication	ICD-10 Code
Plantar fasciitis	M72.2

Relevant Anatomy: (Fig. 11.50)

PATIENT POSITION

- Supine on the examination table with the hip in full external rotation, the knee slightly flexed, and the ankle in a neutral position.
- Alternatively, lying on the examination table on the affected side with the knee slightly flexed and the ankle in a neutral position.
- Rotate the patient's head away from the side that is being injected. This minimizes anxiety and pain perception.

LANDMARKS

1. With the patient lying supine on the examination table, the clinician stands or sits in front of the affected foot.
2. Identify the point of maximal tenderness over the plantar aspect of the foot. This is usually just medial of midline over the medial tubercle of the calcaneus.

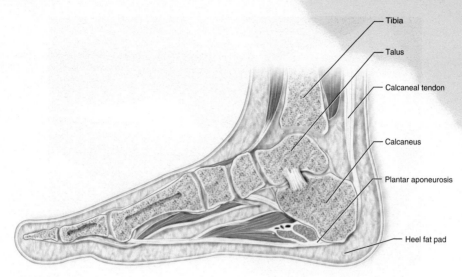

Tibia
Talus
Calcaneal tendon
Calcaneus
Plantar aponeurosis
Heel fat pad

FIGURE 11.50 ● Medial right foot—sagittal section.

3. Draw a vertical line down the posterior border of the tibia.
4. Draw a horizontal line that is above the plantar fat pad. This will be at least one fingerbreadth above the plantar surface.
5. Mark the point where these two lines intersect over the medial aspect of the foot.
6. At that site, press firmly on the skin with the retracted tip of a ballpoint pen. This indention represents the entry point for the needle.
7. After the landmarks are identified, the patient should not move the foot or ankle.

ANESTHESIA

- Local anesthesia of the skin using a topical vapocoolant spray

EQUIPMENT

- Topical vapocoolant spray
- 3-mL syringe
- 25-gauge, 1½-in. needle
- 1 mL of 1% lidocaine without epinephrine
- 1 mL of the steroid solution (40 mg of triamcinolone acetonide)
- One alcohol prep pad
- Two povidone–iodine prep pads
- Sterile gauze pads
- Sterile adhesive bandage
- Nonsterile, clean chucks pad

TECHNIQUE

1. Prep the insertion site with alcohol followed by the povidone–iodine pads.
2. Achieve good local anesthesia by using topical vapocoolant spray.
3. Position the needle and syringe perpendicular to the skin and the intersection of the two landmark lines with the tip of the needle directed laterally.

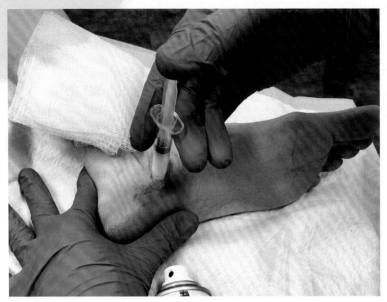

FIGURE 11.51 ● Plantar fasciitis injection.

4. Using the no-touch technique, introduce the needle at the insertion site (Fig. 11.51).
5. Advance the needle toward the medial tubercle of the calcaneus until the needle tip is located at the origin of the plantar fascia.
6. Withdraw the plunger of the syringe to ensure that there is no blood return.
7. Inject the lidocaine/corticosteroid solution as a bolus at the origin of the plantar fascia. The injected solution should flow smoothly into the space. If increased resistance is encountered, advance or withdraw the needle slightly before attempting further injection.
8. Following injection, withdraw the needle.
9. Apply a sterile adhesive bandage.
10. Instruct the patient to massage the area and then take several steps. This movement distributes the lidocaine/corticosteroid solution along the plantar fascia.
11. Reexamine the foot in 5 min to assess pain relief.

AFTERCARE

- NSAIDs, ice, heat, and/or physical therapy as indicated.
- Instruct the patient to perform heel cord static stretching exercises of the gastrocnemius and soleus muscles four times a day.
- Wear proper shoes or orthotics as indicated.
- Consider the use of a tension night splint.
- Consider follow-up examination in 2 weeks.

CPT codes:
- 20550—Injection(s); single tendon sheath, or ligament, aponeurosis
- 76942 (optional)—Ultrasonic guidance for needle placement with imaging supervision and interpretation with permanent recording

PEARLS

- The plantar fascia injection may rarely be quite painful. This is especially true if the injection is performed through the plantar surface of the foot. The medial approach described above minimizes, but may not eliminate the pain of this procedure. Vapo-coolant spray should always be used.
- Notice the thickness of the plantar fat pad in the anatomic drawing. The injection should be placed superior to the fat pad in order to prevent fat atrophy in this critical area.

 A video showing a plantar fasciitis injection can be found in the companion eBook.

REFERENCES

1. Trojian T, Tucker AK. Plantar Fasciitis. *Am Fam Physician.* 2019;99(12):744–750.
2. Ball EM, McKeeman HM, Patterson C, et al. Steroid injection for inferior heel pain: a randomised controlled trial. *Ann Rheum Dis.* 2013;72(6):996–1002.
3. Whittaker GA, Munteanu SE, Menz HB, et al. Corticosteroid injection for plantar heel pain: a systematic review and meta-analysis. *BMC Musculoskelet Disord.* 2019;20(1):378.
4. Chen CM, Chen JS, Tsai WC, et al. Effectiveness of device-assisted ultrasound-guided steroid injection for treating plantar fasciitis. *Am J Phys Med Rehabil.* 2013;92(7):597–605.
5. McMillan AM, Landorf KB, Gilheany MF, et al. Ultrasound guided corticosteroid injection for plantar fasciitis: randomised controlled trial. *BMJ* 2012;344:e3260.
6. Chen CM, Lee M, Lin CH, et al. Comparative efficacy of corticosteroid injection and non-invasive treatments for plantar fasciitis: a systematic review and meta-analysis. *Sci Rep.* 2018;8(1):4033.
7. Johannsen FE, Herzog RB, Malmgaard-Clausen NM, et al. Corticosteroid injection is the best treatment in plantar fasciitis if combined with controlled training. *Knee Surg Sports Traumatol Arthrosc.* 2019;27(1):5–12.
8. Mansiz-Kaplan B, Nacir B, Pervane-Vural S. Effect of dextrose prolotherapy on pain intensity, disability, and plantar fascia thickness in unilateral plantar fasciitis: a randomized, controlled, double-blind study. *Am J Phys Med Rehabil.* 2020;99(4):318–324.
9. Ling Y, Wang S. Effects of platelet-rich plasma in the treatment of plantar fasciitis: a meta-analysis of randomized controlled trials. *Medicine (Baltimore).* 2018;97(37):e12110.
10. Shetty SH, Dhond A, Arora M, et al. Platelet-rich plasma has better long-term results than corticosteroids or placebo for chronic plantar fasciitis: randomized control trial. *J Foot Ankle Surg.* 2019;58(1):42–46.
11. Díaz-Llopis IV, Gómez-Gallego D, Mondéjar-Gómez FJ, et al. Botulinum toxin type A in chronic plantar fasciitis: clinical effects 1 year after injection. *Clin Rehabil.* 2013;27(8):681–685.
12. Elizondo-Rodriguez J, Araujo-Lopez Y, Moreno-Gonzalez JA, et al. A comparison of botulinum toxin a and intralesional steroids for the treatment of plantar fasciitis: a randomized, double-blinded study. *Foot Ankle Int.* 2013;34(1):8–14.

Midfoot Joints

Midfoot joint pain is an unusual presenting complaint in primary care. This may occur following acute trauma or with osteoarthritis, gout, rheumatoid arthritis, or other inflammatory conditions. Conservative treatment of osteoarthritis includes weight loss, physical therapy, bracing, orthoses, and the use of acetaminophen or NSAIDs. A small-diameter needle is employed as this technique is used to inject steroid solution into painful midfoot joints. A recent study shows that corticosteroid injections are a viable diagnostic and short- to mid-term therapeutic option. The results at 4 months were statistically significant for decreased pain and with the additional finding of a difference observed between obese and nonobese patients.[1]

Indications	ICD-10 Code
Foot joint pain	M25.579
Midtarsal joint arthritis	M19.079
Midtarsal joint osteoarthritis, primary	M19.079
Foot osteoarthritis, posttraumatic	M19.179
Foot osteoarthritis, secondary	M19.279

Relevant Anatomy: (Fig. 11.52)

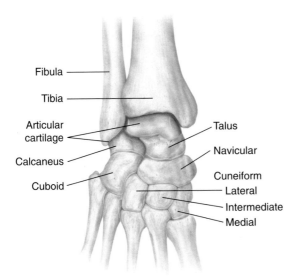

Fibula
Tibia
Articular cartilage
Calcaneus
Cuboid
Talus
Navicular
Cuneiform
Lateral
Intermediate
Medial

FIGURE 11.52 ● Midfoot joints.

PATIENT POSITION

- Supine on the examination table.
- The knee on the affected side is placed in 90 degrees of flexion.
- The ankle is slightly plantar flexed so that the plantar surface is in full contact with the chucks pad covering the exam table.
- Rotate the patient's head away from the side that is being injected. This minimizes anxiety and pain perception.

LANDMARKS

1. With the patient lying supine on the examination table, the clinician stands or sits directly in front of the affected foot.
2. Identify the painful articulation over the dorsal aspect of the midfoot.
3. Mark a point over this articulation. There is normally a soft depression in that area.
4. At that site, press firmly on the skin with the retracted tip of a ballpoint pen. This indention represents the entry point for the needle.
5. After the landmarks are identified, the patient should not move the foot.

ANESTHESIA

- Local anesthesia of the skin using topical vapocoolant spray

EQUIPMENT

- Topical vapocoolant spray
- 3-mL syringe—for injection
- 25-gauge, 5/8-in. needle
- 0.5 mL of 1% mepivacaine without epinephrine
- 0.5 mL of the steroid solution (20 mg of triamcinolone acetonide)
- One alcohol prep pad
- Two povidone–iodine prep pads
- Sterile gauze pads
- Sterile adhesive bandage
- Nonsterile, clean chucks pad

TECHNIQUE

1. Prep the insertion site with alcohol followed by the povidone–iodine pads.
2. Achieve good local anesthesia by using topical vapocoolant spray.
3. Position the needle and syringe perpendicular to the skin with the tip of the needle directed inferiorly into the midfoot joint.
4. Using the no-touch technique, introduce the needle at the insertion site (Fig. 11.53).
5. Advance the needle into the midfoot joint.
6. Withdraw the plunger of the syringe to ensure that there is no blood return.
7. Inject the mepivacaine/corticosteroid solution as a bolus into the midfoot joint. The injected solution should flow smoothly into the space. If increased resistance is encountered, advance or withdraw the needle slightly before attempting further injection.

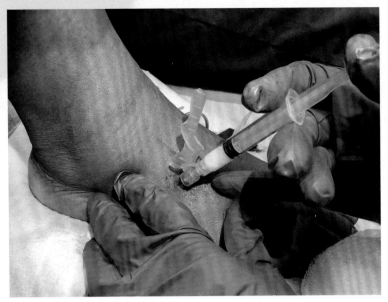

FIGURE 11.53 ● Midfoot joint injection.

8. Following injection, withdraw the needle.
9. Apply a sterile adhesive bandage.
10. Instruct the patient to move his or her foot through its full range of motion. This movement distributes the mepivacaine/corticosteroid solution throughout the midfoot joint.
11. Reexamine the foot in 5 min to assess pain relief.

AFTERCARE

- Consider the use of an ankle–foot orthosis.
- Avoid vigorous use of the foot over the next 2 weeks.
- NSAIDs, ice, and/or physical therapy as indicated.
- Consider follow-up examination in 2 weeks.

CPT codes:
- 20600—Arthrocentesis, aspiration and/or injection, small joint or bursa; without ultrasound guidance
- 20604—With ultrasound guidance, with permanent recording and reporting

 A video showing a midfoot joint injection can be found in the companion eBook.

REFERENCE

1. Protheroe D, Gadgil A. Guided intra-articular corticosteroid injections in the midfoot. *Foot Ankle Int.* 2018;39(8):1001–1004.

First Metatarsophalangeal Joint

Pain involving the first metatarsophalangeal (MTP) joint of the foot is frequently encountered by primary medical providers. It is a common aspiration and injection site for diagnostic and therapeutic purposes. This great toe MTP is the most frequently involved joint by gout and is the most common site of osteoarthritis in the foot. Conservative treatment of osteoarthritis includes weight loss, physical therapy, bracing, orthoses, and the use of acetaminophen or NSAIDs. Sivera et al. described the use of a 29-gauge needle to successfully aspirate this joint.[1] Corticosteroids are effective in the treatment of arthritis of the MTP joint. Ultrasound may be used as a tool to select joints that will benefit from intra-articular injections.[2] Injected corticosteroids are also useful in patients with mild, but not severe, grades of hallux rigidus.[3]

Indications	ICD-10 Code
Pain of first MTP joint	M25.579
Acute gout involving toe	M10.9
First MTP joint arthritis, unspecified	M19.079
First MTP joint osteoarthritis, primary	M19.079
First MTP joint osteoarthritis, posttraumatic	M19.179
First MTP joint osteoarthritis, secondary	M19.279

Relevant Anatomy: (Fig. 11.54)

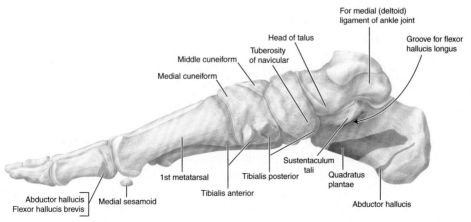

FIGURE 11.54 ● Medial aspect of the right foot—bony anatomy. (Modified from Agur AM, Dalley AF. *Grant's Atlas of Anatomy*, 14th Ed. Philadelphia, PA: Wolters Kluwer, 2016.)

PATIENT POSITION

- Supine on the examination table.
- The knee on the affected side is placed in 90 degrees of flexion.
- The ankle is slightly plantar flexed so that the plantar surface is in full contact with the chucks pad covering the exam table.
- Rotate the patient's head away from the side that is being injected. This minimizes anxiety and pain perception.

LANDMARKS

1. With the patient lying supine on the examination table, the clinician stands or sits medial to the affected foot.
2. Locate the first MTP joint with simultaneous palpation and flexion/extension of the great toe proximal phalanx. The patient will report tenderness in this joint, and there may be associated erythema and swelling.
3. The injection point is directly over the first MTP joint.
4. At that site, press firmly on the skin with the retracted tip of a ballpoint pen. This indention represents the entry point for the needle.
5. After the landmarks are identified, the patient should not move the foot or toe.

ANESTHESIA

- Local anesthesia of the skin using topical vapocoolant spray

EQUIPMENT

- Topical vapocoolant spray
- 3-mL syringe
- 3-mL syringe—for optional aspiration
- 25-gauge, 5/8-in. needle for injection
- 25-gauge, 5/8-in. needle for optional aspiration
- 0.25 to 0.5 mL of 1% mepivacaine without epinephrine
- 0.25 to 0.5 mL of the steroid solution (10 to 20 mg of triamcinolone acetonide)
- One alcohol prep pad
- Two povidone–iodine prep pads
- Sterile gauze pads
- Sterile adhesive bandage
- Nonsterile, clean chucks pad

TECHNIQUE

1. Prep the insertion site with alcohol followed by the povidone–iodine pads.
2. Achieve good local anesthesia by using topical vapocoolant spray.
3. Position the needle and syringe perpendicular to the skin with the tip of the needle directed into the center of the joint.
4. Using the no-touch technique, introduce the needle at the insertion site (Fig. 11.55).
5. Advance the needle until the tip is located in the joint capsule. If the needle contacts bone or cartilage, back up the needle 1 to 2 mm.

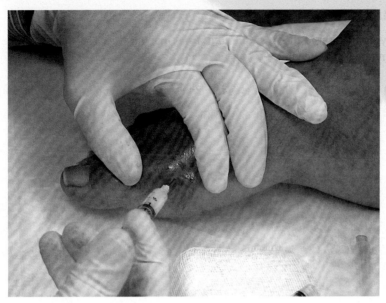

FIGURE 11.55 ● Right first MTP joint injection.

6. If aspirating, withdraw fluid using the 25-gauge, 5/8-in. needle with a 3-mL syringe.
7. If injection following aspiration is elected, remove the 3-mL syringe from the 25-gauge needle and then attach the 3-mL syringe filled with the mepivacaine/corticosteroid solution.
8. If only injecting mepivacaine/corticosteroid solution, use a 25-gauge, 5/8-in. needle with the 3-mL syringe.
9. Inject the mepivacaine/corticosteroid solution as a bolus into the joint capsule. The injected solution should flow smoothly into the space. If increased resistance is encountered, advance or withdraw the needle slightly before attempting further injection.
10. Following injection, withdraw the needle.
11. Apply a sterile adhesive bandage.
12. Instruct the patient to move his or her toe through its full range of motion. This movement distributes the mepivacaine/corticosteroid solution throughout the joint capsule.
13. Reexamine the first MTP joint in 5 min to assess pain relief.

AFTERCARE

- Avoid excessive movement of the first MTP joint over the next 2 weeks.
- NSAIDs, ice, and/or physical therapy as indicated.
- Consider the use of an ankle–foot orthotic or wooden-soled shoe.
- Consider follow-up examination in 2 weeks.

CPT codes:
- 20600—Arthrocentesis, aspiration and/or injection, small joint or bursa; without ultrasound guidance
- 20604—With ultrasound guidance, with permanent recording and reporting

PEARLS

- Applying traction to the great toe in a distal direction may help open up the joint to accommodate the needle.

 A video showing a first MTP joint injection can be found in the companion eBook.

REFERENCES

1. Sivera F, Aragon R, Pascual E. First metatarsophalangeal joint aspiration using a 29-gauge needle. *Ann Rheum Dis.* 2008;67(2):273–275.
2. Nordberg LB, Lillegraven S, Aga AB, et al. The impact of ultrasound on the use and efficacy of intraarticular glucocorticoid injections in early rheumatoid arthritis: secondary analyses from a randomized trial examining the benefit of ultrasound in a clinical tight control regimen. *Arthritis Rheumatol.* 2018;70(8):1192–1199.
3. Solan MC, Calder JD, Bendall SP. Manipulation and injection for hallux rigidus: is it worthwhile? *J Bone Joint Surg Br.* 2001;83:706–708.

Intermetatarsal (Morton's) Neuroma

Compression of the interdigital nerves as they course between the metatarsal bones in the foot can result in a painful condition referred to as a Morton's neuroma. This is a fairly common condition seen by primary care clinicians. The disorder is a compressive neuropathy often causing inflammation, perineural fibrosis, and enlargement of the interdigital nerve. It presents symptoms of significant lancinating pain and dysesthesias with weight bearing—especially when wearing shoes with a narrow toe box. Usually, the neuroma lies between the second and third or the third and fourth metatarsal heads. Conservative treatment strategies include shoe-wear modifications, custom-made orthotics, and corticosteroid injections.

Corticosteroid injections have traditionally been used to provide at least short- to medium-term pain relief.[1,2] Corticosteroid injections and manipulation/mobilization are the two interventions with the strongest evidence for pain reduction.[3] Ultrasound-guided steroid injections in Morton's neuroma lead to a higher percentage of short-term pain relief and fewer skin side effects than do landmark-based injections.[4] However, treatment failures are encountered. The size of the neuroma on ultrasonography is the sole predictor of corticosteroid injection failure.[5] With a cutoff value of 6.3 mm, larger Morton's neuromas are associated with failure of corticosteroid injection.[6]

Sclerosant treatment with ultrasound-guided alcohol injections into the substance of the neuroma is a promising intervention as summarized in a recent systematic review.[7] Perini and colleagues also demonstrated a safe profile and relief of neuropathic symptoms using this technique in a relatively large study.[8] Patients who do not respond to conservative management and injections may require operative intervention with nerve decompression or neurectomy.

Indication	ICD-10 Code
Morton's neuroma	G57.60

Relevant Anatomy: (Fig. 11.56)

PATIENT POSITION

- Supine on the examination table.
- The knee on the affected side is placed in 90 degrees of flexion.
- The ankle is slightly plantar flexed so that the plantar surface is in full contact with the chucks pad covering the examination table.
- Rotate the patient's head away from the side that is being injected. This minimizes anxiety and pain perception.

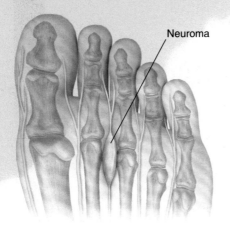

FIGURE 11.56 ● Dorsal aspect of the right foot.

Neuroma

LANDMARKS

1. With the patient lying supine on the examination table, the clinician stands or sits in front of the affected foot.
2. Locate the site of maximal tenderness. This is found between the heads of the metatarsals. The most common sites are located between the second and third or the third and fourth metatarsal heads.
3. The injection point is on the dorsal aspect of the distal foot directly over the area of maximal tenderness. A tender nodule may be palpated occasionally at this site.
4. At that site, press firmly on the skin with the retracted tip of a ballpoint pen. This indention represents the entry point for the needle.
5. After the landmarks are identified, the patient should not move the foot.

ANESTHESIA

- Local anesthesia of the skin using topical vapocoolant spray

EQUIPMENT

- Topical vapocoolant spray
- 3-mL syringe
- 25-gauge, 1-in. needle
- 0.5 mL of 1% lidocaine without epinephrine
- 0.5 mL of the steroid solution (20 mg of triamcinolone acetonide)
- One alcohol prep pad
- Two povidone–iodine prep pads
- Sterile gauze pads
- Sterile adhesive bandage
- Nonsterile, clean chucks pad

TECHNIQUE

1. Prep the insertion site with alcohol followed by the povidone–iodine pads.
2. Achieve good local anesthesia by using topical vapocoolant spray.

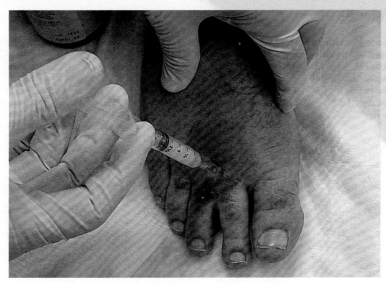

FIGURE 11.57 ● Morton neuroma injection.

3. Position the needle and syringe perpendicular to the skin with the tip of the needle directed inferiorly between the affected metatarsal heads.
4. Using the no-touch technique, introduce the needle at the insertion site (Fig. 11.57).
5. Advance the needle until the needle tip is located in the neuroma between the metatarsal heads.
6. Withdraw the plunger of the syringe to ensure that there is no blood return.
7. Inject the lidocaine/corticosteroid solution as a bolus into or around the neuroma. The injected solution should flow smoothly. If increased resistance is encountered, advance or withdraw the needle slightly before attempting further injection.
8. Following injection, withdraw the needle.
9. Apply a sterile adhesive bandage.
10. Instruct the patient to massage the area of injection. This movement distributes the lidocaine/corticosteroid solution around the neuroma.
11. Reexamine the foot in 5 min to assess pain relief.

AFTERCARE

- Avoid wearing shoes with a narrow toe box.
- NSAIDs, ice, and/or physical therapy as indicated.
- Consider metatarsal pads or custom orthotics.
- Consider follow-up examination in 2 weeks.

CPT codes:
- 64455—Injection(s), anesthetic agent, and/or steroid, plantar common digital nerve(s)
- 76942 (optional)—Ultrasonic guidance for needle placement with imaging supervision and interpretation with permanent recording

 A video showing a Morton neuroma injection can be found in the companion eBook.

REFERENCES

1. Markovic M, Crichton K, Read JW, et al. Effectiveness of ultrasound-guided corticosteroid injection in the treatment of Morton's neuroma. *Foot Ankle Int.* 2008;29(5):483–487.
2. Hassouna H, Singh D, Taylor H, et al. Ultrasound guided steroid injection in the treatment of interdigital neuralgia. *Acta Orthop Belg.* 2007;73(2):224–229.
3. Matthews BG, Hurn SE, Harding MP, et al. The effectiveness of non-surgical interventions for common plantar digital compressive neuropathy (Morton's neuroma): a systematic review and meta-analysis. *J Foot Ankle Res.* 2019;12:12.
4. Ruiz Santiago F, Prados Olleta N, Tomás Muñoz P, et al. Short term comparison between blind and ultrasound guided injection in Morton neuroma. *Eur Radiol.* 2019;29(2):620–627.
5. Park YH, Kim TJ, Choi GW, et al. Prediction of clinical prognosis according to intermetatarsal distance and neuroma size on ultrasonography in Morton neuroma: a prospective observational study. *J Ultrasound Med.* 2019;38(4):1009–1014.
6. Park YH, Lee JW, Choi GW, et al. Risk factors and the associated cutoff values for failure of corticosteroid injection in treatment of Morton's neuroma. *Int Orthop.* 2018;42(2):323–329.
7. Santos, D Morrison G, Coda A. Sclerosing alcohol injections for the management of intermetatarsal neuromas: a systematic review. *Foot (Edinb).* 2018;35:36–47.
8. Perini L, Perini C, Tagliapietra M, et al. Percutaneous alcohol injection under sonographic guidance in Morton's neuroma: follow-up in 220 treated lesions. *Radiol Med.* 2016;121(7):597–604.

Consent for Needle Aspiration and/or Injection

Date: _____

I hereby authorize

_____

(Provider's name)

to perform upon

_____

(Patient's name)

the following procedure(s): _____

_____

_____

The procedure(s) consists of: _____

_____

_____

_____

(Describe in lay language)

Possible risks associated with the performance of a needle injection/aspiration may include but are not limited to:

Bleeding, Infection, Local pain, Fainting, Allergic reaction, or

_____

Possible risks with the use of injected corticosteroids may include but are not limited to:

Feeling flushed	**Flare-up of joint inflammation**
Tendon rupture	**Abnormal thinning of the skin**
Abnormal skin color	**Worsening blood sugars in diabetes**
Impaired immune response	**Disturbance of hormone balance**
Irregular menstrual periods	

The nature of this procedure, methods of diagnosis/treatment, and possible alternatives has been explained to me by _____ or his/her associate. I am aware that there are certain risks associated with this procedure and that the practice of medicine and surgery is not an exact science. I acknowledge that no guarantees have been made to me concerning the results of the procedure or its interpretation.

I certify that I understand the contents of this form:

_____

Signature of patient or authorized representative

_____

Witness

IF THE PATIENT IS UNABLE TO CONSENT OR IS A MINOR, COMPLETE THE FOLLOWING:

The patient is a minor, _____ years of age, or is unable to consent because _____

_____

(strike or define).

The undersigned hereby consents to the performance of the above described diagnostic/therapeutic procedure on the above patient as well as any tests, which are deemed necessary.

_____

Signature of authorized representative

Aspiration and Injection Aftercare Handout

You have just had a procedure done by: _____

Your diagnosis is: _____

The procedure involved placing a needle into the tissues to: _____

withdraw fluid from the _____

inject "cortisone" into the _____

other _____

Please Follow These Instructions:

Recurring Pain:
Injections are usually done using a local anesthetic such as lidocaine or mepivacaine mixed with cortisone. The anesthetic effect of the lidocaine or mepivacaine usually lasts for 30 to 60 minutes and then wears off. At that time, your pain will return. Improvement in pain from the cortisone injection usually takes 24 to 48 hours. So, expect the pain to return after an hour and hopefully go away in 1 to 2 days.

Rest the Area:
Be careful with the affected area/joint. Usually, the injected medication causes the area to feel numb. Because you may not feel pain, it is easy to suffer further injury to the area. Do not use the area for anything more than mild essential movements for the next 2 weeks.

Watch for Infection:
Although every precaution has been taken to prevent infection, be alert for the following signs—fever above 100°F, increased warmth in the area, redness at the injection site, redness moving up the arm or leg, and swelling of the area.

If *any* of these symptoms develop, call this office immediately at (INSERT PHONE NUMBER).

Follow the Directions of Any Checked Boxes:
❑ Apply ice to the area every 4 hours for 20 minutes at a time for _____ day(s).
❑ Apply a heating pad to the area every 4 hours for 20 minutes at a time for _____ day(s).
❑ Apply an elastic compression wrap to the area for _____ day(s).

❑ Perform stretching exercises as instructed.
❑ Wear a splint to the area for _____ day(s).
❑ Referral for physical therapy.
❑ Take the following medicines in addition to your usual medications:

_____

_____

_____

Return to this office in _____ day(s)/week(s) for further evaluation and management of your condition.

Medical Record
Documentation

The following template is an example of documentation that may be used for a knee aspiration and injection procedure. Setting this up as a text template in an electronic medical record allows the practitioner the greatest documentation flexibility to deal with the inevitable variations encountered during the procedure.

Patient name: _____ Date: _____

Ultrasound Guidance of Arthrocentesis/Injection: CPT #20611

Procedure:
The patient was placed in a recumbent position on the examination table. The musculoskeletal probe with the [Brand/Model] ultrasound machine was used. An ultrasound survey of the knee joint structures was performed in the sagittal and transverse planes.

Knee Aspiration and Injection:
Prior to performance of the knee aspiration and injection, a discussion of the nature of this procedure, proposed benefits, material risks, and alternative treatments was conducted with the patient. All questions were answered. After informed consent was obtained, the following procedure was performed:

Lateral Suprapatellar Approach:
A point at the intersection of a line in the axial plane 2 cm above the patella and a line, perpendicular to the first, in the coronal plane at the undersurface of the patella was identified and marked with the retracted tip of a ball point pen. The superior-lateral aspect of the knee was prepped in a sterile fashion with alcohol and Betadine. Topical [Brand] vapocoolant spray was used to achieve good local anesthesia.

Following the no-touch technique:
• For injection only:
 ❑ A 2 in. 25 gauge needle was inserted and directed medially into the knee joint capsule under direct ultrasound guidance with the needle in the long axis and in-plane. The image was documented.
• For aspiration and injection:
 ❑ 4 mL of 1% lidocaine without epinephrine was used to adequately anesthetize the skin and joint capsule.
 ❑ Next, a 1 1/2 in. 18-gauge needle was directed medially into the knee joint capsule under direct ultrasound guidance. The image was documented.

❑ No; ❑ A small amount; ❑ A moderate amount; ❑ A large amount; of fluid was observed.

❑ No; ❑ ____ mL of _____ describe appearance _____ fluid was removed.

Next, a mixture of 1 mL of 1% mepivacaine without epinephrine and 1 mL of Triamcinolone (40 mg) was injected easily into the knee joint through the 18-gauge needle.

The needle was withdrawn. No bleeding was encountered.
The injection site was covered with a sterile bandage.
The patient tolerated the procedure well without complications.
He/she reported complete relief of pain within 5 min.

_____

Signature of medical provider

Index

Note: Page numbers followed by '*f*' indicate figures; those followed by '*t*' indicate tables.